Artificial Intelligence in Neuroradiology

Daniel Thomas Ginat
Editor

Artificial Intelligence in Neuroradiology

A Practical Guide

Springer

Editor
Daniel Thomas Ginat
Co-founder
Rad-Lab.ai
CHICAGO, IL, USA

ISBN 978-3-032-24567-0 ISBN 978-3-032-24568-7 (eBook)
https://doi.org/10.1007/978-3-032-24568-7

This Springer imprint is published by the registered company Springer Nature Switzerland AG
The registered company address is: Gewerbestrasse 11, 6330 Cham, Switzerland

Preface

In 1948, Alan Turing introduced concepts related to artificial intelligence in his report "Intelligent Machinery." The term "artificial Intelligence" was coined by Professor John McCarthy in 1955 and defined as "the science and engineering of making intelligent machines." Since that time, artificial intelligence has progressed substantially and encompasses several categories and techniques. Artificial intelligence has become ubiquitous across many industries including the field of radiology, both for research purposes and clinical applications. Thus, this guide aims to provide an overview of what artificial intelligence research entails, how it is carried out, what current uses include, and what future applications are envisioned specifically for neuroimaging.

Categories of Artificial Intelligence

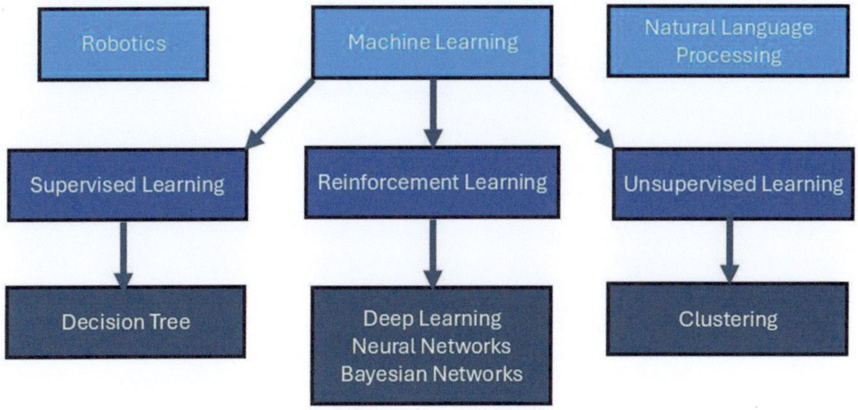

Chicago, IL, USA

Daniel Thomas Ginat

Contents

Contributors

Asim Dhungana Pritzker School of Medicine, University of Chicago, Chicago, IL, USA

Daniel Thomas Ginat Co-founder, Rad-Lab.ai, Chicago, IL, USA

Vrushab Gowda Department of Radiology, Massachusetts General Hospital, Boston, MA, USA

Harvard Medical School, Boston, MA, USA

Harlan Benjamin Harvey Radiology Physicians, Inc., Dayton, OH, USA

Grayson W. Hooper UH Cleveland Department of Radiology, Cleveland, OH, USA

Mathew Illimoottil University of Missouri Kansas City, Kansas City, MO, USA

Andrew Kunz University of Chicago, Chicago, IL, USA

Golnaz Lotfian Department of Diagnostic Radiology and Nuclear Medicine, Rush University Medical Center, Chicago, IL, USA

Yauheniya Makarevich Leiden University, Leiden, The Netherlands

Radhika Rajpurohit University of Delaware, Newark, DE, USA

Ramkumar Rajabathar Babu Jai Shanker Biological Sciences Division, University of Chicago, Chicago, IL, USA

Amogh Shetty Department of Biology, Rensselaer Polytechnic Institute, Troy, NY, USA

Marius Staring Leiden University, Leiden, The Netherlands

Chapter 1
Overview of Machine Learning and Deep Learning Algorithms

Ramkumar Rajabathar Babu Jai Shanker and Daniel Thomas Ginat

Introduction

Why Should We Learn About Machine Learning and Deep Learning?

Artificial Intelligence (AI) has revolutionized the field of medical imaging, and specifically in neuroradiology, it has already helped solve some of the most pressing problems neuroradiologists face. In the field of oncology, AI-based methodologies have been shown to not only automate some of the most manual and tedious tasks, such as tumor segmentation and characterization, but also aid in clinical decision-making, such as predicting treatment response. In the field of emergency neuroradiology, where "time is brain," AI has aided radiologists in accelerating the time to diagnosis. AI tools, for instance, can notify the radiologist of an intracranial hemorrhage within 1–2 min of the scan's completion.

Many of these implementations share a commonality—the symbiotic relationship between human expertise and artificial intelligence. It is essential to emphasize that AI technologies function optimally when they augment the clinical expertise of radiologists. Most use cases can be thought of as utilizing either human expertise only, machine expertise only, or a human-machine interface. While some edge cases still require the use of human knowledge or machine expertise alone, many tasks that fall within the purview of a neuroradiologist can be considered suitable for a

R. R. B. J. Shanker (✉)
Biological Sciences Division, University of Chicago, Chicago, IL, USA

D. T. Ginat
Department of Radiology, Section of Neuroradiology, University of Chicago, Chicago, IL, USA

D. T. Ginat (ed.), *Artificial Intelligence in Neuroradiology*,
https://doi.org/10.1007/978-3-032-24568-7_1

human-machine interface, where human expertise is enhanced using artificial intelligence technologies.

In the field of neuroradiology, while some algorithms have proven effective in clinical practice, a significant portion of algorithms developed in research do not transition to clinical practice. Although it has been established that AI algorithms are sufficiently complex to learn the nuances that radiologists wish them to grasp, AI systems significantly lag in their explanation aspects. To bridge this chasm between performance and understanding, it is essential to enhance existing explainability methods. Although these explainability methods have significantly improved in recent years, truly "explaining" an AI algorithm requires a deep understanding of its subtleties and operations. Practitioners must familiarize themselves not only with what the algorithm accomplishes but also with its limitations. Filling these knowledge gaps could significantly enhance the adoption of AI algorithms in clinical settings. This chapter aims to provide the reader with an overview of machine learning and deep learning algorithms, as well as specific methods that address some of the main challenges to their adoption in real-world practice.

In the subsequent chapters, we discuss the primary applications of AI algorithms for workflow optimization, anatomy and lesion segmentation, radiomics for tumor characterization and prognosis, evaluating neurodegenerative disease, and AI for cerebrovascular disease. The concepts presented in this chapter form the foundation for understanding and appreciating the applications discussed in the following chapters of this book. Additionally, in this chapter, we cover some of the conceptual elements that help clinical practitioners understand the algorithms they encounter in practice. For further reading, relevant texts are highlighted in appropriate sections.

What Has AI Achieved, and What Is Its Potential?

In neuroradiology, AI technologies have been shown to successfully detect stroke, traumatic brain injury, intracranial hemorrhage, brain tumors, and neurodegenerative disease. Their performance in specific tasks, such as lesion detection and segmentation, can match, and in some tasks occasionally exceed, human accuracy in controlled studies though the real-world impact varies. In certain critical care settings, AI-based auto-detection and auto-segmentation algorithms may enable radiologists to triage urgent cases, reduce diagnostic delays, minimize inter-observer variability, and improve efficiency and patient outcomes. AI algorithms are also vital in use cases where medical imaging is integrated with data from other modalities, such as genomic data. This enables noninvasive prediction of tumor subtypes and treatment response, an emerging application that holds promise for personalized medicine and improved prognostic planning.

One of the recurrent themes observed in many AI studies across neuroradiology applications is that AI algorithms often outperform prior non-AI baselines on benchmarks. Still, gains may diminish on external or real-world data. This significant performance improvement can be attributed to three primary factors: increased model complexity, automatic feature extraction, and enhancements in data augmentation. Neural networks contain significantly more parameters than traditional algorithms, typically in the millions or billions. These parameters, when utilized in the right neural network architecture, can learn highly complex concepts from multiple data modalities and nuances, enabling the task to be carried out effectively. The high number of parameters also makes neural networks highly prone to overfitting, where they tend to memorize specific information in the training data and fail to generalize well.

However, the most significant aspect of AI algorithms is their potential to identify novel patterns or imaging features that were previously unknown or undetectable. AI algorithms hold the power to automatically generate features or imaging representations that best explain the prediction. In other words, by looking inside an AI algorithm's inner workings, we can discover novel features, such as radiomic features or biomarkers that were previously unknown.

Why Now? Converging Trends in AI and Medical Imaging

While AI algorithms have been steadily gaining importance across various industries, their rapid adoption within neuroradiology can be attributed to three key factors: the evolution of open-source medical imaging data repositories, advances in medical imaging-specific network architectures, and advances in explainable AI algorithms.

Open-Source Data repositories Medical imaging repositories such as The Cancer Imaging Archive (TCIA) provide annotated datasets spanning multiple modalities (imaging, genomics, clinical notes) and studies. Machine learning challenges such as the Brain Tumor Segmentation (BraTS) and Medical Segmentation Decathlon (MSD) provide a curated set of standardized images acquired from multiple centers. The NIH's mandate for FAIR (Findable, Accessible, Interoperable, and Reusable) data sharing helps access this trend. These datasets have improved the development of novel AI technologies and helped evaluate the generalizability of such developed algorithms to unseen data, thereby enhancing trust in clinical settings. More recently, the datasets that combine medical images and radiological reports, such as Radiology Objects in Context (ROCO), MIMIC-CXR, and PMC-15M, have fundamentally improved the potential applications of vision-language models to operate reliably within the radiology domain. These open-source data repositories also foster collaboration by improving reproducibility and benchmarking the performance of AI algorithms.

Advances in Network Architectures Specialized deep-learning architectures, such as Convolutional Neural Networks (CNNs), Vision Transformers (ViTs), and other hybrid models, have been adapted to work effectively for medical imaging tasks. However, it is the development of novel architectures that take into account some of the distinguishing features of radiological images, such as the standard range of intensity values in computed tomography images and a relatively standard arrangement of anatomies within images, that has led to improvements in accuracy, efficiency, and adaptability. For example, the U-Net algorithm and the nnU-Net adapted the CNN architecture and encoder-decoder architectures for medical imaging settings and continue to be the most widely utilized neural network architecture for most medical imaging segmentation algorithms.

Advances in Explainable AI (XAI) Algorithms AI algorithms were once thought of as "black-box" algorithms, but are now increasingly transparent and interpretable using explainable AI techniques. Algorithms such as the Gradient Class-activation Mapping (GRAD-CAM), Local Interpretable Model-agnostic Explanations (LIME), and Shapley Additive Explanations (SHAP) have been integrated into medical imaging workflows, enabling clinicians to visualize and understand the reasoning behind the predictions made by AI algorithms. These explainable AI algorithms have played a crucial role in building trust and facilitating the clinical adoption of AI.

How to Use This Chapter

This chapter introduces foundational principles without immediate reference to deep learning applications to facilitate a logical progression of conceptual understanding. It is important to clarify that the scope of this chapter is not to provide an exhaustive or highly technical treatise on machine learning. Rather, the aim is to present a focused overview of machine learning (ML) and deep learning (DL) as they pertain specifically to the practice of artificial intelligence (AI) within the field of neuroradiology.

This book is a practical guide, so each section has its accompanying code repository (Fig. 1.1) (hosted on GitHub), featuring concrete examples and applications that readers can follow along. Wherever applicable, the original use cases, along with the corresponding research literature, are referenced. However, some of the examples have been adapted or simplified to make the illustrations more effective. For example, the objective of differentiating gliomas (Glioblastoma from Low-grade glioma) is used to illustrate many concepts in Sect. 2. In some cases, the illustrations contain models built using single features or a small subset of features to explain using 2-dimensional visualizations. Some of the datasets used contain patients from multiple centers; however, for simplicity, the models are built without these center-aware splits.

In addition to outlining the core concepts and practical applications, this chapter critically examines the underlying questions associated with these algorithms: What are the essential concepts, and how do they integrate to enable successful applications in neuroradiology? Why do specific algorithms perform effectively or ineffectively in neuroradiological contexts? How are these networks trained, validated, and implemented in practice?

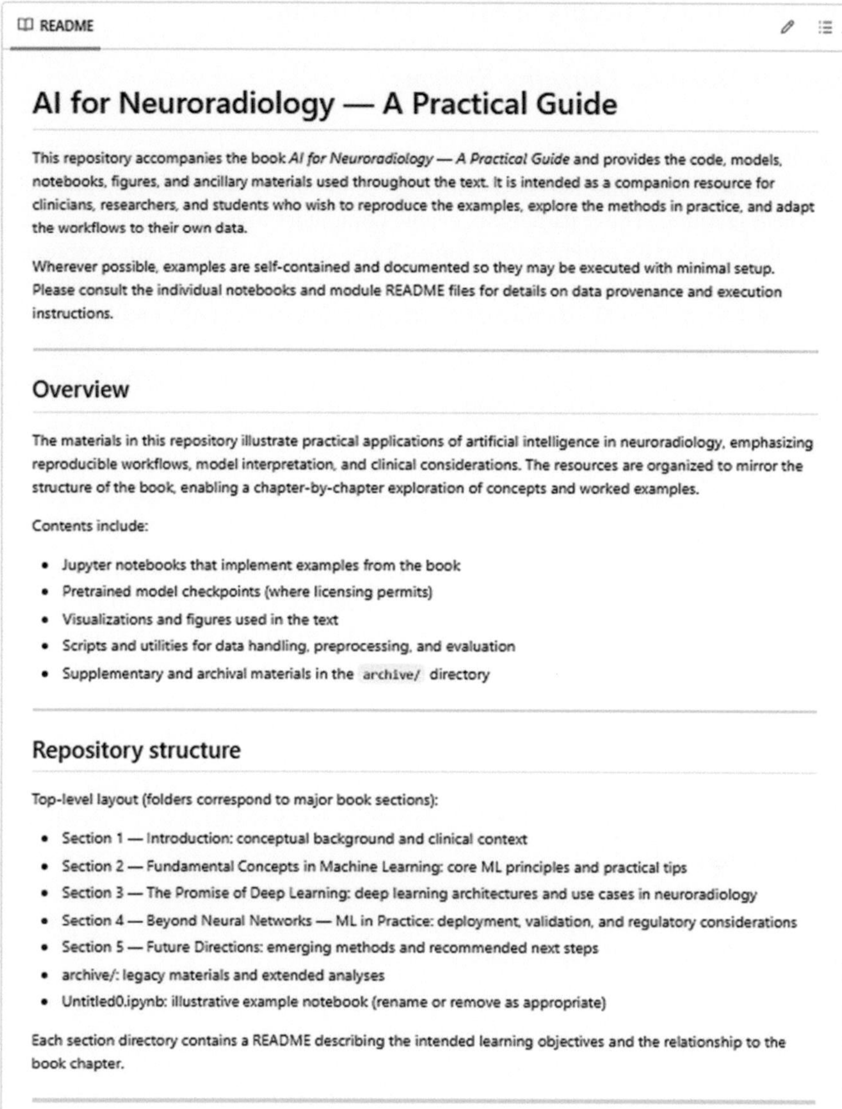

README

AI for Neuroradiology — A Practical Guide

This repository accompanies the book *AI for Neuroradiology — A Practical Guide* and provides the code, models, notebooks, figures, and ancillary materials used throughout the text. It is intended as a companion resource for clinicians, researchers, and students who wish to reproduce the examples, explore the methods in practice, and adapt the workflows to their own data.

Wherever possible, examples are self-contained and documented so they may be executed with minimal setup. Please consult the individual notebooks and module README files for details on data provenance and execution instructions.

Overview

The materials in this repository illustrate practical applications of artificial intelligence in neuroradiology, emphasizing reproducible workflows, model interpretation, and clinical considerations. The resources are organized to mirror the structure of the book, enabling a chapter-by-chapter exploration of concepts and worked examples.

Contents include:

- Jupyter notebooks that implement examples from the book
- Pretrained model checkpoints (where licensing permits)
- Visualizations and figures used in the text
- Scripts and utilities for data handling, preprocessing, and evaluation
- Supplementary and archival materials in the `archive/` directory

Repository structure

Top-level layout (folders correspond to major book sections):

- Section 1 — Introduction: conceptual background and clinical context
- Section 2 — Fundamental Concepts in Machine Learning: core ML principles and practical tips
- Section 3 — The Promise of Deep Learning: deep learning architectures and use cases in neuroradiology
- Section 4 — Beyond Neural Networks — ML in Practice: deployment, validation, and regulatory considerations
- Section 5 — Future Directions: emerging methods and recommended next steps
- archive/: legacy materials and extended analyses
- Untitled0.ipynb: illustrative example notebook (rename or remove as appropriate)

Each section directory contains a README describing the intended learning objectives and the relationship to the book chapter.

Fig. 1.1 The code repository that accompanies this book chapter with the algorithms, visualizations and quick-start Colab execution instructions. (Link to code repository: https://github.com/rbramkumar/Artificial-Intelligence-in-Neuroradiology-A-Practical-Guide)

Furthermore, we address the practical challenges, such as data augmentation, dataset imbalances, and explainability methods, encountered when deploying AI systems in clinical settings. We also discuss contemporary techniques and strategies developed to overcome these obstacles. Through this approach, the chapter seeks to provide both a conceptual framework and practical insights relevant to AI practitioners in neuroradiology.

Fundamental Concepts in Machine Learning

Types of Machine Learning Systems

Machine Learning (ML), as a discipline, employs four core algorithmic paradigms: supervised learning, unsupervised learning, semi-supervised learning, and reinforcement learning. These paradigms enable computers to learn from the provided data without explicitly programming for each specific task. In the context of neuroradiology, the application of Machine learning algorithms depends on the data type and clinical need. Each algorithm discussed below has its strengths, limitations, and technical requirements. They can be conceptualized as tools within the practitioner's toolbox, to be used independently or in combination, depending on the clinical problem and the nature of the available data.

Supervised Learning

In this approach, AI models are trained using labeled datasets, where inputs to the model, such as brain MRI sequences, are paired with corresponding known outputs, such as tumor classification. Considering that most AI systems are developed to address highly specialized problems related to disease classification, automated segmentation, and other tasks that require expert input, supervised learning remains the dominant paradigm in Medical Imaging and Clinical AI.

Key Characteristics

In its most basic form, supervised learning can be used to address two primary tasks: Classification and Regression.

- Classification algorithms make categorical predictions, such as distinguishing between metastatic and benign lymph nodes.
- Regression algorithms estimate continuous values, such as the reduction in tumor volume in response to chemoradiotherapy treatment.

Higher-level tasks, such as segmentation or landmark detection, can be considered pixel-wise classification or coordinate-based regression problems, respectively. During the training process, the algorithms learn the relationship between the input features and output labels. This is achieved by minimizing errors when model predictions align with known labels. These errors typically correspond to an objective function, such as cross-entropy in the case of classification or Mean Squared Error in the case of regression.

Commonly Used Algorithms

Regression (Linear/Logistic) In linear regression, a linear equation is used to model the relationship between input features and a continuous outcome variable. During the training process, the sum of squared errors is minimized. In logistic regression, a logistic (or sigmoid) function is used to transform and fit the linear combination of input features to the outcome variable. During the training, the cross-entropy loss is minimized.

Figure 1.2 illustrates the logistic regression model applied to a tumor classification task: differentiating between Lower-Grade Glioma (LGG) and Glioblastoma Multiforme (GBM) tumors using data from The Cancer Genome Atlas (TCGA). In this specific illustrative example, the model utilizes a single radiomic feature, VOLUME_NET_over_TC, which measures the volume of the non-enhancing (NET) parts of the tumor core relative to the volume of the Tumor Core (TC). A higher value for this feature would indicate that a larger fraction of the tumor core consists of non-enhancing and necrotic tissue. The data points represent individual patient cases, positioned vertically according to their actual diagnosis, i.e., LGG or

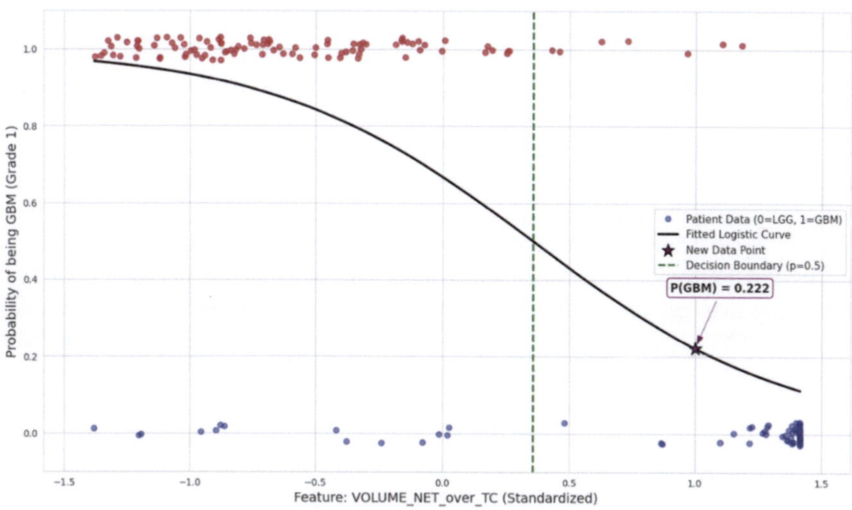

Fig. 1.2 Logistic Regression for LGG vs. GBM Classification. This plot shows the fitted logistic regression curve using the *"VOLUME_NET_over_TC"* feature (the volume of the non-enhancing (NET) parts of the tumor core relative to the volume of the Tumor Core (TC)) to classify LGG and GBM tumors. Patient data points are scattered, colored by their actual grade. The black curve represents the predicted probability of being GBM based on the feature value, and the dashed green line indicates the decision boundary at a probability of 0.5. A new data point is shown with its predicted probability annotated. (The code used to train the logistic regression is available here: supervised_01_logistic_gbm_lgg.ipynb)

GBM, and horizontally by their corresponding feature value. The model's objective is to mathematically describe the relationship between the feature and the probability of a case belonging to the GBM class.

To achieve this, the logistic regression algorithm fits a sigmoid function, represented by the black "S"-shaped curve, to the observed data. This function transforms any input feature value into a corresponding output value constrained between 0 and 1, which serves as the predicted probability, as shown in Fig. 1.2. As the standardized feature value increases, the curve rises, indicating a higher predicted probability of the tumor being a GBM. The vertical dashed line denotes the decision boundary, which is the specific feature value at which the predicted probability is exactly 0.5. This threshold is often used to make a discrete classification: samples with feature values on one side of the boundary would be classified as LGG, and those on the other as GBM, thereby translating the model's probabilistic output into a definitive class assignment. This threshold is typically decided after evaluating the Type-1 and Type-2 errors. For example, choosing a higher threshold may reduce the number of false positives (sample that in truth belongs to the LGG class, but the model predicts as GBM) and increase the number of false negatives (samples that in truth belong to the GBM class, but the model predicts as LGG).

Nearest-Neighbors (kNN) In this algorithm, each sample (usually patients) is plotted in a feature space using a distance metric, usually the Euclidean distance. Then, each sample is assigned the average value (regression) or majority vote (classification) of its k closest training samples.

Figure 1.3 provides a visualization of a KNN classifier with k = 7 applied to the task of differentiating Lower-Grade Glioma (LGG) from Glioblastoma Multiforme (GBM) using two standardized radiomic features from the TCGA dataset. While a typical project would include all radiomic features (after a rigorous feature selection process) and create a multidimensional space, we illustrate the decision boundary using only two features to visualize it on a 2-dimensional graph. The "training process" for KNN is distinct from that of many other machine learning algorithms because it involves simply storing the entire training dataset, including the feature vectors and their corresponding class labels (LGG or GBM). Because the algorithm does not learn explicit model parameters from the data during this phase, but rather uses the data directly during inference, it is often referred to as a "lazy learner." The classification of a new, unlabeled data point, such as the yellow square shown, is determined by identifying the k closest points (its "nearest neighbors") in the stored training set, typically using Euclidean distance. The new point is then assigned the class that constitutes the majority among those k neighbors, a process illustrated in the inset by the seven dashed lines connecting the new point to its closest neighbors and the subsequent vote count.

The resulting decision boundary, seen as the border between the blue and red regions, is a result of this local voting system and is therefore often complex and non-linear. The concept of a "loss function" in the context of KNN differs from that in parametric models, such as logistic regression. KNN does not minimize a global loss function during training to learn parameters. Instead, a loss metric, such as the

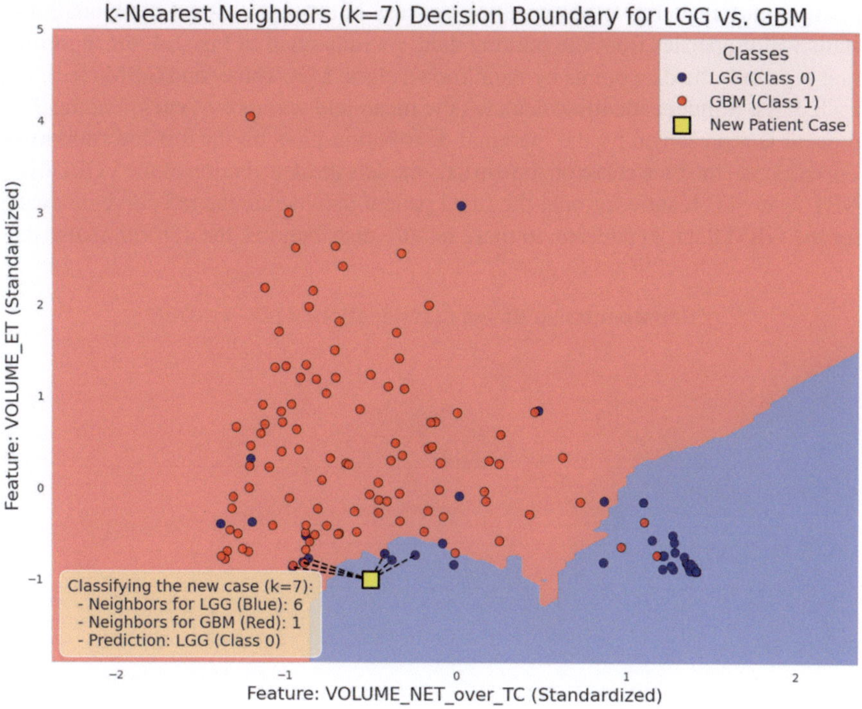

Fig. 1.3 Visualization of the k-Nearest Neighbors (KNN) algorithm for classifying brain tumors. The decision boundary for a k = 7 model is shown, trained on the two most predictive radiomic features (VOLUME_NET_over_TC and VOLUME_ET, which measure the volume of the enhancing (ET) part of the tumor core (TC) from the TCGA LGG-GBM dataset. The background color indicates the predicted class region (blue for LGG, red for GBM). To illustrate the classification process, a new sample case (yellow square) is introduced. The dashed lines connect this new case to its 7 nearest neighbors in the training data. The new case is classified based on a majority vote from these neighbors. (The code used to train the KNN classifier is available here: supervised_02_knn_gbm_lgg.ipynb)

0-1 loss (misclassification rate), is typically used during a separate model selection phase to determine the optimal value for the hyperparameter k. A practitioner would evaluate the performance of the KNN classifier on a validation dataset using several different values of k, and the value that results in the lowest loss (i.e., the fewest errors) is chosen for the final model. This process ensures the model's predictive capabilities are optimized without a traditional, iterative training procedure.

Naïve Bayes The relationship between input features and outcome variable is modeled by computing class posterior probabilities via Bayes' theorem. In this algorithm, the "naïve" assumption that the features are conditionally independent given the class is used. The Gaussian Naive Bayes classifier operates on the principles of Bayes' theorem, combined with a simplifying "naive" assumption that all features are independent of one another, given the class. The algorithm's "training" phase is not an iterative optimization process but rather a direct computation of statistical properties from the training data. As illustrated in Fig. 1.4, the algorithm first separates the data points by their known class: LGG (blue) and GBM (red). For each class, it independently calculates the mean and variance of each feature. This process is represented by the marginal distribution plots on the top and right axes. For example, the blue curve on the top axis models the distribution of the VOLUME_NET_over_TC feature for only the LGG patient data, while the red curve models it for the GBM data. In addition to these feature distributions, the algorithm also cal-

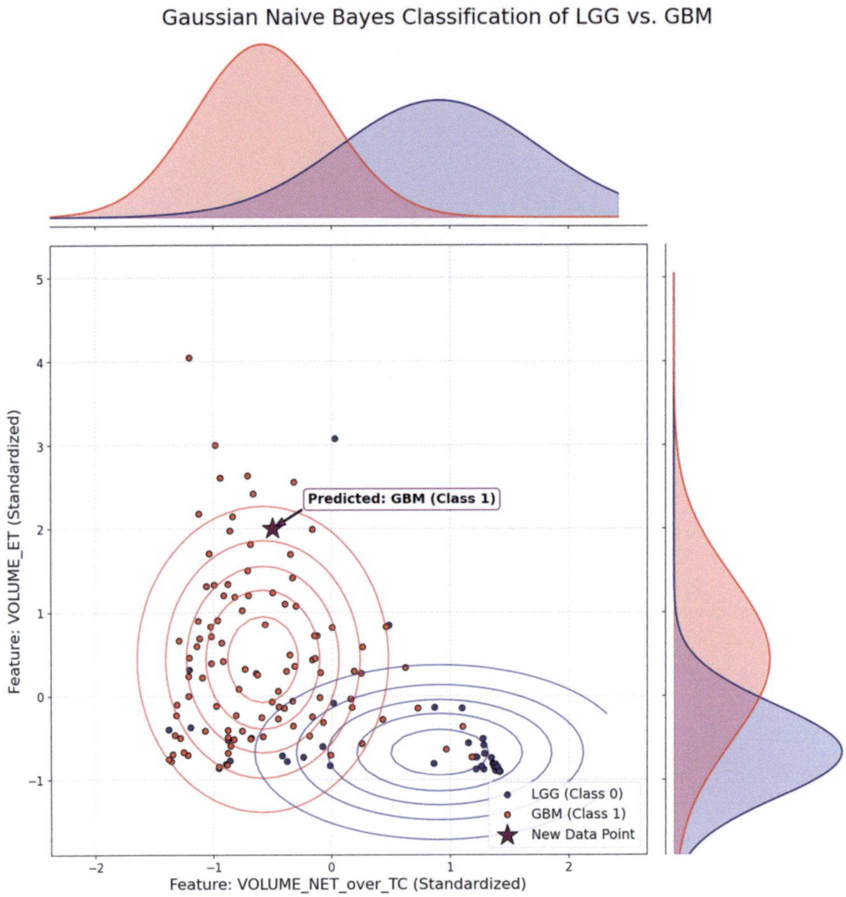

Fig. 1.4 Visualization of the Gaussian Naive Bayes classifier applied to the TCGA LGG-GBM dataset. The central plot shows patient data points for LGG (blue) and GBM (red) classes distributed across a 2D feature space defined by "VOLUME_NET_over_TC" and "VOLUME_ET." The concentric ellipses represent the contour lines of the Gaussian probability distributions that the algorithm has learned for each class independently. The marginal plots along the top and right axes show the corresponding one-dimensional Gaussian distributions for each feature. (Data Source: The Cancer Imaging Archive (TCIA), collections TCGA-LGG and TCGA-GBM. Code Repository: supervised_03_naivebayes_gbm_lgg.ipynb)

culates the overall prior probability of each class based on its frequency in the dataset.

To classify a new, unseen tumor, the classifier uses the learned models to determine which class provides a more probable explanation for the new data's features. It calculates a score for each potential class by first determining the likelihood of the new point's feature values occurring within that class's learned distributions (i.e., the height of the corresponding marginal curves). Because of the "naive" independence assumption, these individual feature likelihoods are simply multiplied together. This combined likelihood is then multiplied by the prior probability of that class to yield a final posterior probability score. This process is repeated for every class, and the new data point is ultimately assigned to the class that returns the highest score, completing the classification.

Discriminant Analysis This algorithm combines dimensionality reduction and feature transformation, maximizing the between-class variance relative to within-class variance.

As illustrated in Fig. 1.5, Linear Discriminant Analysis (LDA) works by first analyzing the distribution of the LGG (blue) and GBM (red) classes in the original two-dimensional feature space, as shown in the top panel (a). It then computes an optimal new one-dimensional axis, the "linear discriminant," which is oriented to simultaneously maximize the distance between the centers of the two classes while minimizing the spread of points within each class. The bottom panel (b) visualizes the core of the LDA process, where every original data point is projected perpendicularly onto this new axis, effectively reducing the data's dimensionality from 2D to 1D. This projection is designed to preserve the maximum amount of class-separating information, resulting in a simplified representation where the two tumor types remain distinctly clustered. The linear decision boundary shown in the left panel is the direct result of this process, representing the classification threshold on the new axis projected back into the original feature space.

Support Vector Machines This algorithm finds the "hyperplane" that maximizes the margin between classes in feature space. This versatile algorithm uses the "kernel-trick," which solves nonlinear problems by mapping data into a higher-dimensional space where the linear decision boundaries are more accurate (Fig. 1.6).

Decision Trees In this algorithm, the feature space is recursively split into subsets using simple thresholding rules, where each final subset (or leaf) predicts a constant value or class. Decision Trees excel at capturing non-linear interactions, but they are prone to overfitting (Fig. 1.7).

The Decision Tree model "learns" to separate LGG from GBM by carrying out a recursive set of splits as below.

1. Root node (RN)
   In the root node (RN), there are a total of **167 samples**, comprising **102 samples from the GBM class** and **65 samples from the LGG class**. One feature that has the highest data separation or the lowest "impurity" is chosen. Gini impurity of

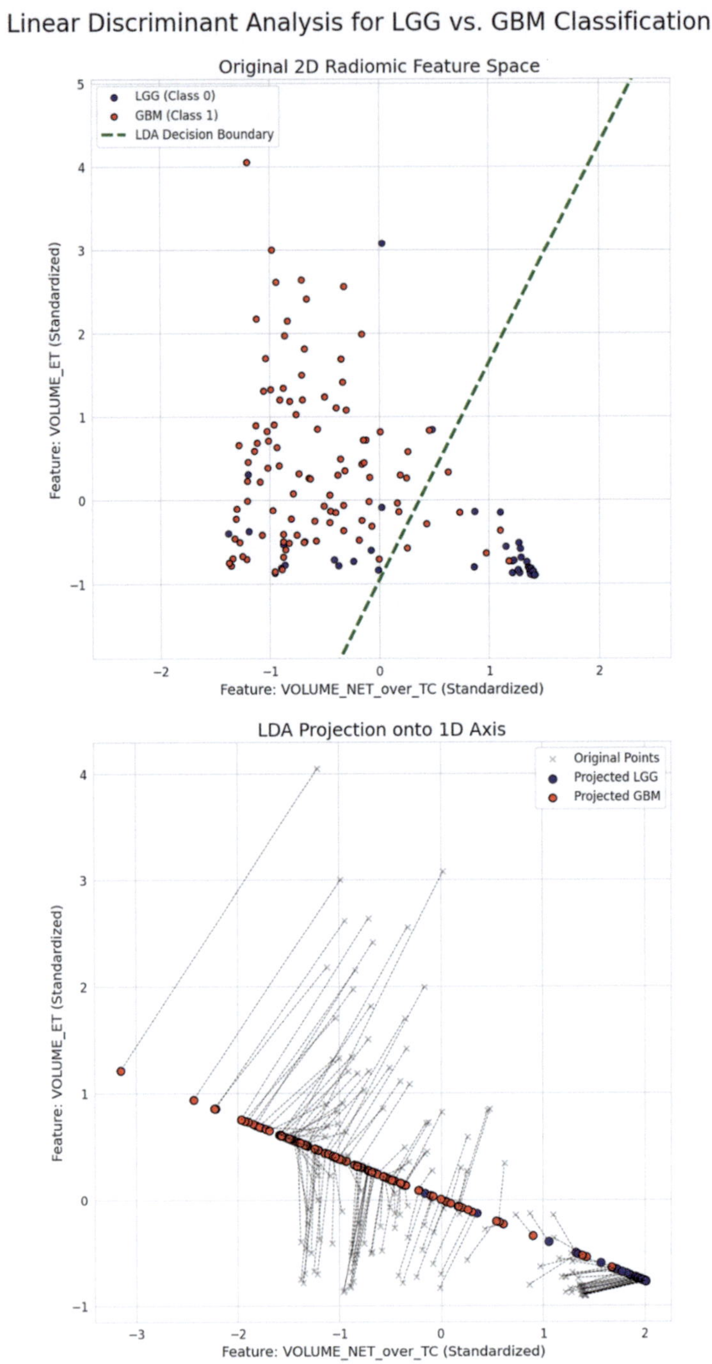

Fig. 1.5 Visualization of Linear Discriminant Analysis (LDA) for dimensionality reduction on the TCGA LGG-GBM dataset. (Data Source: The Cancer Imaging Archive (TCIA), collections TCGA-LGG and TCGA-GBM. Code Repository: supervised_04_discriminant_gbm_lgg.ipynb)

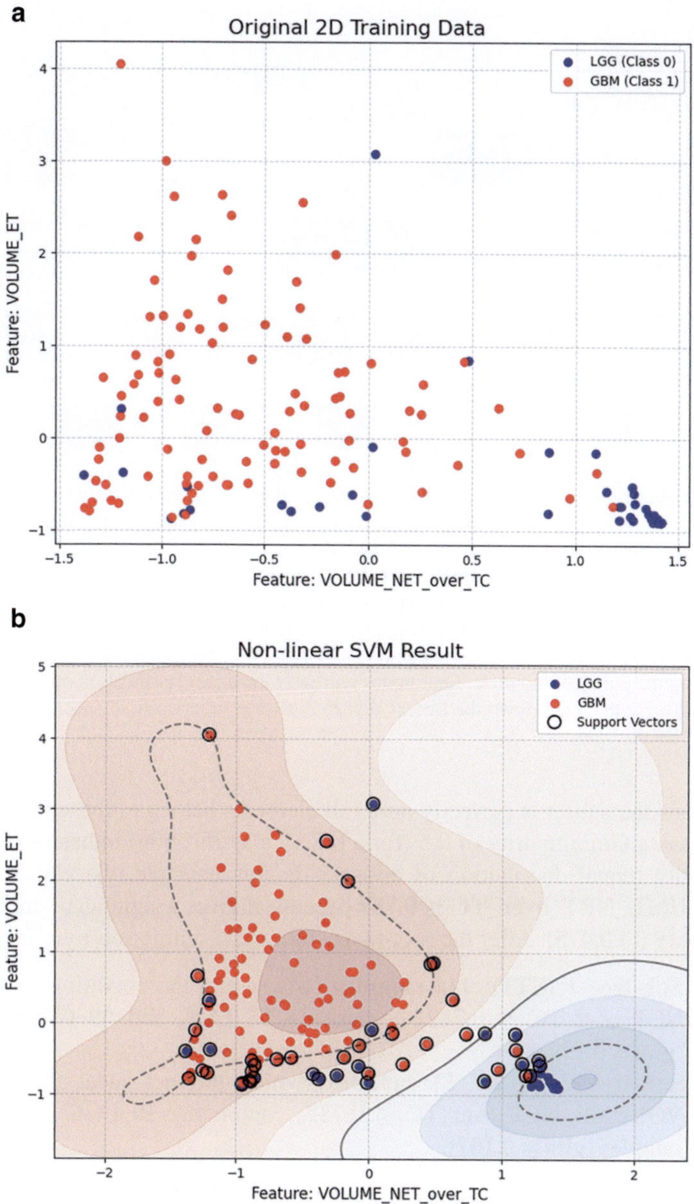

Fig. 1.6 Visualization of a Support Vector Machine (SVM) with a Radial Basis Function (RBF) kernel applied to the TCGA LGG-GBM classification problem. (**a**) The original data is shown in the 2D feature space defined by "VOLUME_NET_over_TC" and "VOLUME_ET," where a linear separation is not optimal. (**b**) To address this, the "kernel trick" conceptually maps the data into a higher-dimensional space using an RBF kernel. This hyperplane, when projected back into the original 2D space, results in a complex, non-linear decision boundary. The solid line represents the final boundary, while the dashed lines represent the margins. The circled points are the support vectors, the critical data points that dictate the position and shape of the boundary. (Code Repository: supervised_05_svm_gbm_lgg.ipynb)

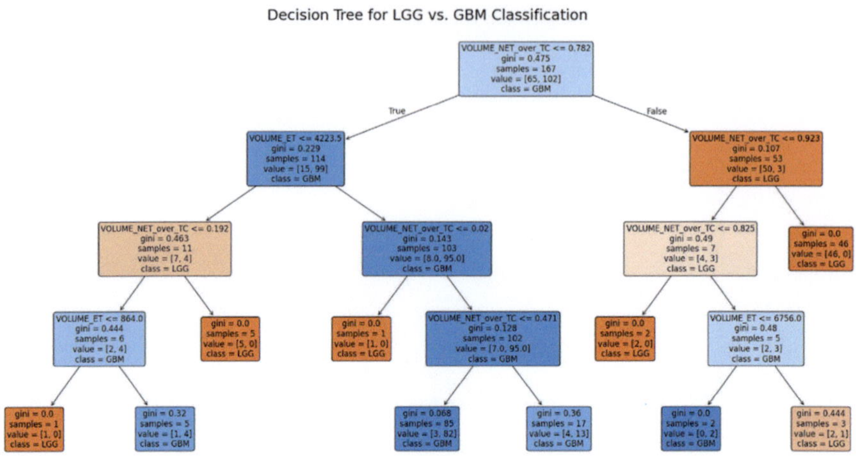

Fig. 1.7 Visualization of a Decision Tree classifier trained to distinguish between Lower-Grade Glioma (LGG) and Glioblastoma Multiforme (GBM). The tree was built using two radiomic features, "VOLUME_NET_over_TC" and "VOLUME_ET," with a maximum depth of 4 to ensure interpretability. Each node in the tree represents a decision rule based on a feature's value. The algorithm starts at the root node and recursively splits the data based on the condition that provides the best separation, measured by the Gini impurity. The color of each node indicates the majority class of the samples it contains (e.g., orange for LGG class, blue for the GBM), with color intensity representing the purity of the node. Leaf nodes represent the final classification outcome for samples that traverse that path down the tree. (Code Repository: supervised_06_decisiontrees_gbm_lgg.ipynb)

0 means the subset is perfectly pure (all elements belong to the same class). In contrast, a Gini impurity of 0.5 (for a binary classification) indicates maximum impurity (equal distribution of classes). In this example, the chosen split is **VOLUME_NET_over_TC ≤ 0.782** because it gives a significant drop in Gini impurity (to **0.475**). After the root-node split, the resulting sub-trees include:

- **Sub-tree 1 (ST1): 114 samples** (which met the condition VOLUME_NET_over_TC ≤ 0.782) comprising **15 LGG** and **99 GBM** samples (**gini = 0.229**)
- **Sub-tree 2 (ST2): 53 samples** (which did not meet the condition VOLUME_NET_over_TC ≤ 0.782) comprising **50 LGG** and **3 GBM** samples (**gini = 0.107**)

Upon observation of the class distribution of samples within the sub-trees, we can intuitively understand that ST1 would predict GBM and ST2 would predict LGG. But, at this level, the resulting nodes still contain misclassifications or still have impurity.

Stopping criteria: Whenever a node has no impurity (gini = 0) or reaches a minimum sample count (e.g., < 2), the algorithm stops growing that branch and assigns the majority class as the leaf prediction. These criteria can be modified to reduce (prune) the tree depth and complexity to reduce overfitting.

2. Sub-tree 1 (ST1)

   In ST1, there are **114 samples** with a gini of **0.229**, so this node is further split. The feature and value threshold chosen at this stage are **VOLUME_ET ≤ 4223.5**. This split yields two groups:

   - **Branch 1 (ST1-B1): 11 samples** (which met the condition VOLUME_ET ≤ 4223.5) comprising **7 LGG**, **4 GBM** (**gini = 0.463**)
   - **Branch 2 (ST1-B2): 103 samples** (which did not meet the condition) comprising **8 LGG** and **95 GBM** samples (**gini = 0.143**)

3. Sub-tree 2 (ST2)

   In ST2, there are **53 samples** with a gini of **0.107**. Depending on the use-case, a gini value of 0.107 would be considered quite low and the tree would not be split further since it may lead to overfitting, where the tree starts memorizing the training values and fails to generalize well. In this example, we split the node and use the feature **VOLUME_NET_over_TC <= 0.923**. This split yields two groups:

   - Branch 1 (ST2-B1): 7 samples (which met the condition) comprising 4 LGG and 3 GBM (gini = 0.49)
   - **Branch 2 (ST2-B2): 46 samples** (which did not meet the condition) comprising **46 LGG** and **0 GMB** (**gini = 0.0**). This node now becomes a leaf node (with no further splits) since the samples in this node have no impurity.

   This recursive process is repeated until all the other sub-trees and branches reach their leaf nodes, or until the stopping criteria are met (maximum depth of tree, minimum samples) that prevent overfitting Fig. 1.8. At the time of inference, the new sample is run through the tree, starting at the root, evaluating each node's feature threshold to follow the corresponding branch, and repeating until a leaf is reached, whose stored class label (or value) is returned.

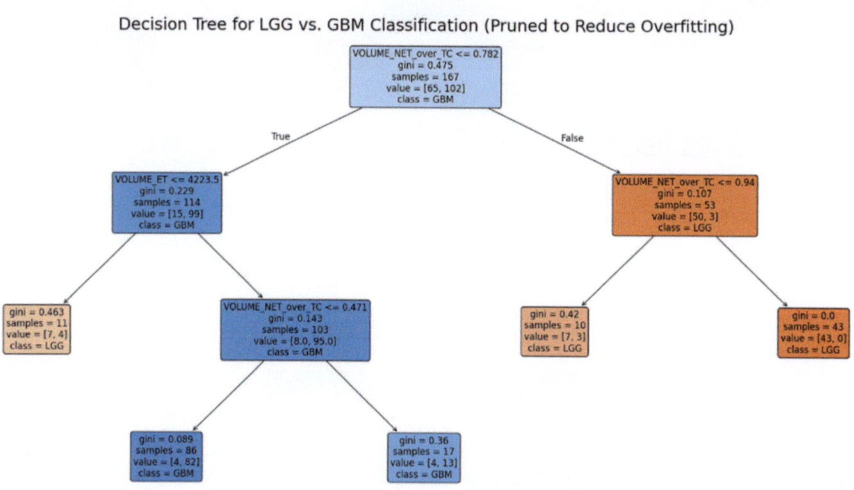

Fig. 1.8 Visualization of a Decision Tree classifier, pruned to reduce overfitting

It is worth noting that, unlike other classifier algorithms, Decision Trees do not need the features to be scaled or standardized. Therefore, the model is easy to interpret, using actual values of the features, which improves model explainability and fosters clinical trust among practitioners. For example, using the attached Decision Tree, we can infer that the model classifies the glioma as GBM when the ratio of the non-enhancing and necrotic tumor volume to the whole tumor volume (VOLUME_NET_OVER_TC) is less than or equal to 0.782 unless the volume of the enhancing tumor is less than 4334 mm^3, in which case the glioma is classified as LGG. Conversely, the model classifies the glioma as LGG if the ratio of the non-enhancing and necrotic tumor volume to the whole tumor volume (VOLUME_NET_OVER_TC) > 0.782. This transparency allows clinicians to validate the model's reasoning against their own expertise, ensuring its predictions are based on clinically sound principles.

Random Forest The Random Forest algorithm builds on the Decision Trees algorithm by creating an ensemble of Decision Trees on selected samples with randomized feature subsets at each split (Fig. 1.9). Intuitively, the Random Forest algorithm builds many weak Decision Trees that perform very well when their predictions are aggregated.

Gradient Boosting Gradient boosting builds on Decision Trees by providing more emphasis to hard-to-learn samples (or incorrectly predicted samples) by sequentially adding a weak learner that fit the residual errors of the existing ensemble. This algorithm is highly flexible but is again prone to overfitting. As illustrated in Fig. 1.10, the Gradient Boosting algorithm typically follows the below process:

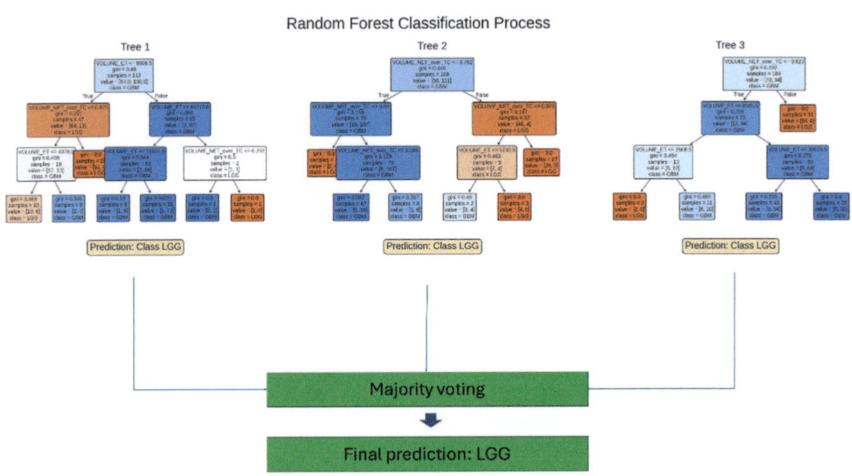

Fig. 1.9 Illustration of a random forest ensemble for LGG vs GBM classification: three Decision Trees, each trained on bootstrapped samples and random subsets of radiomic features, independently predict LGG, and a majority-voting scheme yields the final LGG classification. (Code Repository: supervised_07_rf_gbm_lgg.ipynb)

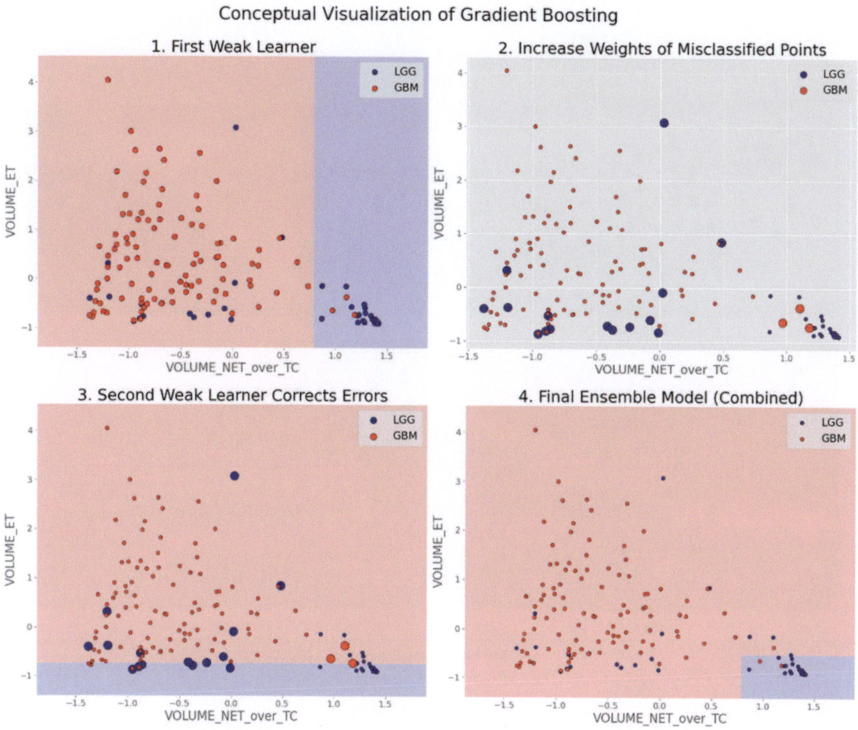

Fig. 1.10 A conceptual visualization of the Gradient Boosting algorithm for classifying LGG vs. GBM tumors. (Data Source: The Cancer Imaging Archive (TCIA), collections TCGA-LGG and TCGA-GBM. Code Repository: supervised_08_gboosting_gbm_lgg.ipynb)

1. A single, "weak" Decision Tree creates an initial, simple decision boundary.
2. The points that this first tree misclassified are identified, and their importance is increased (visualized by larger point sizes).
3. A second weak learner is then trained, which focuses on correctly classifying these previously missed points, creating a new decision boundary. This sequential process, where each new learner corrects the errors of its predecessor, continues for a set number of iterations.
4. The final result is a strong ensemble model that combines the insights from all the weak learners to create a more complex and accurate decision boundary.

Choosing the Right Supervised Learning Algorithm

While all classification algorithms try to identify the decision boundaries in their own way, the model complexity significantly influences how smooth or right each decision surface is. As observed in Fig. 1.11, simple, low-complexity models such as Logistic regression and Linear Discriminant analysis algorithms typically yield

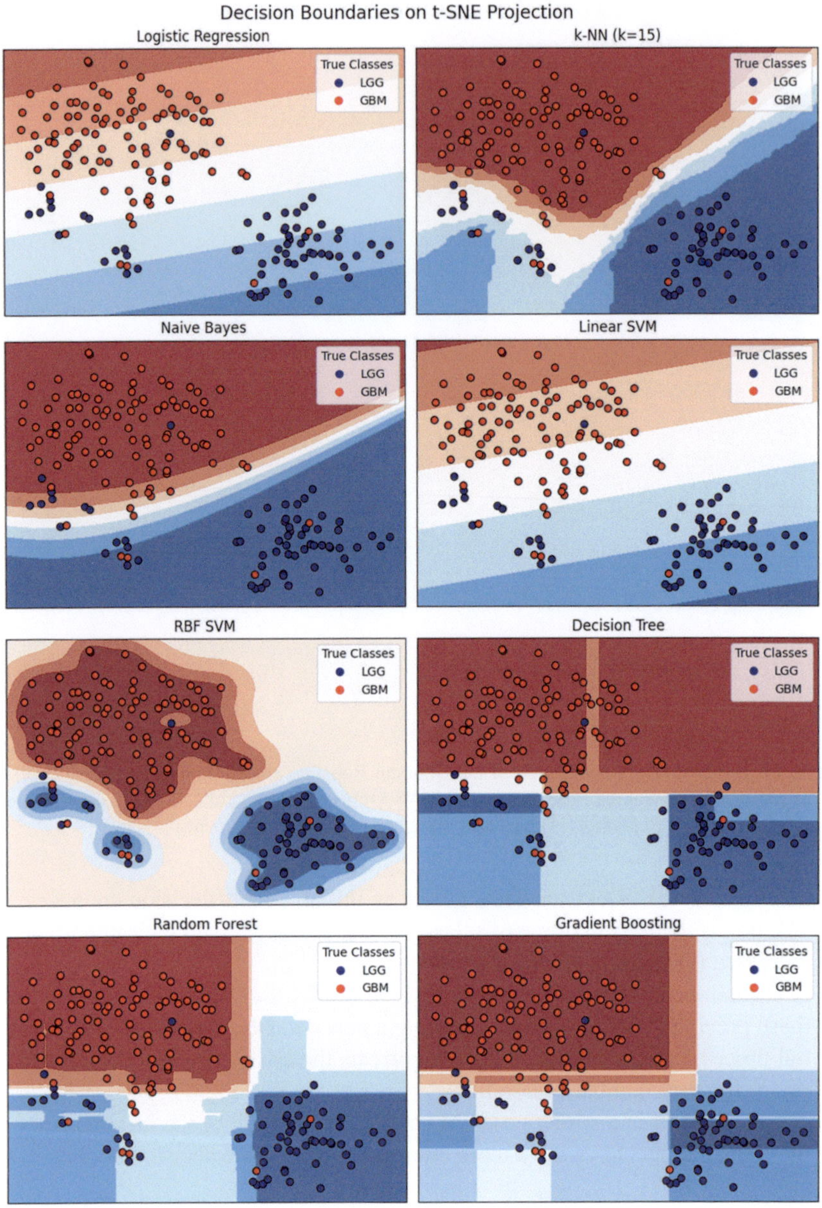

Fig. 1.11 Decision boundaries of various machine learning classifiers on a t-SNE projection of the TCGA-LGG and TCGA-GBM brain tumor datasets. The blue points represent samples of Low Grade Glioma (LGG), and the red points represent samples of Glioblastoma Multiforme (GBM). Each subplot displays the decision surface learned by a different classifier: Logistic Regression, k-Nearest Neighbors (k = 15), Naive Bayes, Linear Support Vector Machine, Radial Basis Function Support Vector Machine, Decision Tree, Random Forest, and Gradient Boosting. The background shading indicates the predicted class region for each model. This visualization illustrates the varying ability of different algorithms to separate these two tumor grades in a reduced-dimensional space (using t-SNE). (Data Source: The Cancer Imaging Archive (TCIA), collections TCGA-LGG and TCGA-GBM. Code Repository: supervised_10_decision_boundaries_viz)

smooth, nearly linear boundaries. Moderately complex algorithms such as KNN, Naive Bayes, and SVM introduce non-linear curves. While smooth, these decision boundaries adapt locally to clusters of points. High-complexity algorithms such as tree-based algorithms (Decision Trees, RF, and Gradient Boosting) produce highly irregular regions that can capture fine-grained patterns. This can also lead to overfitting if not properly addressed.

It is common practice to fit multiple candidate algorithms on a validation set that is further carved out from the training set and select the best-performing algorithm. This algorithm can then be evaluated on the final hold-out test set for generalization performance.

Strengths & Limitations

Supervised learning enables algorithms to learn to perform highly specialized tasks when provided with the right inputs to learn from. One of their biggest strengths lies in the fact that these algorithms excel at making precise predictions when trained on high-quality labeled data, making them suitable for learning highly specialized tasks in neuroradiology. Additionally, they provide transparent decision-making processes that aid trust and debugging. The performance of these algorithms is easily measured using hold-out sets. However, these algorithms are also highly dependent on labeled data, and acquiring adequate, accurately labeled datasets is quite time-consuming. Some highly complex supervised algorithms are highly prone to overfitting, where they perform well on training data but fail to generalize to new, unseen data.

Use-Cases

Table 1.1 below provides an overview of commonly used supervised learning algorithms (not exhaustive), their primary machine learning tasks, and representative neuroradiology use-cases as reported in recent research studies.

Unsupervised Learning

In this approach, the goal of the AI algorithms is to find underlying structures, patterns, or relationships in the data. Therefore, these algorithms are trained without explicit labels. Unsupervised learning algorithms are especially useful for understanding "what the data is trying to tell us". For example, unsupervised learning can be used to train on healthy scans to learn "normal" appearance, which can subsequently be used to flag for deviations such as incidental microbleeds or small infarcts. Generative algorithms are typically defined as unsupervised algorithms, but they are covered in detail in the next section focused on deep learning.

Table 1.1 Summary of supervised learning algorithms and their applications in neuroradiology

Clinical goal	Data used	Features	ML algorithm	Performance
Prediction of *IDH* genotype in gliomas	Preoperative MRIs of 538 glioma patients	Radiomic features (Histogram, shape, and texture features) from CE-T1W	Random forest algorithm	AUC ≈ 0.92
Classification of glioblastomas (GBM), meningiomas, brain metastases, and normal controls (NC).	154 patients (74 GBM, 62 meningioma, 18 brain metastases) and 170 Normal controls	Radiomic features were extracted using gray-level co-occurrence matrix (GLCM) analysis and Curvelet-based transformations	Nine machine learning classifiers, including Random Forest (RF), K-Nearest Neighbors (KNN), Categorical Boosting (CatBoost), Extreme Gradient Boosting (XGBoost), Support Vector Machine (SVM), Logistic Regression (LR), Naive Bayes, AdaBoost, and LightGBM	Accuracy = 95.2%
Distinguishing ruptured from unruptured aneurysms	845 aneurysms in 615 patients. Ruptured aneurysms (n = 309, 37%)	Aneurysm location and size	(random forest, linear support vector machine [SVM], and radial basis function kernel SVM)	AUROC 0.77 (linear SVM), 0.78 (RBF SVM), and 0.81 for the RF
Predict hemorrhagic transformation (HT) in acute ischemic stroke	118 patients diagnosed with acute ischemic stroke (52 developed HT, including 21 cases of hemorrhagic infarct (HI) and 31 cases of parenchymal hematoma (PH))	Radiomics features of the infarct areas on non-contrast-enhanced CT	Logistic regression	AUC in validation = 0.75
Predict Patient Outcome in Acute Ischemic Stroke	512 patients with AIS	Predict modified Rankin scale (mRS) scores at 90 days using biomarkers available at admission and 24 h	XGB and GBM	XGB and GBM had an AUC of 0.746 and 0.748, respectively

Key Characteristics

Unsupervised algorithms identify patterns, such as clusters, latent factors, or data manifolds, without explicit ground-truth labels. The training process often involves monitoring of an objective function, such as the within-cluster sum of squares. Unsupervised algorithms help practitioners better understand their high-dimensional data by creating a 2D visualization.

Commonly Used Algorithms

Clustering (K-means, hierarchical, density-based) In clustering, the sample is divided into groups where samples similar to each other are grouped together. In its basic form, the K-means clustering algorithm randomly picks K points as the cluster centroids, assigns each point to its nearest cluster centroid, recomputes cluster centroids as the mean of assigned points, and iteratively updates assignments until the cluster centroids no longer change.

As illustrated in Fig. 1.12,

1. The process begins with the unlabeled data and two randomly initialized centroids.
2. In the first "assignment" step, each data point is assigned to its closest centroid, forming initial clusters. The dashed lines from a few sample points illustrate this distance calculation.
3. In the first "update" step, the centroids are moved to the mean position (center of mass) of all the points assigned to them.
4. Steps 2 and 3 are repeated iteratively until the centroid positions no longer change, resulting in the final, stable cluster assignments.

The Elbow Method plots the Within-Cluster Sum of Squares (WCSS) against the number of clusters (K). WCSS is the sum of squared distances of data points to their assigned cluster center. As K increases, WCSS generally decreases because points are closer to their own cluster center. (Figs. 1.13 and 1.14). The "elbow point" is the value of K where the rate of decrease in WCSS sharply changes, forming an "elbow" shape. This point is often considered a good indicator of the optimal number of clusters, as adding more clusters beyond this point provides diminishing returns in terms of reducing variance within clusters. As with many real-world datasets, the "elbow point" is not well-pronounced because there's no single, clear point where adding another cluster stops providing a significant reduction in the Within-Cluster Sum of Squares (WCSS). In this case, the curve is smooth and gradual, indicating that each additional cluster offers a similarly incremental improvement.

The Silhouette Score measures how similar a data point is to its own cluster (cohesion) compared to other clusters (separation). It ranges from −1 to 1, where a score near +1 indicates that the data point is well inside its own cluster and far from other clusters. A score near 0 indicates that the data point is close to the decision

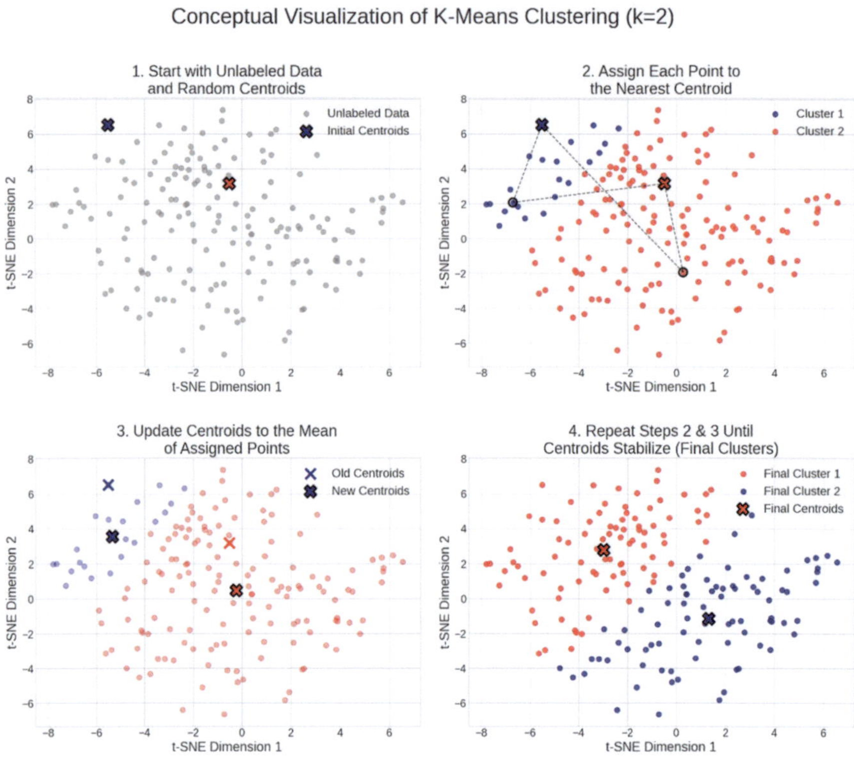

Fig. 1.12 A conceptual visualization of the K-Means clustering algorithm (k = 2) applied to the TCGA LGG-GBM dataset after dimensionality reduction with t-SNE. (Data Source: The Cancer Imaging Archive (TCIA), collections TCGA-LGG and TCGA-GBM. *Code Repository:* unsupervised_01_k-means_gbm_lgg.ipynb)

boundary between two neighboring clusters. A score near −1 indicates that the data point is likely assigned to the wrong cluster. A higher average Silhouette Score across all data points suggests a better clustering configuration. We typically look for the value of K that maximizes the average Silhouette Score. Based on the plot above, the highest silhouette score is observed at K = 3.

Dimensionality reduction (Principal Component Analysis) Principal Component Analysis (PCA) solves the problem of high dimensionality. It's a technique used to simplify complex datasets by reducing the number of features (or dimensions) while retaining the most important information. This technique addresses several challenges, such as data sparsity and multicollinearity, by transforming the original, high-dimensional data into a lower-dimensional space by creating a new set of uncorrelated variables called principal components. The principal components are ranked by the amount of variance they explain in the original data, and the first few principal components are selected based on the total amount of variance they explain from the original dataset. In this manner, the number of features can be

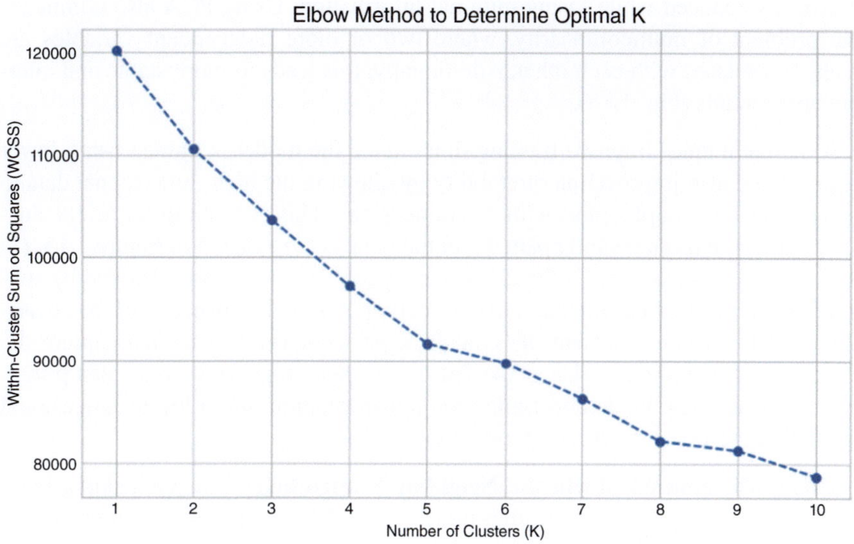

Fig. 1.13 Illustration of the elbow method to select the number of clusters (k). The within-cluster sum of squares is plotted as a function of the number of clusters k ranging from 1 to 10. The curve begins to flatten ("elbow") when the decrease in WCSS provides diminishing improvements with an increasing number of clusters

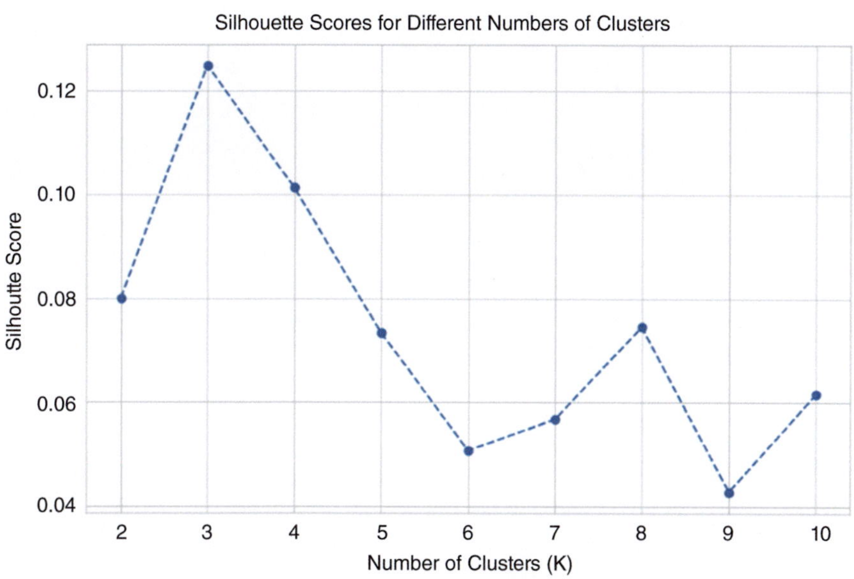

Fig. 1.14 An illustration of the Silhouette Score plot to select the number of clusters (k). Higher values of the mean silhouette score indicate better-defined clusters (greater separation between clusters relative to within-cluster cohesion)

drastically reduced while losing minimal information. Using PCA also eliminates the problem of multicollinearity, where two or more independent variables are highly correlated with each other. Additionally, this leads to more stable and interpretable models (Fig. 1.15).

PCA techniques improve training times since the model is trained using fewer features and also improve interpretability by allowing the high-dimensional data to be visualized in simpler plots with 2–3 dimensions. This can intuitively reveal clusters, outliers and other subtle patterns in the data. As visualized in Figure 1.15, (1) the original data is shown in the 2D feature space. (2) The data is centered by subtracting the mean of each feature. (3) PCA computes the eigenvectors of the covariance matrix, which represent the new principal component axes that capture the directions of maximum variance. (4) The data is then projected onto the first principal component (PC1), demonstrating the transformation into a lower-dimensional space that preserves the most important information.

t-SNE (t-Distributed Stochastic Neighbor Embedding) This embedding technique helps compress complex, high-dimensional data into just two or three dimensions, thereby enabling the creation of intuitive visualizations that facilitate understanding of highly complex data. In these visualizations, similar points are

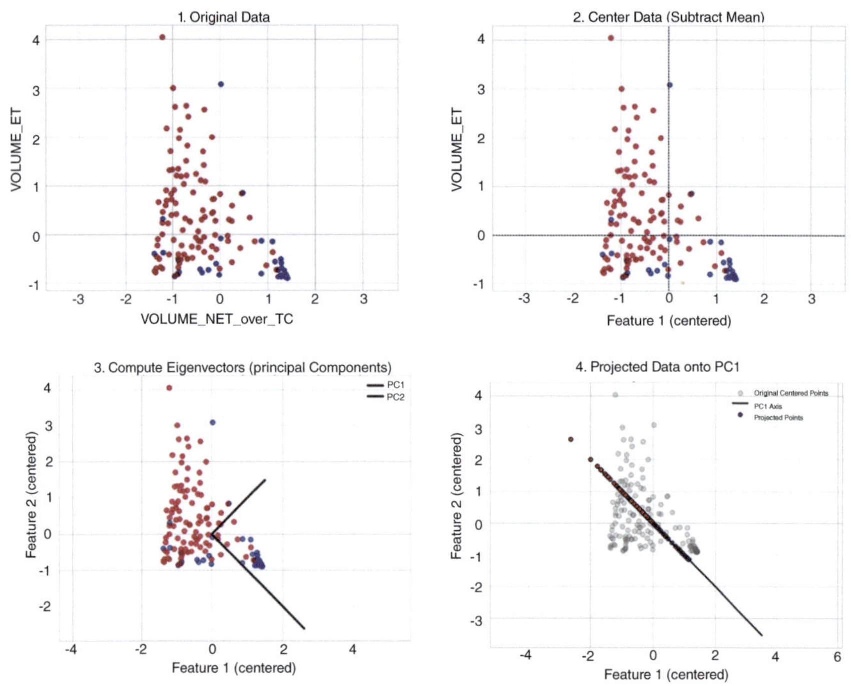

Fig. 1.15 A step-by-step visualization of the Principal Component Analysis (PCA) procedure on the TCGA dataset. (Data Source: The Cancer Imaging Archive (TCIA), collections TCGA-LGG and TCGA-GBM. Code Repository: unsupervised_02_PCA_gbm_lgg.ipynb)

placed closer together, and dissimilar ones are pushed further apart. Perplexity is a parameter that controls the balance between local and global aspects of the data when visualizing high-dimensional data in a lower-dimensional space. It defines the effective number of neighbors a point considers when constructing its similarity map, influencing how tightly clusters are formed in the final visualization. The comparison shown in Fig. 1.16 illustrates how the perplexity hyperparameter affects the resulting structure, with lower values emphasizing local relationships and forming smaller, tighter clusters, while higher values consider more neighbors and tend to reveal broader, more global patterns in the data.

Gaussian Mixture Models (GMM) These unsupervised models help identify hidden groups within the dataset. In this method, each group is assumed to follow a normal distribution (bell curve), and then the combination of these curves is fitted to explain the overall distribution. The final output for each sample is a probability of belonging to each group. As illustrated in Fig. 1.17, in this case, with two components (k = 2), the algorithm has identified two primary clusters in the data, visualized by the blue and red points. The overlaid contour ellipses represent the probability density of each learned Gaussian component, showing their mean, variance, and orientation. This demonstrates GMM's ability to identify and model non-spherical clusters, which correspond well to the underlying structure of the two distinct tumor types.

Choosing the Correct Algorithm

Choosing an unsupervised algorithm largely depends on the analytical objective. Unsupervised algorithms can be used to discover clusters, reduce dimensionality, or model data density. Additionally, the decision also relies on the underlying geometry of your data. For example, simple, fast methods like K-means or PCA work well when clusters are roughly spherical or structure is linear and interpretability is paramount. Techniques such as density-based clustering, GMM, or t-SNE/UMAP handle arbitrarily shaped clusters, overlapping distributions, or nonlinear manifolds at the cost of additional tuning. The size and noise within the dataset must also be taken into account. For example, density-based and model-based methods tend to be more robust to outliers.

Strengths & Limitations

Unsupervised algorithms are quite useful when it comes to generating hypotheses, exploring data, and discovering new biomarkers. However, cluster assignments and principal components are examples of results that often lack direct clinical interpretation and require validation against external standards. Furthermore, the dimensionality of the data, the number of clusters, or the choice of similarity metrics can all impact the performance of unsupervised models.

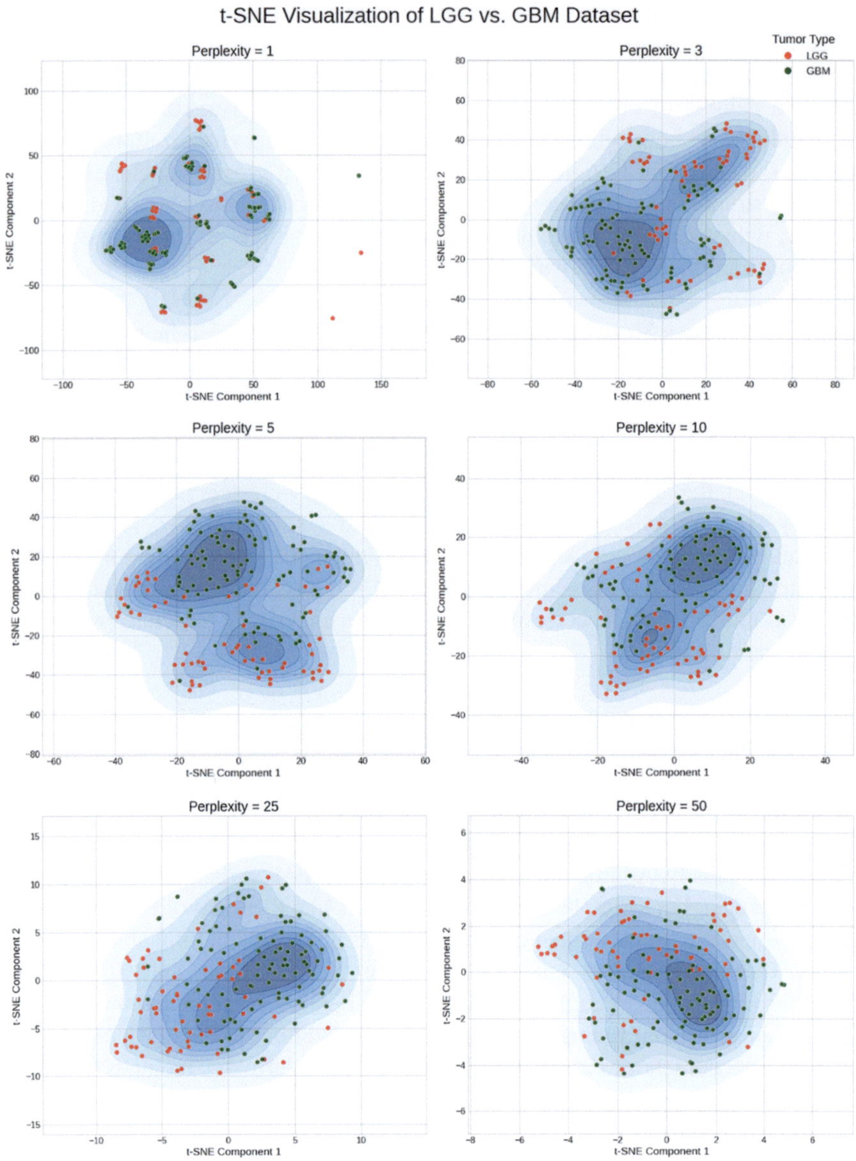

Fig. 1.16 A multi-panel visualization exploring the t-SNE embedding of the high-dimensional TCGA LGG-GBM radiomics dataset using all available features. Each panel represents a different "perplexity" value used during the t-SNE computation, ranging from 1 to 50. The points are colored by their ground-truth tumor type (LGG vs. GBM), and a kernel density estimate is overlaid to show the distribution of the clusters. (Data Source: The Cancer Imaging Archive (TCIA), collections TCGA-LGG and TCGA-GBM. Code Repository: unsupervised_03_tsne_gbm_lgg.ipynb)

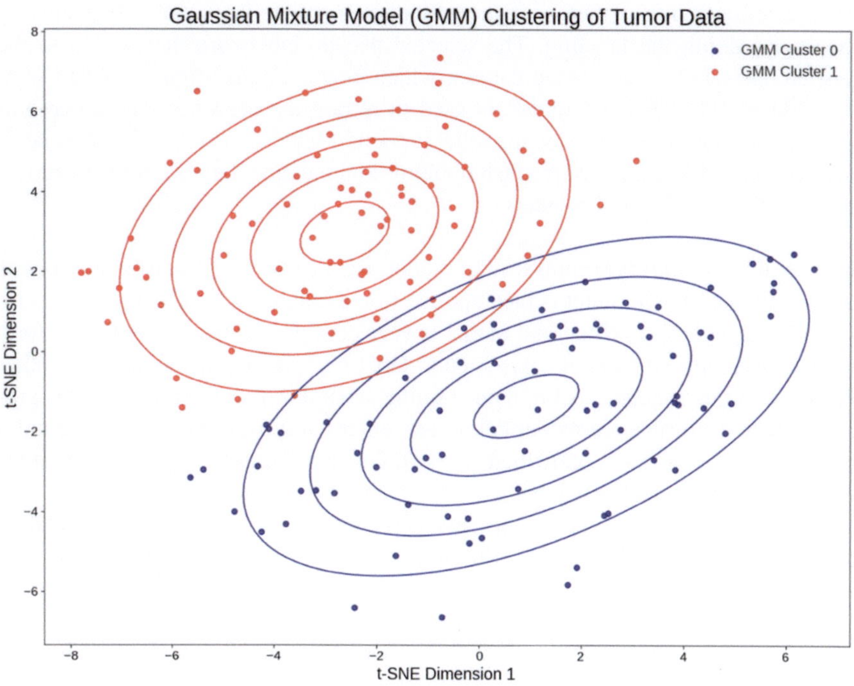

Fig. 1.17 A visualization of a Gaussian Mixture Model (GMM) applied to the t-SNE embedding of the TCGA LGG-GBM radiomics dataset. (Data Source: The Cancer Imaging Archive (TCIA), collections TCGA-LGG and TCGA-GBM. Code Repository: unsupervised_04_GMM_gbm_lgg.ipynb)

Semi-supervised Learning

Key Characteristics

Semi-supervised learning addresses the limitations of supervised and unsupervised algorithms by using both labeled and unlabeled data during training. It uses a hybrid training process, where the initial part focuses on training the supervised learning algorithm using the limited labeled data. The latter part of the training process focuses on refining the trained model from the previous step using the unlabeled dataset. These algorithms can achieve better model performance in settings where limited data is a pervasive challenge, especially in neuroradiology.

Common Algorithms

Self-Training In this method, the model is first trained using labeled data, and this trained model is applied to the unlabeled data to produce pseudo-labels. In the second step, the most reliable labels are selected from the generated pseudo-labels.

This selection is done either using the prediction's probability score or manually by the expert doing the labeling. The selected pseudo-labels are then added to the labeled dataset. This combined dataset, which now contains original labeled samples and pseudo-labeled samples, is used to retrain the classifier. The process of generating pseudo-labels, selecting reliable pseudo-labels, and retraining the classifier is carried out in an iterative fashion until no unlabeled data is left or the model stops finding confident new labels.

Co-training In the algorithm, several models are first trained on different sections of labeled data. Each model is then applied to the unlabeled data and the "pseudo-labels" are generated. When one model is very confident about its prediction for a particular sample, it "shares" this pseudo-label with the other models. The other models add this pseudo-label to their training set and retrain themselves. This process, where each separate model helps each other learn from more and more unlabeled data, is continued until there is no unlabeled data left or the model stops finding more confident new labels.

As shown in Fig. 1.18, (1) the process starts with a small, labeled set and a large, unlabeled pool. (2) Classifier 1 is trained on the labeled set using only the first

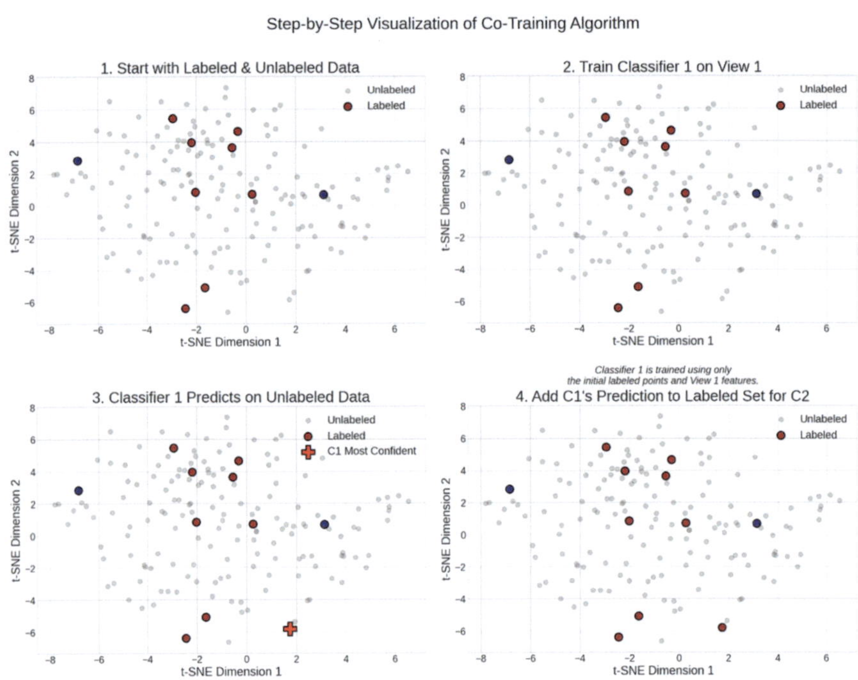

Fig. 1.18 A step-by-step visualization of one iteration of the Co-Training semi-supervised algorithm. (Data Source: The Cancer Imaging Archive (TCIA), collections TCGA-LGG and TCGA-GBM. Code Repository: semisupervised_02_co-training.ipynb)

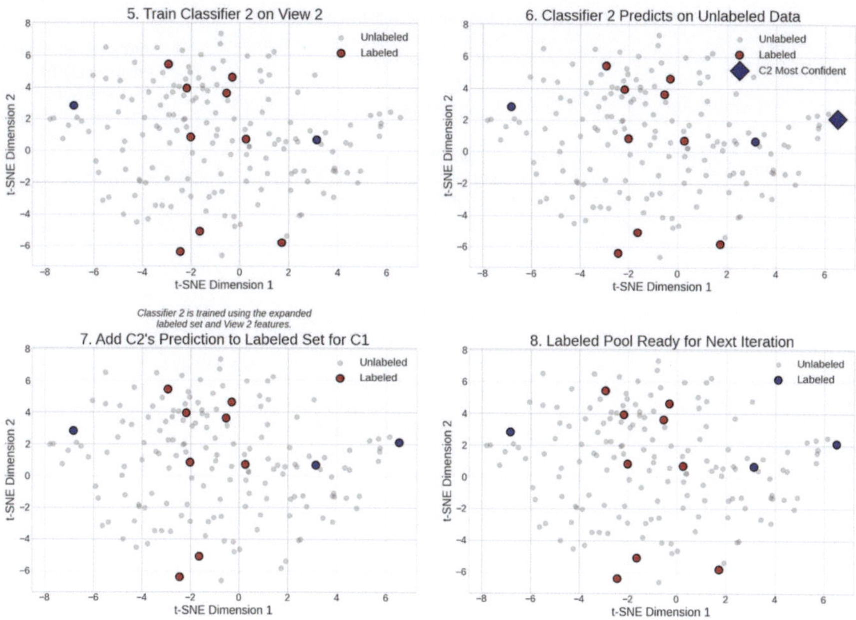

Fig. 1.18 (continued)

feature view. (3) It then predicts labels for the unlabeled data and selects its most confident prediction. (4) This new prediction is temporarily added to the labeled set. (5) Classifier 2 is trained on this expanded set using the second feature view. (6) It then makes its own confident prediction on the remaining unlabeled data. (7) Its prediction is added to the labeled set. (8) The final labeled pool is now larger and ready to be used for the next iteration of training, demonstrating how the classifiers teach each other.

Graph-Based Techniques (Label-Spreading, Label Propagation) Graph-based techniques, like label spreading and label propagation, create a graph with edges that indicate similarity and nodes that represent data points. Using the premise that similar data points will likely have the same label, labels are spread from labeled to unlabeled nodes in the graph. These techniques work especially well when spatial or temporal continuity can be used in imaging applications.

As illustrated in Fig. 1.19, the algorithm begins with a small subset of known data, shown as large circles with a yellow border. The gray arrows illustrate the "spreading" process, where label information is propagated from the initial labeled points to their closest unlabeled neighbors. The final plot shows the predicted class for all the initially unlabeled points (blue and red "x"s), demonstrating how the algorithm has inferred the tumor type for the entire cohort based on both the initial labels and the underlying structure of the data.

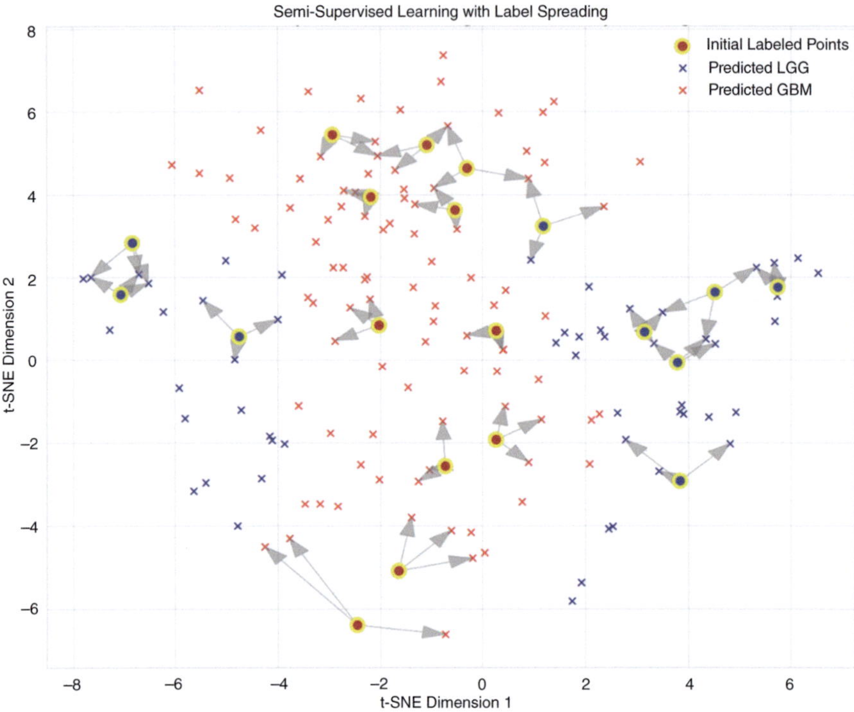

Fig. 1.19 A visualization of the Label Spreading algorithm, a semi-supervised learning technique, applied to the t-SNE embedding of the TCGA LGG-GBM dataset. (Data Source: The Cancer Imaging Archive (TCIA), collections TCGA-LGG and TCGA-GBM. Code Repository: semisupervised_01_label_spreading.ipynb)

Choosing the Right Algorithm

The primary considerations to account for while choosing the right semi-supervised algorithm are data availability, availability of ground truth labels, computational cost, noise robustness, and feature assumptions.

While self-training algorithms are preferred for unified feature spaces, such as single MRI sequence analysis, co-training algorithms require at least two conditionally independent feature views, such as Structural MRI + fMRI features. While both self-training and co-training algorithms are computationally lighter than graph-based methods, they are also sensitive to noise within the input datasets. Co-training typically uses double the model training, but those computations can also be parallelized. Graph-based algorithms (label spreading, label propagation) excel when neighborhood relationships matter. Similar samples influence each other's labels, thereby spreading label information that effectively identifies clusters or groups.

Self-training works best when the dataset involves only a single imaging modality, such as CT or MRI. Typically, self-training algorithms need at least 10% of the dataset to be labelled by an expert practitioner. Co-training performs best for datasets with natural feature splits, such as multi-modal data. For example, if radiology reports are combined with imaging features, co-training is a powerful tool in this situation. Graph-based methods work best when computational costs are not a significant concern. Within Graph-based methods, label propagation is preferred over label spreading when the dataset may contain label noise in the form of noisy annotations.

Strengths & Limitations

Semi-supervised learning algorithms reduce dependence on extensive labeled datasets. They also learn underlying patterns from unlabeled data, improving their final generalization performance. These algorithms are not computationally complex and can be trained without an extensive computing setup (Table 1.2).

However, mislabeled or unrepresentative data labels adversely affect model performance. Errors can be propagated since incorrect pseudo-labels can reinforce misclassifications. To reduce these risks, thorough validation and the application of uncertainty estimation methods are crucial.

Reinforcement Learning

Unlike supervised learning, which relies on labeled examples, or unsupervised learning, which relies on pattern identification, reinforcement learning algorithms train using sequential decision-making and trial and error.

Key Characteristics

At their core, RL algorithms train an ***agent*** to make decisions by interacting with an ***environment*** with the goal of maximizing a ***cumulative reward***. At each step, the agent inputs a ***state*** of the environment, takes an ***action***, which causes the environment to transition into a new state, and receives a ***reward***. Over time, the agent learns an optimal ***policy***, which is a decision strategy that provides the highest rewards.

Table 1.2 Strengths and limitations of Self-supervised learning algorithms

Comparison factor	Strengths	Limitations
Labeled data	Reduces costs by 70–90%	Requires high-quality initial labels
Unlabeled data	Improves generalization	Sensitive to noise/distribution shifts
Computational resources	Scalable for large datasets	Graph methods are impractical beyond 10k samples
Theoretical foundation	Effective in practice	Few performance guarantees

Components of an RL system Reinforcement learning systems comprise several important components. The Agent is the decision maker or learner that interacts with the environment. The Environment is the external system with which the agent interacts. A State is the environment's condition at a given point in time. The Action is the step that the agent takes to navigate the environment. The Reward is the feedback provided to the agent based on its action. The Policy is the strategy that determines how the agent selects actions given a current state. The Value function estimates the expected future reward from a given state. It is important to understand that while policy tells the agent what to do in a given state, the value function estimates the worth of the agent being in a certain state.

Model-Based vs. Model-Free Algorithms It is important to note that RL algorithms can either be model-based, where agents build internal models of the environment dynamics, or model-free, where agents learn directly from interactions without explicit modeling of the environment dynamics. Model-based algorithms simulate future state trajectories, thinking ahead and evaluating actions before actually taking them. Model-free algorithms are especially suited for cases where comprehensive modeling may be impractical, or the environment does not conform to known data distributions. For example, imagine that the goal for an AI system is to identify brain tumors in MRI scans. If we were to use the model-based learning paradigm, the AI system would first learn or be given knowledge about brain anatomy and typical growth patterns. This knowledge is used to build an internal model of tumors' appearance and development. The RL algorithm would use this model to more efficiently search for tumors in new scans. There is minimal trial-and-error in this approach. On the other hand, model-free RL algorithms would try many different ways to analyze the images using trial-and-error. While it may sometimes focus on irrelevant regions, it may derive the patterns that lead to correct tumor detection. Model-based algorithms are, therefore, more sample-efficient than model-free algorithms, but with adequate training data, model-free algorithms are easier to train.

Exploration vs. Exploitation Balance RL algorithms also frequently balance discovering new actions (exploration) and leveraging already known high-reward actions (exploitation). A highly exploratory model doesn't leverage the information it has about the environment, while an overly exploitative model relies too much on the information it already has and doesn't learn other potential solutions.

Temporal Difference (TD) RL systems usually operate in complex situations where there are multiple steps to perform to arrive at the optimal solution, so the consequences of their actions at a given step aren't immediately apparent. Temporal Difference is a method that addresses this by coming up with an estimate of future rewards at a given step rather than waiting for final outcomes.

On-Policy vs. Off-Policy Learning RL agents are configured to either learn from their actions while following a certain strategy or learn from actions taken across different strategies (off-policy). On-policy methods update their policy using data generated only by their current strategy. Off-policy approaches separate data collection from policy optimization, so these algorithms can learn from historical or external datasets while pursuing optimal decision-making.

State vs. Action Value Function State-value functions are used to quantify the expected return (cumulative future reward) an agent can achieve from a given state and following a specific policy thereafter. On the other hand, action value functions (or Q-functions) are used to estimate the expected return of taking a particular action in a given state and then following the policy for subsequent steps. So, while the state-value function provides a measure of the long-term desirability of states under a policy, the action-value function provides a measure of the quality of individual state-action pairs.

Common Algorithms

At its core, Reinforcement learning can be categorized into three types: Value-based, Policy-based, and Actor-Critic algorithms. While value-based methods focus on predicting the long-term value of specific actions, policy-based methods learn optimal behavior patterns without explicitly calculating values. Actor-critic algorithms utilize a hybrid approach, where the elements of value-based and policy-based methods are combined.

Value-Based Algorithms Q-learning is a model-free algorithm that estimates, in an iterative manner, the expected return (value) of taking specific action in given states. Deep-Q-Networks (DQN) utilize deep neural networks to handle high-dimensional states. State-Action-Reward-State-Action (SARSA) is another value-based algorithm that adopts an on-policy approach where the value estimates are updated based on actual actions taken.

Policy-Based Algorithms Unlike value-based methods that learn value functions and derive policies indirectly, policy-based methods focus on learning the policy itself directly. The core idea behind such algorithms, the Policy Gradient, is to use an optimization algorithm, such as the gradient ascent, to update the policy parameters that increase the probability of actions leading to higher rewards. The REINFORCE algorithm uses the policy gradient method to directly optimize a policy by updating its parameters at the end of each interaction based on the cumulative reward received. While simple, the REINFORCE algorithm suffers from high variance, which would exacerbate instability in sensitive tasks such as lesion segmentation. To address these issues, the **Trust Region Policy Optimization (TRPO)** method uses a KL Divergence constraint to ensure the policy updates remain within a "trust region." While this method makes the methodology highly stable for clinical applications, it is very computationally complex. The Proximal Policy Optimization (PPO) algorithm addresses the instability problem of REINFORCE and high computational complexity of TRPO by using a clipped objective function. The clipping function restricts the policy changes from making overoptimistic updates and approximates the trust region instead of calculating the KL divergence, which is quite computationally complex.

Actor-Critic Algorithms These hybrid algorithms combine policy-based action selection with value-based evaluation to achieve stable, sample-efficient learning, often outperforming isolated policy-based or value-based algorithms. The Actor (policy-network) decides what action the agent should take in a given state. The Critic (value-network) evaluates how good that action was by estimating the expected future rewards from that state. After each action, the critic provides feedback using the "advantage" metric, which measures how much better (or worse) the action was compared to the average expected outcome in that state. The Actor uses this feedback to adjust its decisions so that it makes good actions more likely in the future. For example, in the context of MRI scan parameter optimization, one of the potential proposals from the Actor would be to adjust slice thickness or contrast timing (continuous actions). The Critic would use these proposals to estimate how these changes affect diagnostic accuracy.

Advanced Actor-Critic (A2C) algorithms use parallel training environments to update the networks at every step, thereby making the learning process faster and more stable. In neuroradiology, A2C has been applied to real-time lesion tracking in dynamic contrast-enhanced MRI, where the critic evaluates tracking accuracy frame-by-frame while the actor refines region-of-interest adjustments. Deep Deterministic Policy Gradient (DDPG) combines the key ideas of Actor-Critic architectures and Q-learning, which makes it more suitable for continuous-control tasks. For example, in optimizing 3D brain scan reconstruction parameters, the actor network in DDPG proposes voxel-intensity thresholds for tissue segmentation, while the critic evaluates segmentation quality against ground truth masks, creating a feedback loop that stabilizes training in high-dimensional medical imaging environments.

Choosing the Right Algorithm

Different reinforcement algorithms have distinct strengths and weaknesses. Value-based algorithms, such as DQNs, work well for tasks involving discrete navigation through image space. On the other hand, policy-gradient or actor-critic algorithms are better suited for tasks with continuous action spaces. For example, let's take the case of brain lesion detection on brain MRI scans. In this case, the RL task can be defined in such a way that each state represents the current viewing position or region of interest, and discrete actions determine which direction to move the viewing position or the direction of adjustment of bounding boxes. For such tasks where the action spaces are discrete, value-based methods such as DQNs are more appropriate. However, these algorithms are quite computationally intense and may require careful designing of the reward function to avoid unwanted behaviors. Let's take another example of an RL task where the goal of the algorithm is to optimize MRI acquisition strategies. This is a continuous action space since the parameters include balancing scan time, image quality, and downstream diagnostic performance. In this case, where the actions are in a continuous space, policy-gradient or actor-critic methods are more appropriate since they are able to carry out fine-grained adjustment of acquisition parameters without the need to discretize the action space artificially.

On-policy algorithms, such as PPO and A2C, learn from data that is sampled according to the current policy. They are beneficial in settings where algorithms require greater stability and robustness in non-stationary environments. However, these algorithms are also not sample-efficient, as they require numerous interactions to converge. On-policy algorithms are better suited when the task requires the agent's behavior to remain safe and converge reliably during training. An example of this task is the optimization of acquisition parameters, where the agent must sequentially choose parameters based on intermediate reconstructed images, without running the risk of taking wildly off-distribution actions. On-policy approaches perform well when safety, stability, and direct alignment with complex clinical objectives are paramount, even if that comes at the cost of requiring more environment interactions or higher sample complexity. By constraining learning to what the agent does, they provide a controlled, interpretable path toward deploying RL agents in sensitive neuroradiology workflows. On the other hand, off-policy algorithms, such as DQN and DDPG, are more sample-efficient since they can reuse past experiences from other strategies. They excel in tasks that utilize large, pre-existing datasets or simulated datasets. They also work well with heterogeneous data sources and multi-task learning. For example, an off-policy DQN trained on archived 3D CT brain scans can learn to propose optimal slice orientations for intracranial hemorrhage detection without requiring fresh on-scanner trials for every policy update. Off-policy algorithms are also better suited for parallel experimentation, as they are not constrained by on-policy data collection.

The Promise of Deep Learning

Traditional machine learning algorithms still rely on manually engineered features and shallow representations, which limit their ability to capture complex, hierarchical patterns. Deep Learning introduced neural networks composed of multiple processing layers that automatically learn successive feature abstractions directly from raw inputs, obviating the need for bespoke feature engineering. Deep neural networks perform well with both structured and unstructured datasets, making them well-suited for many applications within neuroradiology, which involves dealing with medical images and written reports. Additionally, advances in high-performance computing, including GPU-accelerated computing, have helped deep-learning-based tools become increasingly integrated into neuroradiology workflows, supporting tasks such as lesion delineation, differential diagnosis, and prognosis. This section provides a structured overview of deep learning, elucidating the mechanics of neural network learning, reviewing major architectures, and examining their impact in computer vision, generative AI, and multimodal systems. Since Convolutional Neural Networks and Transformer networks have been widely used for AI in neuroradiology tasks, more in-depth discussions with network architectures, codes, and visualizations have been included for these specific sections.

How Neural Networks Learn

A neural network is a parametric model defined by an architecture, a directed acyclic graph of computational nodes (neurons) organized into layers, where each neuron computes a weighted sum of its inputs plus a bias and then applies a nonlinear activation function. Formally, given an input vector $x \in R^n$, the network implements a function $f(x; \theta)$, where the parameter set θ consists of all weight matrices $\{W^l\}$ and bias vectors $\{b^l\}$ across layers l.

Hyperparameters are a set of values, such as the number of layers, units per layer, choice of activation functions, learning rate, batch size, and regularization coefficients, that govern the architectural design and the training process of the model. Unlike parameters, which are learnt during the training process, hyperparameters are not learnt but instead set by the user while training the network.

During training, a loss function $L(f(x; \theta), y)$ measures the discrepancy between the network's predictions and true labels y; an optimization algorithm (e.g., stochastic gradient descent) then adjusts the weights and biases by following loss gradients to minimize L. Over successive epochs on labeled data, this iterative updating of parameters enables the network to learn hierarchical, task-relevant representations directly from raw inputs.

Weights, Biases and Activation

Each neuron within the neural network contains a weight, a bias, and an activation parameter. Weights and Biases are the learnable parameters of the neural network. These parameters are adjusted during the training process to minimize the discrepancy between the network's prediction and the ground truth values as provided in the labeled data. The weight parameter determines how much influence each input signal has on the neuron's output. Inputs with larger weights have a greater influence on the neuron's output. Biases are constant values that are added to the neuron's output after the weighted inputs are summed. Biases act as thresholds, allowing neurons to activate even when inputs are zero (Figs. 1.20 and 1.21).

Activation functions are mathematical functions that are applied to the output of a neuron's weighted sum plus biases. They introduce non-linearity to the network, which is important for the network to learn complex, non-linear relationships in the

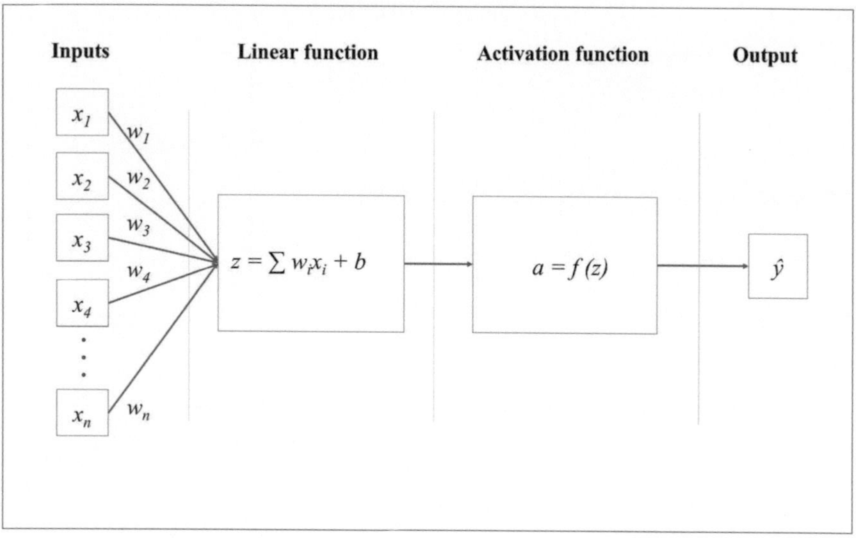

Fig. 1.20 A single-neuron schematic showing how inputs x_i are scaled by weights w_i, summed with a bias term, and passed through an activation function *f(x)* to produce the output $\hat{y}$

data. Commonly used activation functions are Sigmoid, Rectified Linear Unit (ReLU), Tanh and Softmax.

Hidden Layers

Deep Neural networks contain many layers between the input layer and the output layer, which are responsible for extracting features from the input data and transforming them into a form that the output layer can then use to make predictions (Fig. 1.22). These intermediate layers, also known as hidden layers, enable neural networks to learn complex patterns and relationships. Each hidden layer can contain a different number of neurons. A "deeper" network has more hidden layers, while a "wider" network has more neurons per layer. Wider layers can learn more varied features at the same level of abstraction and increase the network's overall capacity. However, a network that may be too wide may overfit or become computationally expensive without necessarily improving generalization.

Loss Functions

Loss functions, which quantify the difference between a model's prediction and the actual ground truth label, are used to guide the training process to minimize errors and improve model performance. Choosing the right loss function depends on the specific task at hand. For example, in regression tasks, the commonly used loss

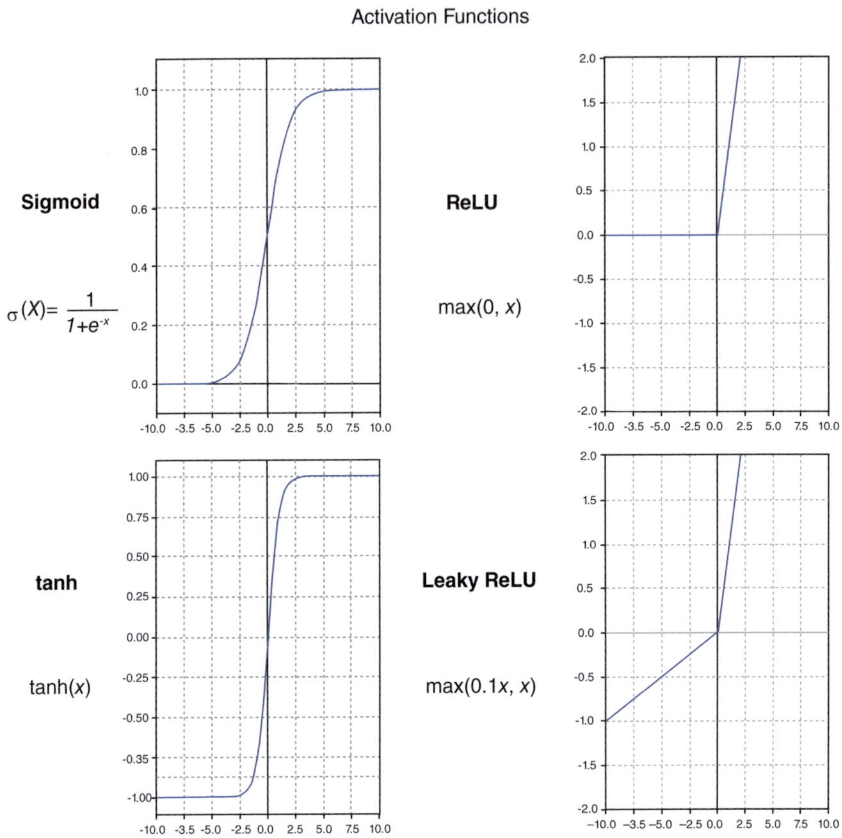

Fig. 1.21 Illustration of commonly used activation functions

functions are Mean Squared Error (MSE), and in classification, the Cross-Entropy (CE) loss is commonly used (Fig. 1.23).

Loss functions need to be differentiable, continuous, and ideally convex to ensure their effectiveness via an optimization algorithm such as gradient descent Table 1.3.

Parameters and Hyperparameters

Parameters are the weights and biases that are adjusted during the training process and are internal to the neural network. Hyperparameters are values that control the training process itself and are external to the neural network (Fig. 1.24).

Learning Rate This hyperparameter determines how much a model's parameters are adjusted during each iteration of the training process. A well-chosen learning is important for efficient and effective model training. A learning rate that is too high can cause the model to oscillate around the minimum, while a learning rate that is too low can result in unnecessarily slow or long training duration.

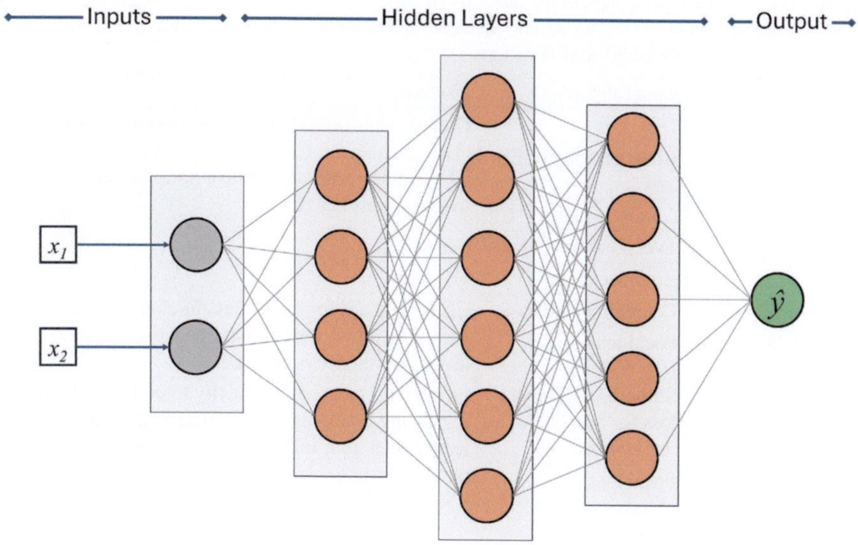

Fig. 1.22 A feedforward neural network with one Input layer (2 units), three hidden layers (depth = 3), the first of width 4 units, the second of width 6 units, and the third of width 5 units, transforming two inputs into a single output

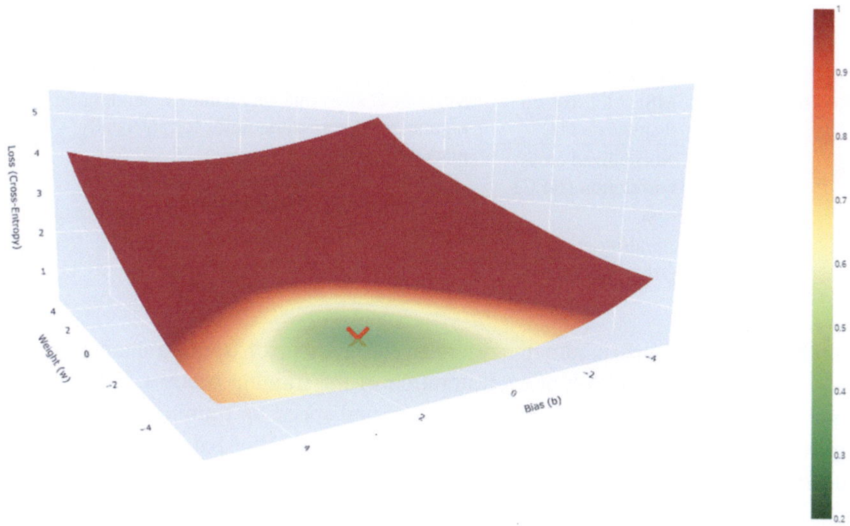

Fig. 1.23 3D visualization of the loss landscape for a logistic regression model trained on the TCGA LGG-GBM dataset. The surface represents the binary cross-entropy loss calculated for a range of possible values for the model's weight (w) and bias (b) parameters. The goal of the training algorithm (e.g., gradient descent) is to navigate this surface to find the combination of parameters that corresponds to the lowest point on the surface, indicated by the red "x," which represents the minimum possible loss and the optimal model configuration. (Data Source: The Cancer Imaging Archive (TCIA), collections TCGA-LGG and TCGA-GBM. Code Repository: nn_02_importance_of_learning_rate.ipynb)

Table 1.3 Common loss functions used in deep-learning-based neuroradiology applications across segmentation, classification, detection/localization, reconstruction/denoising, and registration tasks, with usage considerations

Task	Loss function(s)	Use/notes
Segmentation	Dice loss	Dice variants directly optimize overlap (robust to class imbalance); CE stabilizes training; Tversky adjusts false-positive/negative trade-off; boundary loss sharpens edges.
	Cross-entropy (CE) loss	
	Combined Dice + CE	
	Tversky loss	
	Boundary loss	
Classification	Categorical CE loss	CE is standard for multi-class/bi-class decisions; focal loss down-weights easy negatives to address lesion prevalence imbalance.
	Focal loss	
Detection/ localization	Smooth L1 (Huber) loss for box regression	Smooth L1 balances sensitivity to outliers when regressing bounding boxes; focal loss handles sparse lesion detection; IoU-based losses improve spatial overlap.
	Focal loss for objectness/class confidence	
	IoU / GIoU loss	
Reconstruction/ denoising	Mean squared error (MSE) loss	MSE/MAE for pixel-wise fidelity; SSIM preserves structural similarity; perceptual losses encourage high-level feature consistency in super-resolution or artifact removal.
	Mean absolute error (MAE) loss	
	SSIM loss	
	Perceptual (VGG-based) loss	
Registration	MSE / L2 loss on displacements	MSE/NCC align intensity patterns; bending-energy regularizes deformation fields for physically plausible warps.
	Normalized cross-correlation (NCC) loss	
	Bending-energy (smoothness) penalty	

Batch Size This hyperparameter refers to the number of training examples provided to the neural network at each iteration of the training process. While larger batch sizes utilize hardware more effectively and speed up training, they can also get stuck in suboptimal areas of the loss landscape. Smaller batch sizes have been shown to provide more generalization ability.

Epochs Epochs represent the number of times a model's entire training dataset is passed through during training. During each epoch, the model's parameters are updated in batches. A higher number of epochs can lead to better accuracy as the model learns more complex patterns from the training data. However, too high a number of epochs may lead to overfitting, where the model starts to memorize the training data and performs poorly on unseen validation data. With too

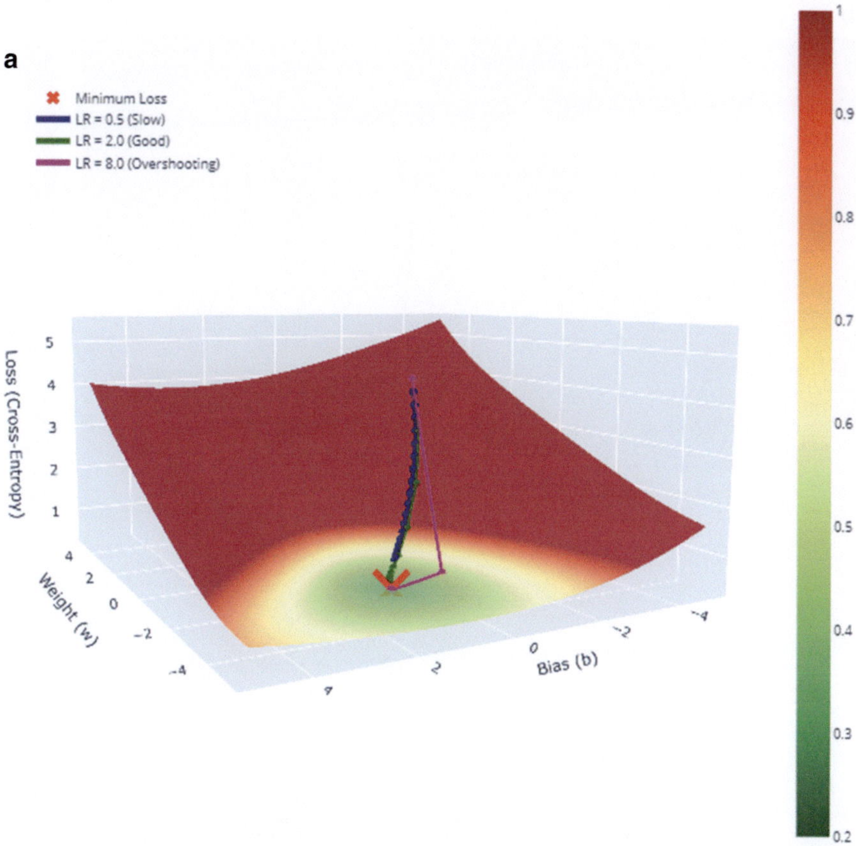

Fig. 1.24 The effect of the learning rate hyperparameter on gradient descent optimization. (**a**) A 3D representation of the cross-entropy loss surface as a function of a model's weight and bias. The paths show that a low learning rate (LR = 0.5, blue) converges slowly, an optimal rate (LR = 2.0, green) converges efficiently, and a high rate (LR = 8.0, magenta) overshoots the minimum loss (red "x"). (**b**) A 2D contour plot of the same landscape, providing a zoomed-in perspective of the optimization paths and illustrating the trajectory of the high learning rate

b

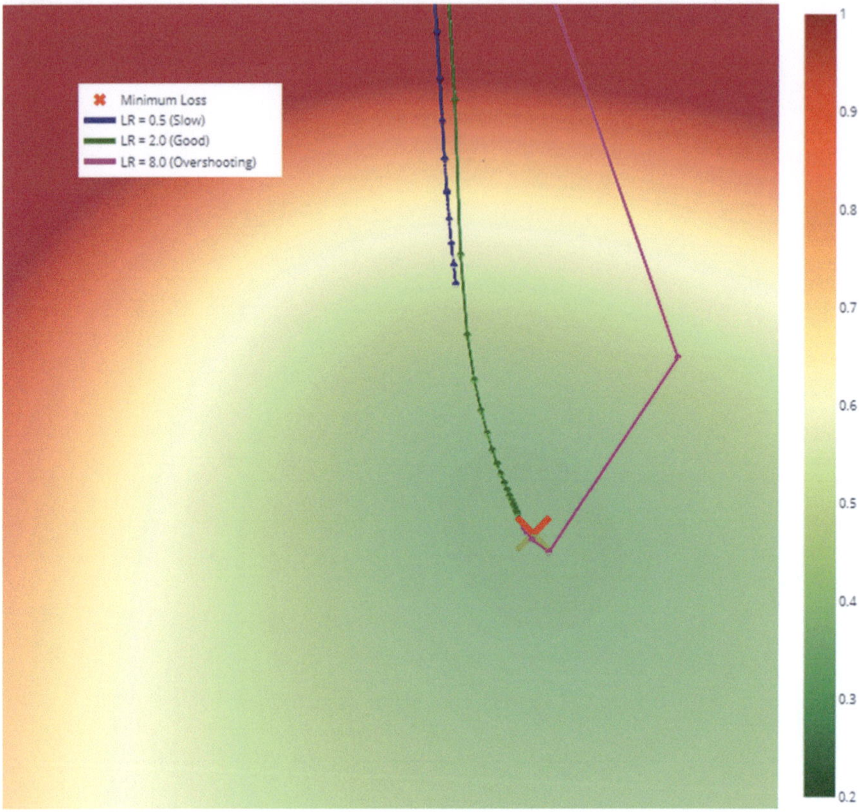

Fig. 1.24 (continued)

few epochs, on the other hand, the model would not have learned enough from the training data and may perform poorly on both the training data and the validation data.

As illustrated in Fig. 1.25, the blue curve represents the training error, which continuously decreases as the model learns from the training data. The orange curve represents the testing error (or validation error), which initially decreases but then starts to increase. The point where the testing error begins to rise while the training error continues to decrease indicates the onset of overfitting. Overfitting occurs when the model learns the training data too well, including noise and specific patterns unique to the training set, leading to poor generalization performance on unseen data (the test set). This plot illustrates the classic behavior of overfitting in machine learning models.

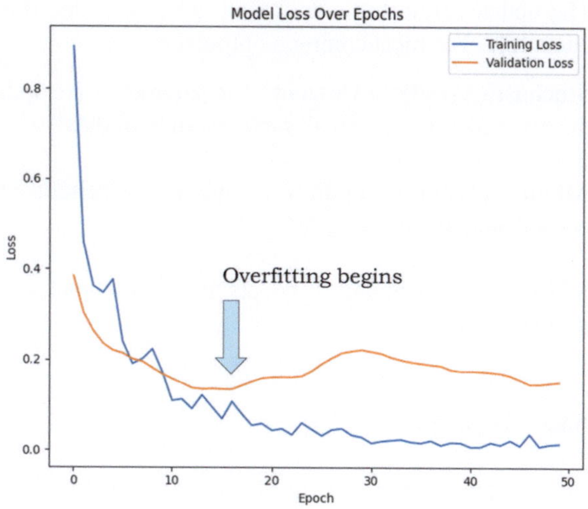

Fig. 1.25 The plot shows the training and testing error (loss) curves of a neural network model trained on a radiomic feature dataset for classifying brain tumors (LGG vs GBM). (Data Source: The Cancer Imaging Archive (TCIA), collections TCGA-LGG and TCGA-GBM. Code Repository: nn_03_overfitting_and_epochs.ipynb)

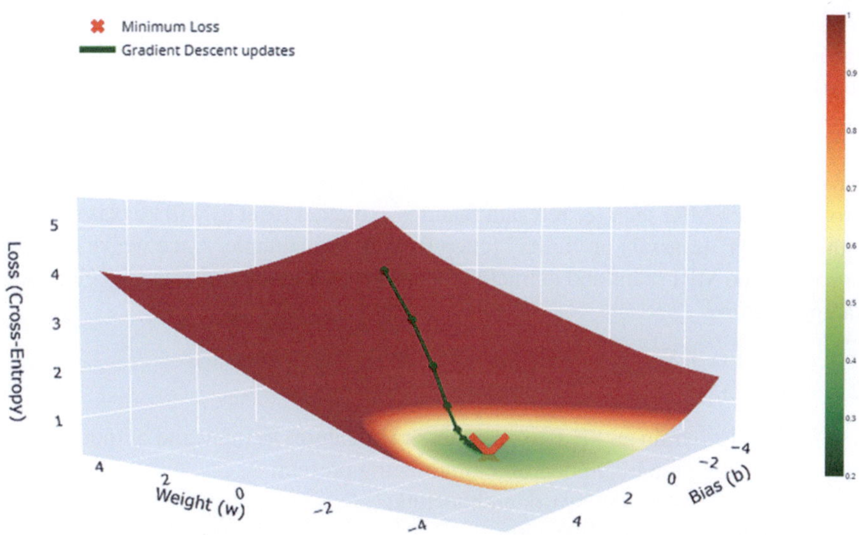

Fig. 1.26 Illustration of stochastic gradient descent, showing how successive small, gradient-guided weight updates computed from individual (or mini-batch) samples iteratively move the model from an initial weight toward the cost function's minimum

Optimizer

Optimizers are algorithms used to minimize the loss function during model training. These functions use the gradient of the loss function, which indicates the direction and magnitude of the steepest descent in the loss landscape. The learning rate determines the magnitude of parameter adjustments during each iteration (Fig. 1.26).

The updates from the output later are propagated through the network using the chain rule. The most common optimizers are:

Stochastic Gradient Descent The parameters are updated based on the gradient of the loss function on a small random batch of data.

Adam This popular optimizer combines the benefits of momentum-based optimizers and adaptive learning rates.

RMSProp This optimizer adapts the learning rate for each parameter based on the historical gradients.

Back Propagation

Backpropagation is the core training algorithm that uses the chain rule of calculus to calculate how much each weight in the network contributed to the error. In this approach, the forward pass first makes a prediction using the input data. The predicted output is then compared with the actual output (ground truth), and the loss is computed. The gradient of the loss with respect to the network's parameters is propagated back through each layer via backpropagation.

Let's refer to use-case where we want to develop an AI system to help identify the differentiation of GBM from LGG on MRI scans. This is a binary classification problem: each MRI scan (or relevant features extracted from it) will be classified as either "GBM" (class 1) or "LGG" (class 0). For our example, since we've already processed the MRI scans and extracted the relevant radiomic features, we select two sample features:

1. Feature 1 (x_1): Volume_NET_over_TC
2. Feature 2 (x_2): Volume_ET

Our goal is to train an MLP to take these two features as input and output a probability indicating the likelihood of a tumor being present.

Step 1: Define neural network architecture:

Let's define a simple MLP with:

1. An **input layer** with 2 neurons (for x_1 and x_2)
2. One **hidden layer** with 2 neurons (h_1 and h_2)
3. An **output layer** with 1 neuron (o_1), which will give the probability of a tumor being present (Fig. 1.27)

We'll use the **sigmoid activation function** for the hidden and output layers. The sigmoid function,

$$\sigma(z) = \frac{1}{1+e^{-z}}$$

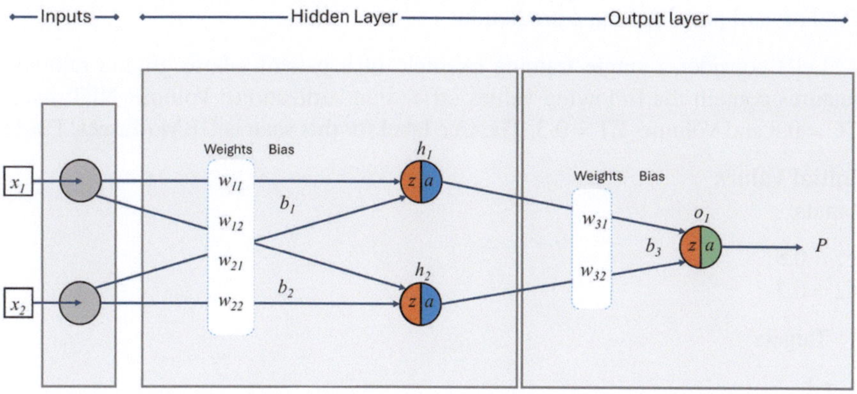

Fig. 1.27 Schematic of a fully connected feed-forward neural network. Two inputs (x_1, x_2) connect to a hidden layer with two neurons (h_1, h_2), which feed into a single output neuron (o_1) producing the prediction P. Edges are weighted by w_{ij}; b_1, b_2, b_3 denote biases. For each neuron, z is the pre-activation and is defined as $z = w^{\mathrm{T}}x + b$, and a is the activated output

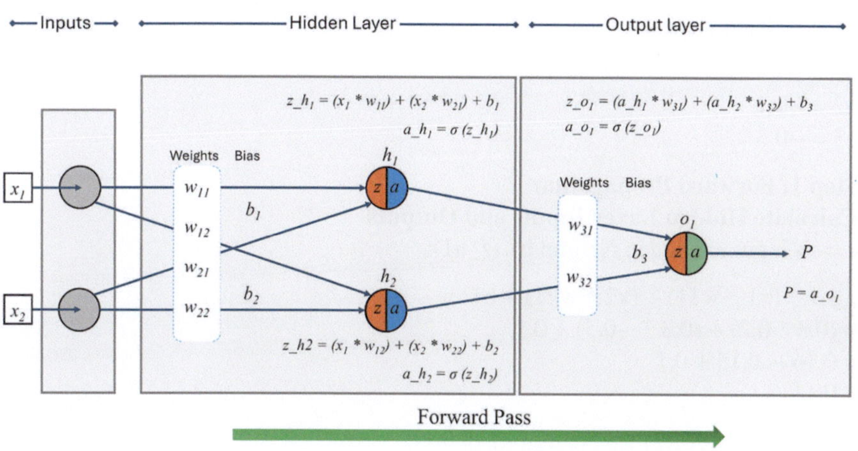

Fig. 1.28 Illustration of forward pass with the calculation of hidden layer inputs and outputs

squashes its input into a range between 0 and 1, which is suitable for probabilities. The connections between neurons have **weights** where the weights from input to hidden layer are defined as w_{11}, w_{12} (to h_1) and w_{21}, w_{22} (to h_2) and weights from hidden to output layer are defined as w_{31} (from h_1 to o_1) and w_{32} (from h_2 to o_1). Each neuron in the hidden and output layers also has a **bias**: b_1 (for h_1), b_2 (for h_2), and b_3 (for o_1).

Step 2: Training process: forward and backward propagation

The training process involves two main steps that are repeated iteratively: forward propagation and backpropagation (Fig. 1.28).

(a) Forward pass: making a prediction

Let's consider a single training example of a patient whose glioma radiomic features contain the following values (after standardization): Volume_NET_over_TC = 0.8 and Volume_ET = 0.3. The true label for this scan is GBM (Target, T = 1).

Initial Values
Inputs:

x1 = 0.8
x2 = 0.3

Target:

T = 1

Initialized weights:

w11 = 0.2 w12 = 0.4
w21 = −0.5 w22 = 0.1
w31 = −0.8 w32 = 0.5

Initialized biases:

b1 = 0.1
b2 = −0.1
b3 = −0.3

Step 1: Forward Propagation
Calculate Hidden Layer Inputs and Outputs
--> Input to Hidden Neuron h1 (z_h1):

z_h1 = (x1 * w11) + (x2 * w21) + b1
= (0.8 * 0.2) + (0.3 * −0.5) + 0.1
= 0.16 − 0.15 + 0.1
= 0.11

--> Output of Hidden Neuron h1 (a_h1):

a_h1 = σ(z_h1)
= σ(0.11)
= 1 / (1 + e^(−0.11))
≈ 0.527

--> Input to Hidden Neuron h2 (z_h2):

z_h2 = (x1 * w12) + (x2 * w22) + b2
= (0.8 * 0.4) + (0.3 * 0.1) − 0.1
= 0.32 + 0.03 − 0.1
= 0.25

--> Output of Hidden Neuron h2 (a_h2):

$$
\begin{aligned}
a\_h2 &= \sigma(z\_h2)\\
&= \sigma(0.25)\\
&= 1 / (1 + e^{\wedge}(-0.25))\\
&\approx 0.562
\end{aligned}
$$

Calculate Output Layer Input and Output

--> Input to Output Neuron o1 (z_o1):

$$
\begin{aligned}
z\_o1 &= (a\_h1 * w31) + (a\_h2 * w32) + b3\\
&= (0.527 * -0.8) + (0.562 * 0.5) - 0.3\\
&= -0.4216 + 0.281 - 0.3\\
&= -0.4406
\end{aligned}
$$

--> Output of o1 (Predicted Probability, P):

$$
\begin{aligned}
P &= a\_o1\\
&= \sigma(z\_o1)\\
&= \sigma(-0.4406)\\
&= 1 / (1 + e^{\wedge}(-(-0.4406)))\\
&\approx 0.3917
\end{aligned}
$$

So, for this input, our network predicts a 39.17% probability of the glioma being a GBM.

Calculate the Error

We use the binary cross-entropy (BCE) loss function.

--> Error (E):

$$E = -\ (T * \log(P) + (1 - T) * \log(1 - P))$$

Since the target T = 1, the formula simplifies to:

$$
\begin{aligned}
E &= -\ \log(P)\\
&= -\ \log(0.3917)\\
&\approx -\ (-0.937)\\
&\approx 0.937
\end{aligned}
$$

Our goal is to adjust weights and biases to reduce this error.

Step 2: Backpropagation

Backpropagation calculates the gradient of the error with respect to each weight and bias using the chain rule. The gradient tells us how a small change in a parameter will affect the error.

A. **Gradients for Output Layer (w31, w32, b3)**

We find the partial derivative of the error E with respect to each parameter.

For w31: $\partial E/\partial w31 = (\partial E/\partial P) * (\partial P/\partial z\_o1) * (\partial z\_o1/\partial w31)$

--> Component 1: $\partial E/\partial P$

$$
\begin{aligned}
\partial E/\partial P &= -\ (T/P - (1 - T)/(1 - P))\\
&= -1 / P = -1 / 0.3917\\
&\approx -2.553
\end{aligned}
$$

--> Component 2: ∂P/∂z_o1 (Derivative of sigmoid)

∂P/∂z_o1 = P * (1 – P)
= 0.3917 * (1–0.3917) = 0.3917 * 0.6083
≈ 0.2382

--> Component 3: ∂z_o1/∂w31

∂z_o1/∂w31 = a_h1
= 0.527

--> Final Gradient for w31:

∂E/∂w31 = −2.553 * 0.2382 * 0.527
≈ −0.3205

To simplify, let's define the error signal for the output neuron, δ_o1:

δ_o1 = (∂E/∂P) * (∂P/∂z_o1)
= −2.553 * 0.2382
≈ −0.6081

Now we can calculate all output layer gradients more easily:

∂E/∂w31 = δ_o1 * a_h1
= −0.6081 * 0.527
≈ −0.3205

∂E/∂w32 = δ_o1 * a_h2
= −0.6081 * 0.562
≈ −0.3418

∂E/∂b3 = δ_o1 * 1
= −0.6081

B. **Gradients for Hidden Layer (w11, w21, b1, w12, w22, b2)**

We propagate the error signal δ_o1 back to the hidden layer.
For w11:

∂E/∂w11 = (∂E/∂a_h1) * (∂a_h1/∂z_h1) * (∂z_h1/∂w11)

--> Component 1: ∂E/∂a_h1 (How h1's output affects the total error)

∂E/∂a_h1 = (∂E/∂z_o1) * (∂z_o1/∂a_h1)
= δ_o1 * w31
= −0.6081 * -0.8
≈ 0.4865

--> Component 2: ∂a_h1/∂z_h1 (Derivative of sigmoid for h1)

∂a_h1/∂z_h1 = a_h1 * (1 – a_h1)
= 0.527 * (1 – 0.527)
≈ 0.249

--> Component 3: ∂z_h1/∂w11

∂z_h1/∂w11 = x1
= 0.8

--> Final Gradient for w11:

∂E/∂w11 = 0.4865 * 0.249 * 0.8
≈ 0.0969

Let's define the error signal for hidden neuron h1, δ_h1:

δ_h1 = (∂E/∂a_h1) * (∂a_h1/∂z_h1)
= (δ_o1 * w31) * (a_h1 * (1 − a_h1))
= 0.4865 * 0.249
≈ 0.1211

Now we can find the gradients for the first set of hidden weights/bias:

∂E/∂w11 = δ_h1 * x1
= 0.1211 * 0.8
≈ 0.0969

∂E/∂w21 = δ_h1 * x2
= 0.1211 * 0.3
≈ 0.0363

∂E/∂b1 = δ_h1 * 1
= 0.1211

Similarly, for neuron h2, the error signal δ_h2 is:

δ_h2 = (∂E/∂a_h2) * (∂a_h2/∂z_h2)
= (δ_o1 * w32) * (a_h2 * (1 − a_h2))
= (−0.6081 * 0.5) * (0.562 * (1 − 0.562))
= −0.3041 * 0.246
≈ −0.0748

And the gradients for the second set of hidden weights/bias are:

∂E/∂w12 = δ_h2 * x1
= −0.0748 * 0.8
≈ −0.0598

∂E/∂w22 = δ_h2 * x2
= −0.0748 * 0.3
≈ −0.0224

∂E/∂b2 = δ_h2 * 1
= −0.0748

Step 3: Weight and Bias Updates

We update the parameters using the gradient descent rule with a learning rate (η) of 0.1. Rule: New Weight = Old Weight − η * Gradient

Output Layer Updates

w31_new = w31 − η * (∂E/∂w31) = −0.8 − (0.1 * −0.3205) = −0.76795
w32_new = w32 − η * (∂E/∂w32) = 0.5 − (0.1 * −0.3418) = 0.53418
b3_new = b3 − η * (∂E/∂b3) = −0.3 − (0.1 * -0.6081) = −0.23919

Hidden Layer Updates

w11_new = w11 − η * (∂E/∂w11) = 0.2 − (0.1 * 0.0969) = 0.19031
w21_new = w21 − η * (∂E/∂w21) = −0.5 − (0.1 * 0.0363) = −0.50363
b1_new = b1 − η * (∂E/∂b1) = 0.1 − (0.1 * 0.1211) = 0.08789

w12_new = w12 − η * (∂E/∂w12) = 0.4 − (0.1 * −0.0598) = 0.40598
w22_new = w22 − η * (∂E/∂w22) = 0.1 − (0.1 * −0.0224) = 0.10224
b2_new = b2 − η * (∂E/∂b2) = −0.1 − (0.1 * −0.0748) = −0.09252

After this single step of backpropagation, the weights and biases have been slightly adjusted. If we were to perform forward propagation again with the same input (x1 = 0.8,x2 = 0.3) using these new weights, the predicted output P would be slightly closer to the target T = 1, and the error E would be smaller.

This process of forward propagation, error calculation, backpropagation (using the chain rule to find gradients), and weight/bias updates is repeated for many training examples (epochs) until the MLP's performance on the classification task (e.g., accurately detecting brain tumors) is satisfactory. The chain rule is fundamental to backpropagation because it provides an efficient way to determine how each individual weight and bias, no matter how deep in the network, contributes to the final error, allowing the network to "learn" from its mistakes.

Model Training

Model training is the iterative process by which a neural network learns how to perform its task. During its first iteration, the model parameters are initialized either randomly or using an initialization scheme such as Glorot or He. These initialized weights are used to process a batch of input data through a forward pass. Using the outputs from the forward pass, the loss is computed, and this loss is propagated backward through each layer via the calculus chain rule. The gradients of the loss function with respect to each parameter are computed and used by the Optimizer, such as Adam or SGD, and the parameters are updated in the direction that most rapidly reduces errors, after scaling by the learning rate. This entire cycle of forward pass and backward propagation is repeated over many epochs (Fig. 1.29).

One significant challenge that needs to be addressed during model training is Overfitting. Since neural networks have a high number of parameters and the algorithms are highly complex, they are especially prone to overfitting. Overfitting

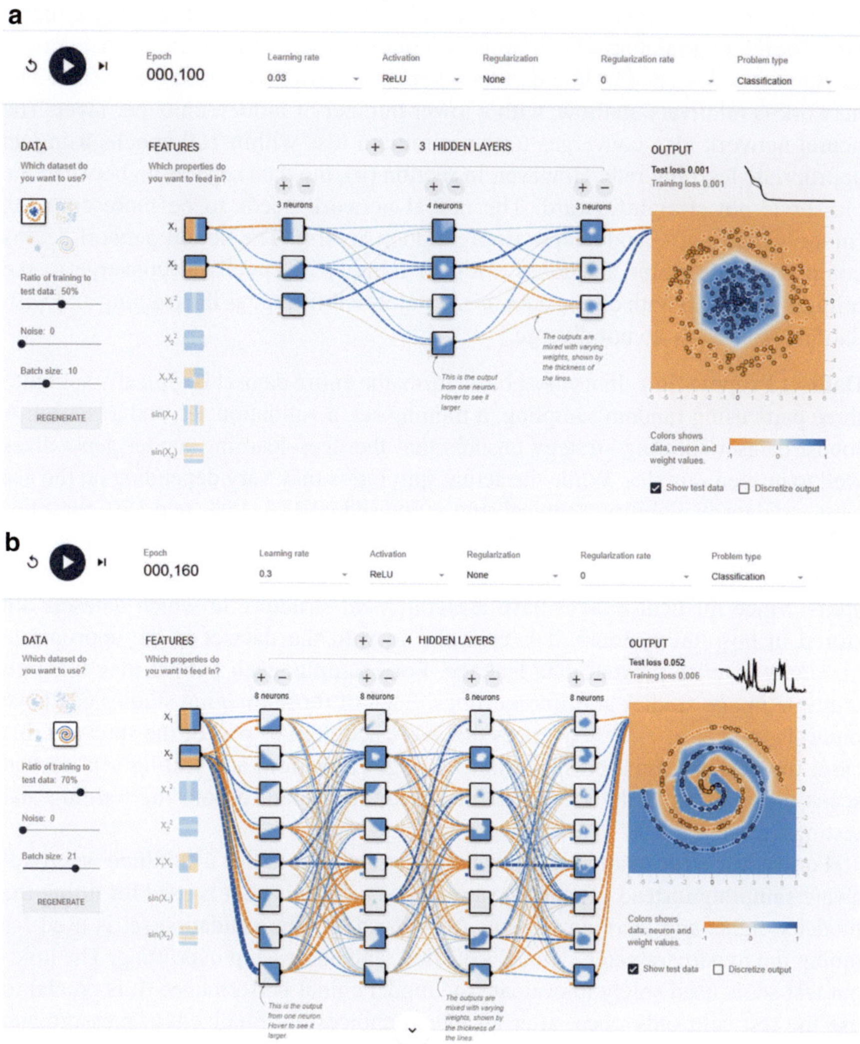

Fig. 1.29 Visualization of two distinct neural network classifiers. (**a**) A shallower network with 3 hidden layers and fewer neurons successfully classifies a simple, linearly separable dataset. (**b**) A deeper network with 4 hidden layers and more neurons per layer is required to learn the complex, non-linear boundary of a spiral dataset. (Image generated using TensorFlow Playground 2016. The TensorFlow Authors, licensed under Apache 2.0. https://playground.tensorflow.org)

occurs when neural networks perform really well with the seen training set but fail to generalize well with unseen validation of test data. The goal is to produce a model that generalizes well to new data, capturing the underlying structure of the problem.

As illustrated in Fig. 1.28, the model training process is a series of iterative updates to the neural network weights. The method of selecting hyperparameters is a more nuanced process, where individual values are selected using either a Grid Search or a random search process. For example, in Fig. 1.28, the network in section (a) is designed to fit a dataset where it is easy to separate the classes. The network is relatively shallow, with a lower number of hidden units per layer. The neural network also converges to the minimum loss within 100 epochs using an appropriate learning rate. However, in section (b), the data separation between the classes is not straightforward. The neural network needs to be more complex (more hidden units) and deeper (more hidden layers). The neural network learns complex relationships and takes a higher number of epochs to converge to the minimum loss. In both cases, there is no major overfitting, as the training and validation loss curves do not diverge.

Dataset Preparation In its most basic form, the entire dataset is typically split into three parts using random sampling: a training set, a validation set, and a test set. A robust dataset splitting strategy ensures that the deep-learning model generalizes well to unseen samples. While the actual split ratios may vary depending on the use case and data availability, a typical split ratio used is 70%, 15%, and 15% for training, validation, and testing, respectively.

During this step, it is crucial to ensure that no data leakage occurs between the splits. Since medical images have a hierarchical structure in which datasets are stored in hospital systems, it is essential to split the dataset at the appropriate hierarchy level to prevent data leakage. For example, each patient may undergo multiple image studies at different times. Each of those imaging studies can have multiple image series or sequences that were acquired as part of the study. In this case, the patients must be split into training, validation, and testing sets so that scans or series from the same patient are not allocated to both the training and testing sets.

For certain classification tasks, it may be important to use a stratified or group-aware sampling instead of random sampling. The training set is used for fitting the model weights and learning patterns from the data. The validation set is used for tuning the hyperparameters, model selection, and addressing overfitting. The hold-out test set is used solely to evaluate the model's final performance. It is crucial to use the test split only once, after all model choices are finalized, to measure and report the model's performance.

Hyperparameter Search Tuning a neural network is still a trial-and-error process since what works well in one use-case may not transfer to another use case. These hyperparameters must be discovered through experimentation. Common approaches for hyperparameter search include *grid-search* (exhaustively evaluating each combination of values within the search space), random search (evaluating combinations of values in the search space at random), Bayesian optimization, or Hyperband (which uses a performance landscape or dynamically allocates computational resources).

Cross-Validation Cross-validation is a resampling strategy used to measure how a predictive model will generalize to a hold-out test dataset or data from an independent source. In this process, the dataset is first partitioned into multiple complementary subsets for training and evaluation.

Cross-validation improves model reliability since it demonstrates that the model performance is not sensitive to the train-test split. By testing the model on multiple data splits, the model can be evaluated for robustness and consistent performance (Fig. 1.30) (Table 1.4).

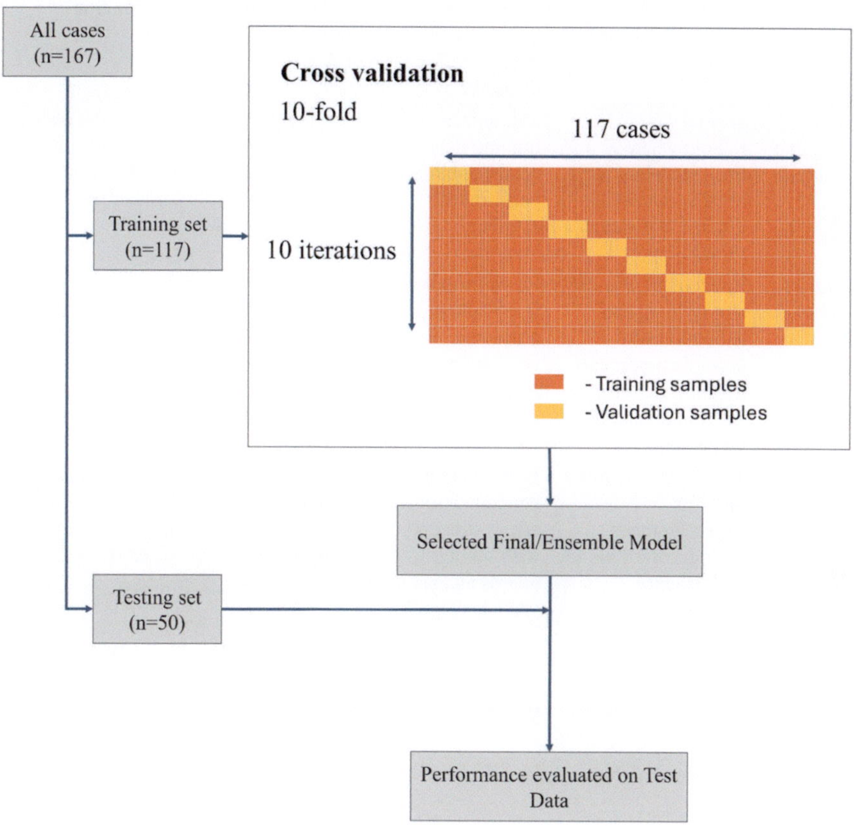

Fig. 1.30 Illustration of Five-Fold Cross-Validation. The TCGA GBM-LGG dataset, which has a combined set of 167 patients, is first split into a training set (70%) and a testing set (30%). The training set is later split into ten equal parts (folds), where each row represents one iteration of training and validation. In each fold, nine subsets (in orange) are used for training, and one distinct subset (in yellow) is used for validation. This process is repeated ten times, ensuring that each subset is used exactly once as the validation set. This technique helps evaluate model performance more reliably by averaging results across multiple folds.

Table 1.4 Cross-validation methods

Method	Description	Advantages	Disadvantages	Typical use case
K-Fold	Data is split into K equal folds. Each fold is held out in turn for validation, while the remaining K-1 folds are used for training.	Efficient at balancing bias/variance; uses all data for both training and evaluation.	Results can vary with K; not stratified by default.	General-purpose model evaluation
Stratified K-Fold	Extension of K-Fold for classification: preserves class proportions in each fold.	Ensures representative class balance, especially for imbalanced datasets.	Slightly more complex to implement; still sensitive to choice of K.	Classification tasks with skewed class distribution
Leave-One-Out (LOO)	Special case of K-Fold where $K = N$. Each sample is used once as the validation set, and N-1 samples for training.	Maximizes training data; nearly unbiased performance estimate.	Extremely computationally expensive; high variance in estimates when N is small.	Very small datasets where maximum training data is critical
Shuffle-Split	Randomly splits data into training and validation sets multiple times; each iteration samples a fraction of data for validation.	Flexible choice of train/validation sizes; can generate many random splits.	Validation sets may overlap; less structured coverage of all points.	Scenarios requiring customized train/test proportions or repeated random subsampling
Nested CV	Two-layer CV: inner loop for hyperparameter tuning, outer loop for performance estimation.	Provides unbiased generalization error estimate with tuning; guards against "data leakage."	Very high computational cost; complex to configure correctly.	Hyperparameter optimization in small-to-medium-sized datasets

Comprehensive Review of Neural Network Architectures

Feedforward Neural Networks

Feed-forward neural networks (FFNNS), also known as multi-layer perceptrons (MLPs), consist of one input layer, one output layer, and one or more hidden layers in the middle. FFNNs are the foundational neural network architecture that excel at modeling complex, non-linear relationships in low-dimensional feature spaces. Despite their simplicity, they form the backbone of deep learning.

FFNNs are effective at handling nonlinear data relationships and work well for both classification and regression tasks. However, deeper FFNNs are more susceptible to overfitting, especially with small datasets. Additionally, FFNNs lack the memory mechanisms to adequately model sequential or time-series data.

In neuroradiology, FFNNs are particularly well-suited for tasks where the domain-expert features or radiomic descriptors are already extracted. For example, in recent works, FFNNs have been used in conjunction with other deep-learning-based segmentation or registration architectures where the FFNNs serve as the final decision-making component. In neuroradiology, FFNNs have been used to classify tumor subtypes based on texture and spatial metrics or to predict patient prognosis from quantitative MRI markers (Fig. 1.31).

FFNNs have multiple limitations. They lack spatial awareness since they treat each input feature independently, making them poorly suited for image data. Additionally, the number of weights increases rapidly with input size, resulting in high memory usage for medical imaging data. FFNNs also have a high model capacity, making them more prone to overfitting. FFNNs also lack memory or feedback connections, which makes them ineffective for tasks involving sequences. Additionally, in deep FFNNs, the gradients may diminish as they are backpropagated, which leads to the early layers learning very slowly or not at all. The neural network architectures presented in the following sections aim to address these challenges by utilizing various architecture designs that work better for medical imaging data.

Recurrent Neural Networks

Feed-forward neural networks don't work well for all types of data. If our ML task involves tracking the progression of white matter lesions in multiple sclerosis or analyzing the dynamic patterns in an fMRI time series, traditional neural network architectures, such as FFNNs, would fail since they lack the design to capture

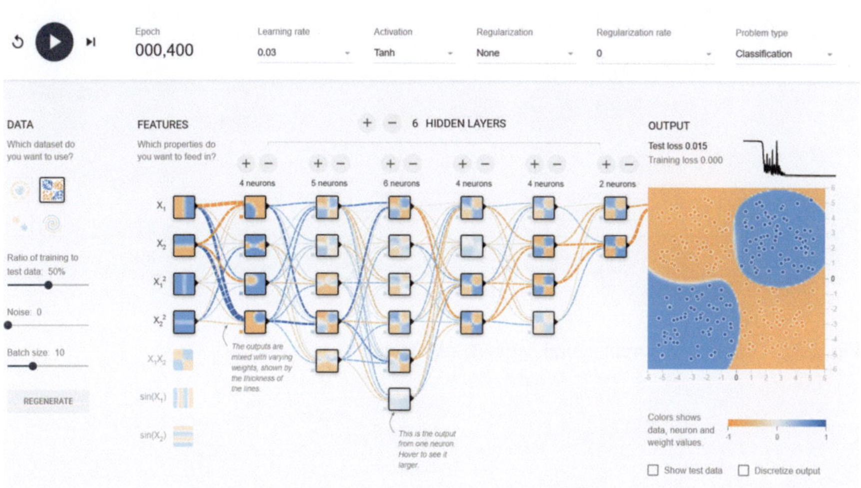

Fig. 1.31 A FFNN model visualizing the classification of a circular dataset. (Image generated using TensorFlow Playground, © 2016 The TensorFlow Authors, licensed under Apache 2.0. https://playground.tensorflow.org)

temporal context in these data types that involve time series. One of the most important differences in sequential data is that the inputs are not assumed to be independent of each other, as is the case with any time series data.

Recurrent Neural Networks (RNNs) are a class of AI algorithms specifically designed to work with sequential data. The core intuition behind an RNN is its inherent "memory." At each step of the input sequence, the neuron receives new input as well as its own output from the previous time step. This loop allows information to be passed from one time step to the next time step, effectively creating a memory of past events. This internal memory, or hidden state, is updated at each time step, incorporating new information while retaining relevant past events.

The trainable parameters within an RNN are the weights and biases associated with connections between the current input, hidden and output layers and within the hidden layer itself. These parameters are updated during the training process to minimize a loss function that is decided based on a task. RNNs use a modified version of back-propagation called Back-propagation through time (BPTT) to adjust the parameters. At its essence, BPTT "unrolls" the RNN over time and applies the typical backpropagation process to each step, propagating the error signal back through the network using the chain rule (Fig. 1.32).

Let's take an example of a sequential text input from a neuroradiology input and follow how an RNN would process this sequence for a classification task.

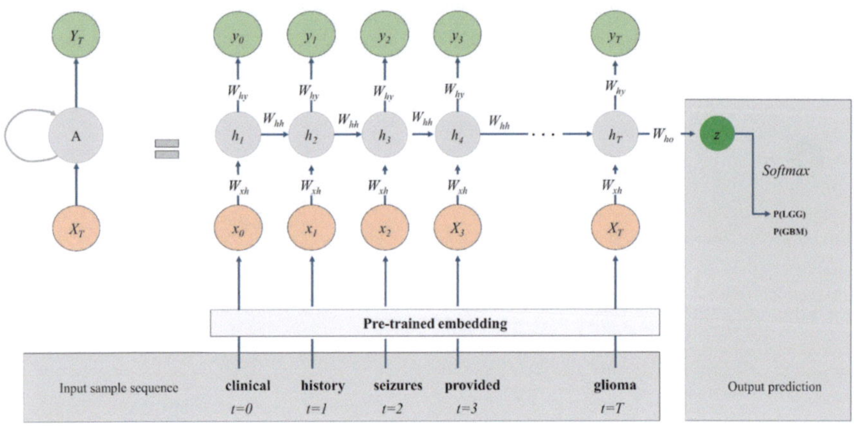

Fig. 1.32 Unrolled recurrent neural network architecture

Example Neuroradiology Report (From Han YT et. al. 2025)
HISTORY: A clinical history of seizures has been provided.

TECHNIQUE: Sagittal T1, axial FLAIR, axial conventional diffusion, axial T2, and postgadolinium sagittal and coronal T1-weighted sequences were obtained.

FINDINGS: The caliber of the ventricular system is within normal limits and appears stable. A fairly well-defined lesion, which demonstrates diminished signal on both T1 and T2-weighted sequences as well as questionable restricted diffusion and fairly homogeneous enhancement, is present involving both gray and white matter (but predominantly subcortical white matter) centered within the postcentral gyrus on the left side. ... To the extent visualized, the orbits are unremarkable.

IMPRESSION: A well-defined, homogeneously enhancing lesion is present centered within the postcentral gyrus on the left side, the etiology of which is uncertain. From an imaging standpoint lymphoma is a definite possibility. An intermediate-grade glioma is an alternate possibility.

An RNN would process the above example report, which is in a sequential text format, using the following steps.

Step 1—Tokenization & Embedding

In this step, the text in the report is split into "tokens." A token, in language modeling, is simply one unit of input that the network processes at each time step. It could be a single word, or clinical phrases or terms such as "enhancing." Tokens typically correspond to words or sub words, though specialized tokenizers can capture domain-specific clinical phrases. In this case the report is split into the tokens as below:

"A" → "clinical" → "history" → "of" → "seizures" → ... → "lymphoma" → ...

Each token is mapped to a dense vector x_t (e.g., via pretrained radiology-domain embeddings). These x_t vectors serve as the RNN's inputs at time steps t = 1 to T. This is because neural networks operate on numerical data, so textual inputs must be converted into numerical form (i.e., vectors) using embedding techniques. Embeddings are trained in a specific domain or for a specific task and typically place semantically related terms closer together in the embedding space.

Step 2—Hidden State Updates (Weights & Biases in Action)

In this step, the hidden states at each time step are computed. For example, if h_{t-1} is the hidden state after reading the token at t-1, the hidden state at token t can be computed as

$$h_t = \tanh\left(W_{ih} x_t + W_{hh} h_{t-1} + b_h \right)$$

where W_{ih} (weight matrix from input to hidden state at current time step) and W_{hh} (weight matrix from hidden state at previous time step to hidden state at current time step) and b_h (bias of hidden state) are the trainable weights and biases.

For example, in this sequence, at $t = 5$, when processing the token "seizures," the RNN uses W_{ih} to interpret that symptom. When it later encounters the tokens "lymphoma" or "glioma" at the end of the sequence, the same W_{hh} ensures it recalls both the patient's seizure history and tumor-related features.

Step 3—Predicted Classification and Loss Computation

After the final token ("glioma"), the RNN takes h_T and applies an output weight matrix W_{ho} and bias b_o to produce logits $z = W_{ho}\, h_T + b_o$. A softmax over z gives predicted probabilities $\hat{y}$ for labels such as {"low-grade glioma," "intermediate-grade glioma," "high-grade glioma," "lymphoma," etc.}.

If the true label is "lymphoma," the cross-entropy loss is

$$L = -\log\left(\hat{y}_{\text{lymphoma}}\right)$$

In this step, the network learns to assign a high probability to "lymphoma" only if its hidden state h_T has successfully integrated all critical cues (e.g., "homogeneous enhancement," "post central gyrus").

Step 4—Back-Propagation Through Time (BPTT)

To update W_{ih}, W_{hh}, W_{ho} and biases, we "unroll" the RNN over all T tokens. The gradient $\partial L/\partial h_t$ at step t flows backward into the same shared weights W_{ih}, W_{hh}. Concretely, at each time step t, we compute

$$\frac{\partial L}{\partial W_{ih}} = \sum_{t-1}^{T} \frac{\partial L}{\partial h_t} \frac{\partial h_t}{\partial W_{ih}}$$

and similarly for Whh, bh, Who, bo.

Essentially, in this step, when the model sees "diminished signal" and later "homogeneous enhancement," it learns that those phrases often correlate higher with "lymphoma" and "intermediate-grade glioma." If on token 50 the network's prediction is wrong, the error signal travels back through all prior tokens ("clinical," "history," … "post central gyrus"), adjusting the same W_{ih} and W_{hh} at each step so that next time "post central gyrus" plus "homogeneous enhancement" more reliably point toward the correct label.

In summary, the steps followed by the RNN are:

- As the RNN reads "A clinical history of seizures…" it uses its weights and biases to build a hidden memory.
- Each subsequent token or phrase ("…lesion…homogeneous enhancement…") updates that memory via the same shared parameters.
- Upon reading "intermediate-grade glioma," it makes a prediction.

- BPTT then sends the final error back through each time step, tweaking those shared weights so that, in the future, "homogeneous enhancement centered in post central gyrus" more strongly triggers "lymphoma" or "intermediate-grade glioma."

In this way, the RNN's trainable weights and biases gradually adjust, based on updates propagated by BPTT, to minimize classification errors on neuroradiology reports.

One of the main challenges with training deep RNNs with BPTT is that, as gradients are propagated back through many time steps, they become too small to make meaningful updates to the network's trainable parameters. This results in the network not learning dependencies between inputs that are far apart in the sequence. Additionally, early layers learn very slowly or not at all. The converse of this situation is also true, where gradients can become excessively large, leading to unstable training and wild swings in each weight update.

Long short-term memory (LSTM) networks address the vanishing gradient problem by using a "memory cell" and three gates, the input gate, the output gate, and the forget gate, which allow LSTMs to selectively remember or forget information over long sequences. The forget gates decide which information to discard from the cell state. The input gates decide which new information to store in the hidden cell state. The output gate decides what to output from the cell state.

Gated recurrent unit (GRU) networks are a more recent variant of RNNs that also use gates to control information flow, but are computationally less expensive than LSTMs. In this architecture, the Forget and Input gates of an LSTM are effectively combined into a single Update gate, and also the cell state and hidden state are merged into one unified hidden state vector. The Reset gate determines how to combine the new input with the previous memory, and the update gate decides how much of the previous memory to keep and what new information (from the current input and reset gate output) to add (Fig. 1.33).

Bi-directional RNNs address an important challenge when it comes to working with sequential data, where bidirectional context is crucial. For example, in a radiology report, the meaning of a phrase or term in a sentence is often disambiguated by the words that follow it as much as by those that precede it. BiRNNs can also be implemented with recurrent units such as LSTMs and GRUs to implement BiLSTMs and BiGRUs, respectively. These bi-directional RNN architectures combine the advantages of bidirectional processing with enhanced memory capabilities of LSTMs and GRUs.

Let's use the sample MRI report again to get an intuitive understanding of how LSTMs work. In this example, we can follow the process of how an LSTM network "reads" the report and builds a representation that lets it assign one or more disease labels at the end. The RNN methodology (word embeddings, sequential encoding, BPTT) follows Lee et al., AJR 2019 approach to automated disease annotation (AJR). The report excerpt is taken from Han YT et al. 2025.

Sample Report Excerpt (Han YT et al. 2024)

HISTORY: A clinical history of seizures has been provided.

TECHNIQUE: Sagittal T1, axial FLAIR, axial conventional diffusion, axial T2, and postgadolinium sagittal and coronal T1-weighted sequences were obtained.

FINDINGS: The caliber of the ventricular system is within normal limits and appears stable. A fairly well-defined lesion, which demonstrates diminished signal on both T1 and T2-weighted sequences as well as questionable restricted diffusion and fairly homogeneous enhancement, is present involving both gray and white matter (but predominantly subcortical white matter) centered within the postcentral gyrus on the left side. … To the extent visualized, the orbits are unremarkable.

IMPRESSION: A well-defined, homogeneously enhancing lesion is present centered within the postcentral gyrus on the left side, the etiology of which is uncertain. From an imaging standpoint lymphoma is a definite possibility. An intermediate-grade glioma is an alternate possibility.

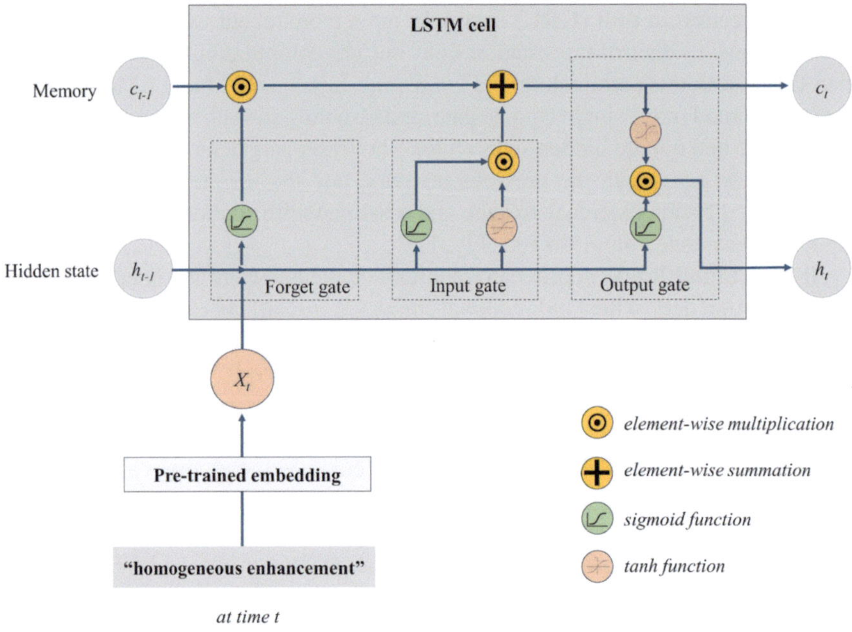

Fig. 1.33 LSTM schematic

A radiologist reading these lines instantly notes that "fairly well defined lesion,", "homogeneous enhancement," and "enhancing lesion centered in postcentral gyrus" would likely indicate lymphoma or intermediate-grade glioma. The LSTM performs a similar process, but token by token, maintaining a hidden "memory" vector that accumulates what it's seen so far. We can break up the full text into chunks to highlight the distinct processes in earlier stages and compare it with those at later stages.

1. First chunk ("A clinical history of seizures has been provided.")

   Each token, "A," "clinical," "history," "of," "seizures," "has," "been," "provided," is embedded into a numeric vector. After reading "clinical history of seizures," the LSTM's hidden state h_t already encodes two key facts: (a) the patient has a seizure history and (b) the context is neurology.
2. Second chunk ("The caliber of the ventricular system … centered within the postcentral gyrus on the left side.")

   As it processes tokens like "ventricular," "system," "well-defined," "diminished signal," "restricted diffusion," "homogeneous enhancement," "subcortical," and "postcentral gyrus," the LSTM's gates decide which previously stored elements to keep (e.g., "seizures") and which to attenuate (e.g., "ventricular system is stable" is background). Simultaneously, it injects new information: lesion location (postcentral gyrus, left side), imaging characteristics (diminished T1/T2 signal, questionable restricted diffusion, homogeneous enhancement).

   Internally, this is implemented by making repeated updates where the LSTM briefly "forgets" less critical tokens (e.g., "ventricular system is stable") and "remembers" core disease-related phrases ("homogeneous enhancement," "postcentral gyrus").
3. Third chunk ("IMPRESSION: A well-defined homogeneous appearing enhancing lesion … most suggestive of low-grade glioma.")

   Upon reading "well-defined," "homogeneous," "enhancing," "lesion," "postcentral gyrus," "most," "suggestive," "of," "low-grade," "glioma," the network's hidden state is already primed with location ("postcentral gyrus") and imaging features ("homogeneous enhancement"). When it reaches "low-grade glioma," its gates allow that decisive phrase to flow through strongly, overwriting any lingering ambiguity (e.g., questionable diffusion). By the end of "glioma," the hidden vector is a compact summary encoding:

   (a) Patient: seizure history
   (b) Imaging: well-defined, homogeneous enhancement, postcentral gyrus location
   (c) Impression: "lymphoma" or "intermediate-grade glioma"

      Because the final hidden state contains all of that compressed information, a simple classification head (fully connected layer + softmax or sigmoid per code) can look at it and output "lymphoma" and "intermediate-grade glioma" (and potentially additional classes if multiple labels apply).

In this example, it is important to recognize that the ***hidden states*** act as a rolling summary. At each timestep t, the LSTM's hidden state h_t acts like a short checklist of "what matters so far." When a new token arrives (e.g., "homogeneous"), the LSTM asks "Should I add this to my list?" and "Should I let go of anything old?"

After reading "clinical history of seizures," the network stores that fact. But once it sees "ventricular system is within normal limits," the model knows that detail is background, so the ***forget gate*** down-weights it.

As the model processes "homogeneous enhancement," it recognizes that this phrase is a strong indicator of tumor grade. The ***input gate*** allows the embedding to enter the hidden state almost unfiltered, ensuring "homogeneous enhancement" isn't lost.

At the last token ("glioma"), the hidden state is transformed into the final vector for classification. The ***output gate*** decides which pieces of the cell's memory (e.g., "postcentral gyrus," "homogeneous enhancement," "intermediate-grade glioma") should influence that final decision.

Because LSTMs carry forward only the most relevant bits of information, by the time the network finishes reading the entire report, it has effectively built up a distilled representation that strongly points to "low-grade glioma."

Convolutional Neural Networks

Convolutional neural networks (CNNs) are a class of deep learning algorithms that work well with data that has a grid-like topology such as images. CNN networks are composed of multiple sequentially applied convolution operations, with each operation expressed as,

$$s = (x * w),$$

where the input x and a convolution kernel w are combined using the convolution operation to obtain the resulting feature map s. For a 2-dimensional input image I and 2-dimensional kernel K (with dimensions m and n), the convolution operation resulting in output matrix Z, implemented mathematically (in many neural network libraries) using a cross-correlation operation, can be formulated as,

$$Z(i,j) = (K^* I)(i,j) = \sum_m \sum_n I(i+m,j+n) K(m,n)$$

where i and j represent the element in the ith row and jth column of the matrix. The only difference between the convolution and cross-correlation operations is that, in the first case, the kernel is flipped (along all spatial dimensions) before being applied. This operation can be visually expressed as shown in Fig. 1.33. A 3 × 3 window (green) is first slid over the input image; each element of this patch is then multiplied by the corresponding filter weight (in yellow) denoted ×1 for non-zero weights and ×0 for zero weights. The products are summed to yield one output activation (right). In this example, the sum product yields an output value of 0. Whether or not the kernel is flipped is typically a matter of implementation since these kernels are eventually learned parameters (Fig. 1.34).

As illustrated in Fig. 1.35, a typical CNN layer typically combines the convolution operation with an activation function and a pooling function applied in that order. In each layer, the convolution operation applies many kernels so that many different feature maps are extracted. These feature maps (Z) are then input into an

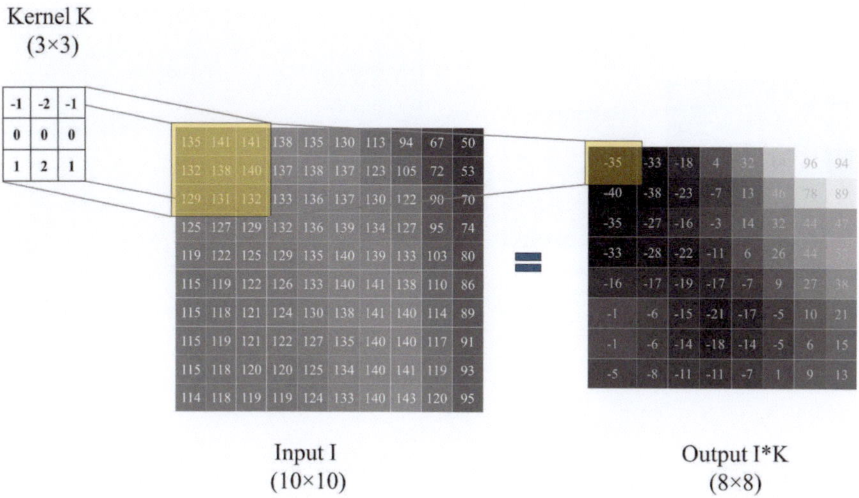

Fig. 1.34 A single 2D convolution step, illustrating the implementation using the correlation operation that moves the filter over the input image and computes the sum of products at each location

activation function, which outputs the non-linear activation A. As noted in Sect. 3.1.1, activation functions introduce non-linearity within the model. This is followed by a pooling function that replaces the output at a certain location of the feature map with a summary statistic, usually the maximum, of the nearby outputs (Fig. 1.36). Pooling functions help make the network approximately invariant to minor translations or scales of the input.

Stacking many convolutional layers sequentially yields deep hierarchical representations, where the early layer captures edges or textures, while deeper layers capture higher-level abstractions and concepts. In a typical CNN, the trainable parameters are usually the weights and biases of the convolutional kernels within each layer. During model training, these parameters are trained using an optimization algorithm such as gradient descent to arrive at the optimized set of values. Depending on the task at hand, convolutional layers are often combined with dense layers from feed-forward neural networks. For example, when CNNs are used to perform a classification task, they are concatenated with dense layers from feed-forward neural networks, followed by a softmax layer to provide class probabilities.

Sequential (Vanilla) CNN

The core concept of a sequential CNN is to simply concatenate a series of convolutional layers with a set of dense layers at the end. The output from the last convolutional layer is flattened and provided as input to the fully-connected (dense) layer. The fully-connected layers at the end of the network make this type of architecture well-suited for classification or object detection tasks.

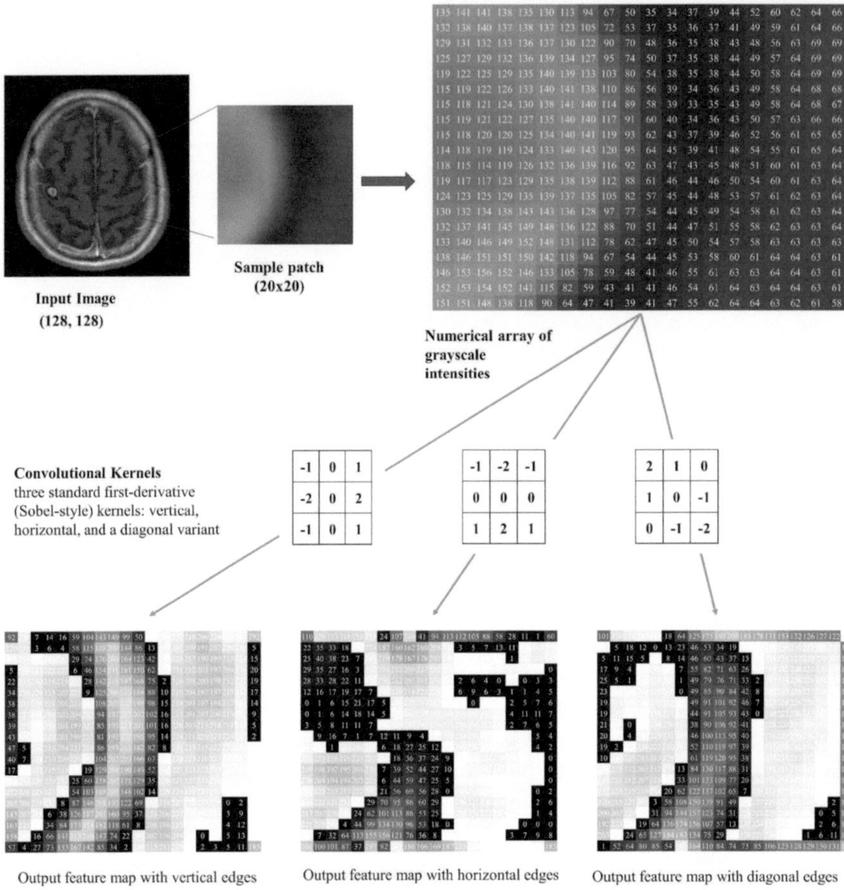

Fig. 1.35 Illustration of 2D convolution in neuroradiology: a 20 × 20 grayscale patch (captured at the edge of brain metastasis voxels) is extracted from a 256 × 256 MRI slice and represented as an intensity matrix (top right). Three 3 × 3 Sobel-style kernels (vertical, horizontal, diagonal; center) convolve over this patch to produce orientation-specific edge maps (bottom), accentuating local gradients along the boundary of the brain metastasis. (Input image from the authors' brain metastasis study IRB14-0749)

In neuroradiology, sequential CNNs have been widely used in image-level tasks such as classification or detection (e.g., Pathology vs. normal) in brain imaging (Fig. 1.37). Commonly used architectures that belong to this design are the AlexNet, VGG-16 / VGG-19. As is the case with most deep learning algorithms, increasing the depth of the neural network increases the complexity, thereby improving performance. In the case of VGG 16, the number denotes the total number of trainable "weight layers." This includes 13 convolutional layers and three fully connected layers. Similarly, in the case of VGG19, the trainable layers include 16 convolutional layers and three fully-connected layers. Due to its relatively simple design, this architecture is often used as a baseline model to learn hierarchical features. In

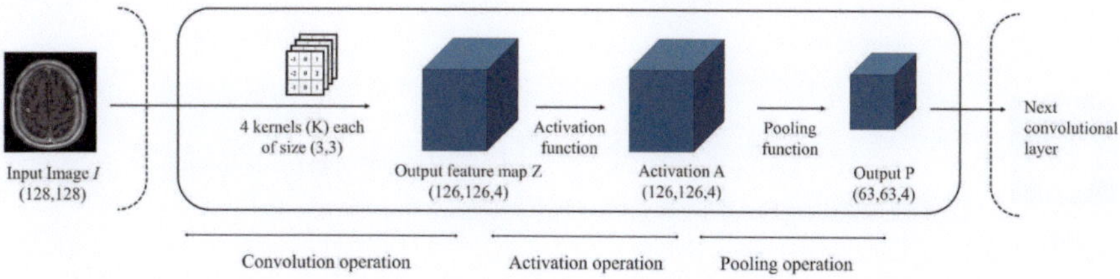

Fig. 1.36 Schematic of a single convolutional layer, which consists of a convolution operation, followed by an activation operation and a pooling operation. (Input image from the authors' brain metastasis study IRB14-0749)

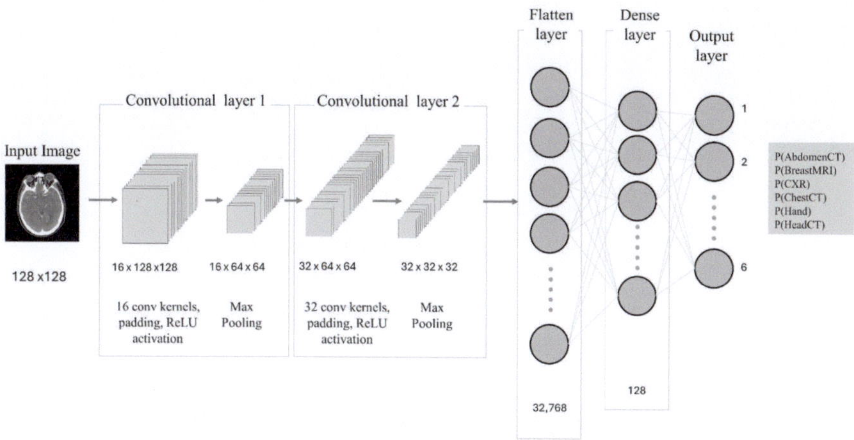

Fig. 1.37 Schematic of a sequential convolutional neural network for image classification. The input image of size 128 × 128 is processed by two Conv+ReLU blocks (3 × 3 kernels, padding = 1, stride = 1), yielding 16 × 128 × 128 and 32 × 64 × 64 feature maps, each followed by 2 × 2 max pooling (stride = 2). The resulting 32 × 32 × 32 activations are flattened into a 32,768-dimensional vector, passed through a 128-unit dense layer, and finally mapped to 6 output units for classification. (CT slice from authors' research study under IRB14-0749)

other cases, these architectures serve as the "backbone" architecture, where more complex neural networks utilize these architectures as one of their components (Fig. 1.38). For example, as stand-alone classifiers, VGG networks have been used to classify brain MRI scans as tumor vs. non-tumor, and, as a backbone network, AlexNet was used as a feature extractor where the inputs from AlexNet's last fully-connected layer were used as inputs to a feed-forward neural network.

In order to intuitively understand how this architecture works, let's refer to an example machine learning task where we train the CNN to classify Head CT images from other types of medical images (Fig. 1.39). For this use-case we use the MedNIST dataset. The MedNIST dataset was gathered from several sets from TCIA, the RSNA Bone Age Challenge (https://www.rsna.org/education/ai-resources-and-training/ai-image-challenge/rsna-pediatric-bone-age-challenge-2017), and the NIH

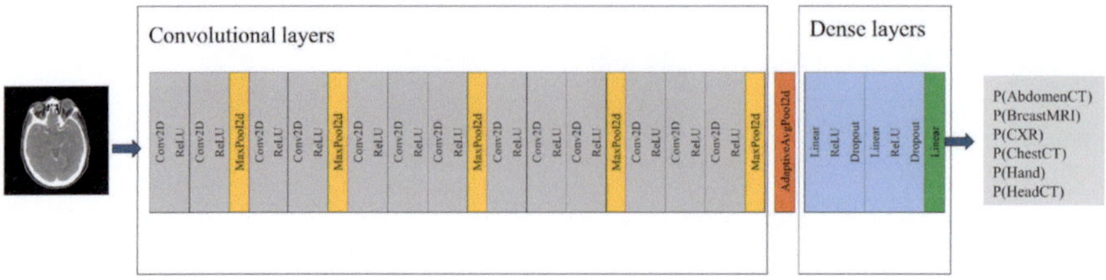

Fig. 1.38 Schematic of VGG-16 adapted to the MEDNIST use-case (CT slice from authors' research study IRB14-0749)

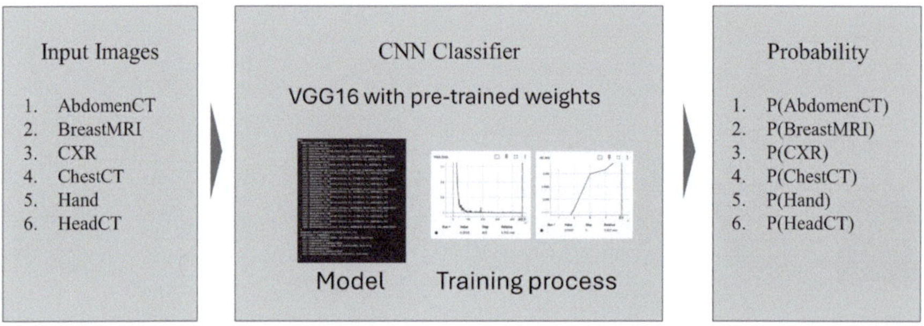

Fig. 1.39 Workflow of a convolutional neural network (CNN)-based image classification pipeline using VGG16 with pre-trained weights

Chest X-ray dataset. The dataset is made available by Dr. Bradley J. Erickson M.D., Ph.D. (Department of Radiology, Mayo Clinic) under the Creative Commons CC BY-SA 4.0 license. In this dataset, there are 6 classes, i.e., "AbdomenCT," "BreastMRI," "CXR," "ChestCT," "Hand," "HeadCT."

Clinically, such a classifier holds promise as a decision support system but would require extensive validation and regulatory steps before being used to guide patient care. Below is a visual schematic of our ML task:

The model takes input images from six medical imaging modalities (Abdomen CT, Breast MRI, chest radiographs [CXR], Chest CT, Hand X-ray, and Head CT), processes them through the CNN classifier, and outputs the corresponding class probabilities for each modality. The training process is monitored using loss and accuracy curves to optimize model performance (Fig. 1.39).

Saliency maps help provide insight into an AI algorithm's decision-making process by visually representing parts of the input that are most important in a model's prediction. These visual explanations are generated from the gradients, which help train the model by adjusting the model parameters. In the context of multi-layer CNNs, activations are the output of a particular layer after the convolution/up-sampling operation is carried out, and gradients are the derivatives of the loss function that are propagated back to the layer under consideration. So, while activations can be thought of as the "state" of a layer, gradients are the "direction and magnitude" of updates that need to be made to the convolutional layer's weights. Gradient-weighted Class Activation Mapping

(Grad-CAM), as the name indicates, uses the gradients to weight the activations within a particular layer to create a visual heat map that highlights the regions of the image that are important to that layer (Fig. 1.40). Early convolutional layers (1–6) capture low-level, modality-agnostic edge and texture information, with diffuse activations along high-contrast anatomical boundaries. Intermediate layers (8–15) transition toward organ-centric representations, emphasizing the intracranial compartment in HeadCT, but we also note that there are some layers where the activations are higher for the background areas. Such findings warrant deeper exploration and failure analysis to identify if the model is not using the anatomically relevant regions for prediction. Deep layers (18–29) concentrate on compact, class-discriminative regions, such as focal intracranial regions in HeadCT. This hierarchical progression illustrates how spatial attention within VGG16 evolves from general structural features to task-specific discriminative patterns, providing interpretable insight into the network's decision-making process in a neuroradiological context.

Overall, these Grad-CAM sequences illustrate a hierarchical representation learning process within VGG16, progressing from low-level edge maps to mid-level organ-centric features, and ultimately to high-level, task-specific discriminative regions (Fig. 1.41). This layer-resolved analysis provides a transparent account of how spatial attention evolves through the network to support modality classification in a neuroradiological context.

Residual Network (ResNet)

One of the challenges with sequential CNNs is that increasing the depth beyond a certain point often results in worse performance. This "degradation" problem occurs in very deep networks where adding more layers leads to higher training

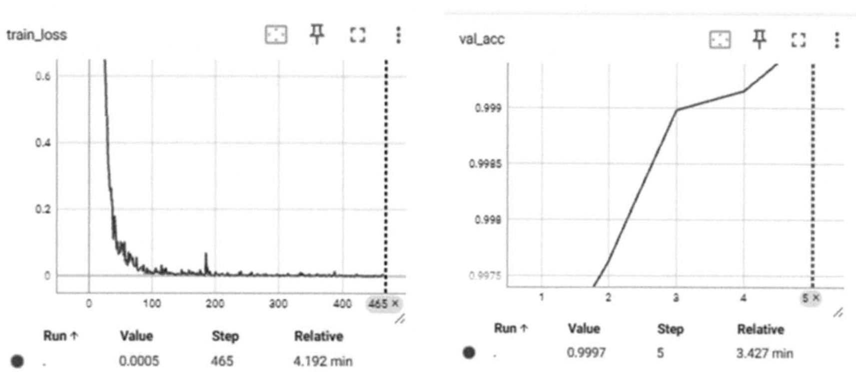

Fig. 1.40 Training performance of the VGG16 classifier on the custom MEDNIST dataset. *(Left)* Training loss curve showing a rapid decrease and stabilization near zero, indicating effective convergence. *(Right)* Validation accuracy curve demonstrating near-perfect performance, with accuracy exceeding 99.9% within the first few epochs. (Code: conv_01_mnist_classification_vgg.ipynb)

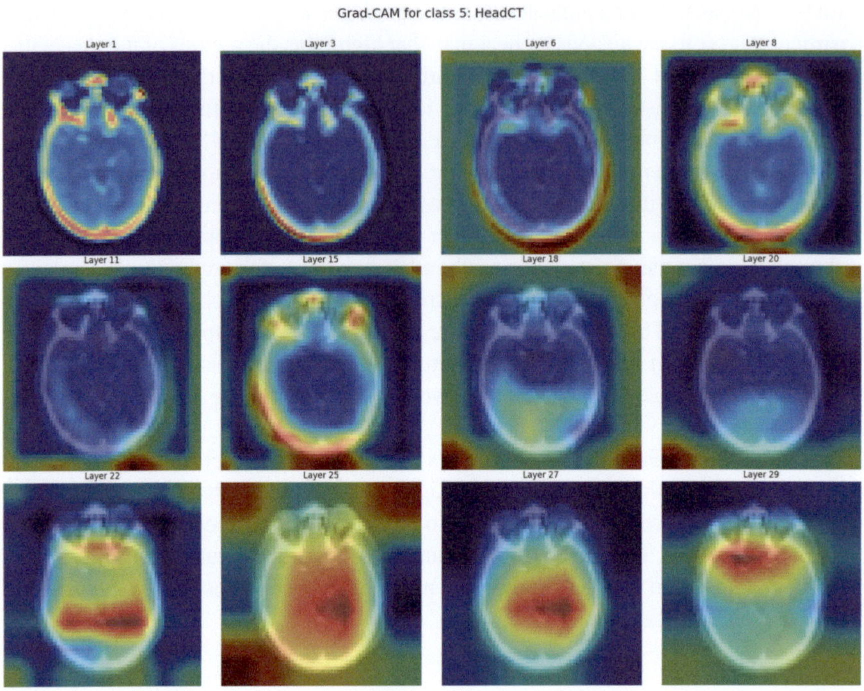

Fig. 1.41 Grad-CAM visualizations across the VGG layers for the HeadCT class (class 5) at multiple convolutional layers of the trained classifier. Warmer colors indicate regions that most strongly increase the class score. For the Head CT images, this corresponds to cranial/skull-associated features. It is important to note that while Grad-CAM images provide an interpretable qualitative view of where the model is focusing on at a given layer, it is not a segmentation of anatomy. A de-identified axial head CT slice from the author's research cohort is shown (IRB14-0749). (Code: conv_01_mnist_classification_vgg.ipynb)

error due to vanishing or exploding gradients. In this situation, the updates propagated to the earlier layers are so small that these layers either learn very slowly or not at all.

The core innovation in ResNet is the introduction of residual connections, or "skip connections," which add or concatenate input from earlier layers to later layers. This allows the network to learn residual functions with reference to the layer inputs, rather than learning unreferenced functions directly. In a residual block, the output is defined as

$$Output = F\left(x\right) + x$$

where $F(x)$ is the residual mapping to be learned and x is the input that is directly added to the output via the skip connection. This diagram illustrates a fundamental residual unit used in ResNet, where the input x is passed through two stacked weight layers (each typically consisting of a convolution, batch normalization, and ReLU activation). The output of the block *F(x)* is then added element-wise to the original input *x* via a shortcut connection (identity mapping), forming the output *F(x)* + *x*. This residual connection enables more effective gradient flow during backpropagation, addressing the vanishing gradient problem in deep neural networks and allowing for the successful training of very deep architectures.

Another benefit of these residual connections is ease of optimization. The identity mapping enables the network to preserve information across layers. This enables the model to learn only the residual refinements instead of entirely new representations, thereby helping the model converge faster and generalize better (Fig. 1.42). Additionally, these residual blocks allow the network to reuse features learned in earlier layers. This helps the model become more efficient and beneficial in image tasks involving subtle or diffuse pathology, common in neuroradiology. Commonly used neural networks that belong to the ResNet architecture are ResNet-18, ResNet-34, ResNet-50, ResNet-101, ResNet-152, where the number after ResNet refers to the number of learnable (convolutional and fully connected) layers the network contains.

With the deeper ResNet architectures, such as ResNet-50, ResNet-101, and ResNet-152, the basic ResNet block is replaced with the "bottleneck" block, which lets them go deeper without blowing up the computation requirements (Fig. 1.43). It does this by using a 1x1 convolution that reduces the dimensions of the feature maps before processing them through the 3 × 3 convolution, followed by another 1 × 1 convolution that expands the dimensions to the original number of channels. The identity shortcut connection adds the original input back to the output to facilitate residual learning.

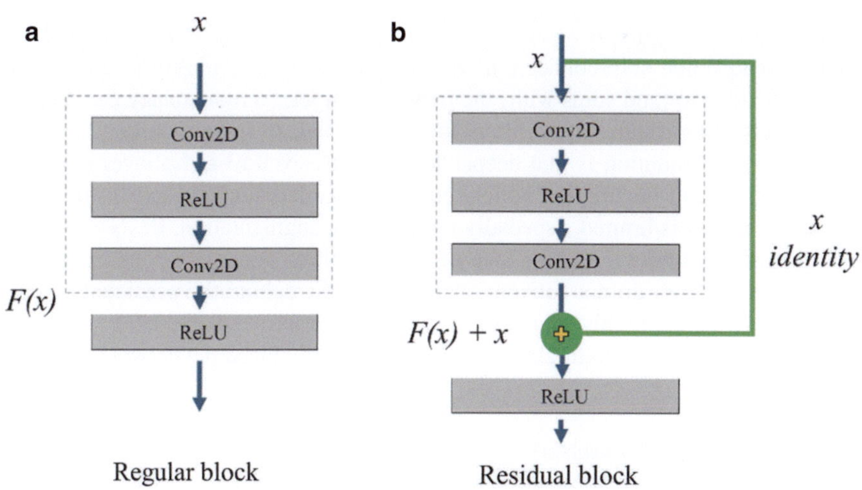

Fig. 1.42 Illustration of a residual connection using an example of a convolutional layer with 2D convolution operations. In a regular block (**a**), the portion within the dotted-line box must directly learn the mapping f(x). In a residual block (**b**), the portion within the dotted-line box needs to learn the residual mapping $g(x) = f(x) - x$, making the identity mapping $F(x) = x$ easier to learn

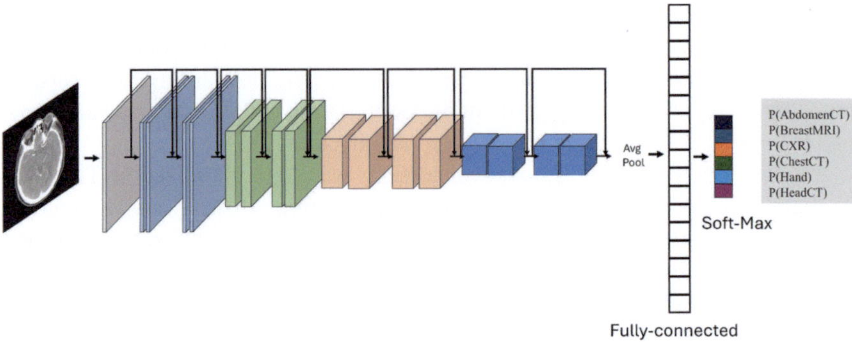

Fig. 1.43 The ResNet-18 architecture. De-identified axial head CT slice from the author's research cohort (IRB14-0749)

In neuroradiology, the deep representations within ResNet can help capture subtle MRI/CT patterns (small lesions, fine texture) that shallower network architectures would miss. The ResNet architecture is commonly used either as a direct classifier or as a backbone network that carries out feature extraction in hybrid architectures, making it well-suited to a wide range of ML tasks, including detection, classification, and segmentation. ResNet-based architectures often outperform shallower sequential CNNs in both accuracy and robustness. ResNet architectures (e.g., ResNet-18/50) have been applied across neuroradiology for tumor classification, lesion segmentation, hemorrhage detection, and Alzheimer's staging. Used either as fine-tuned classifiers or backbones in segmentation models (Fig. 1.44, 1.45, and 1.46),

Despite its strengths, ResNets still face important challenges in neuroradiology applications. While skip-connections improve the network's ability to train, each layer only adds to (and sums with) the previous output, so redundancy can persist, and models often require more filters to perform well in neuroradiology applications. Another limitation is that deeper ResNets (ResNet 50 and above) typically contain millions of parameters, which require large annotated datasets for training. When the dataset is limited, especially without data augmentation, ResNets tend to overfit. Another limitation is the lack of explainability. While ResNets can detect useful patterns, they do not natively explain the logic behind the predicted output. Deeper ResNets are highly reliant on methods that improve explainability such as Grad-CAM, which can highlight regions that most influenced the network's logic.

Dense Connectivity (DenseNet)

In this approach, a structural block containing a series of convolutional layers is defined, where each layer is connected to all following layers. For example, in the Dense block shown in Fig. 1.47, every layer l takes all preceding feature maps as input. Formally, if x_l is the output of layer l, then DenseNet defines

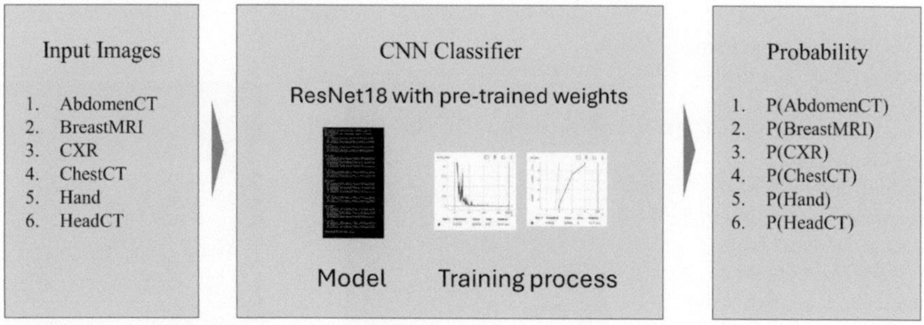

Fig. 1.44 Workflow of a convolutional neural network (CNN)-based classification pipeline using ResNet18 with pre-trained weights. The model processes input images from six medical imaging modalities (Abdomen CT, Breast MRI, chest radiographs [CXR], Chest CT, Hand X-ray, and Head CT) and outputs the corresponding class probabilities. The central panel illustrates the model architecture and the training process, including loss and accuracy curves used to monitor convergence and performance

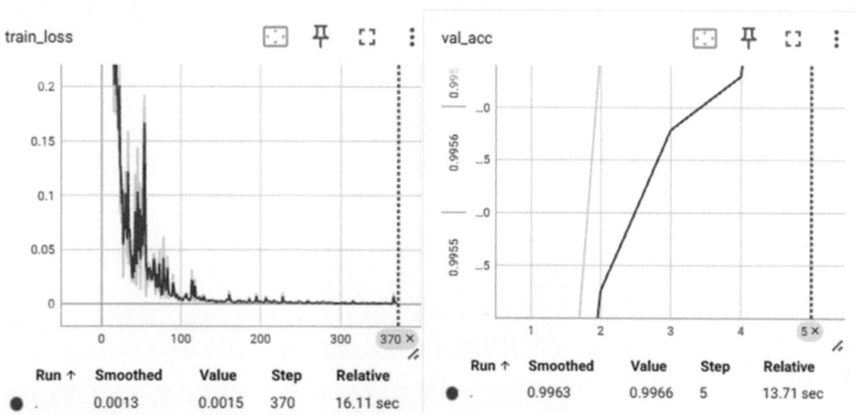

Fig. 1.45 Training performance of the ResNet18 classifier on the custom medical imaging data-set. *(Left)* Training loss curve showing rapid reduction and stabilization near zero, indicating efficient convergence. *(Right)* Validation accuracy curve demonstrating consistently high performance, exceeding 99.6% within the first few epochs. (Code: conv_02_mnist_classification_resnet.ipynb)

$$x_l = H_l\left(\left[x_{0,}x_{1,}x_{2,}\ldots\ldots,x_{l-1,}\right]\right)$$

where $[x_0, x_1, x_2, \ldots\ldots,]$ denotes concatenation of the feature-maps from layers 0 through l-1.

Within each dense block, the channel dimension is set to grow as layers accumulate more features. For example, if the block input has $k0$ channels, then the ℓth layer has $k0+k\times(\ell-1)$ input channels, where k is the growth rate. The growth rate k is a key hyperparameter in DenseNet. In practice, smaller k limits parameter counts where DenseNet layers are quite narrow while still leveraging a large "collective" set from earlier layers. The overall neural network is constructed by

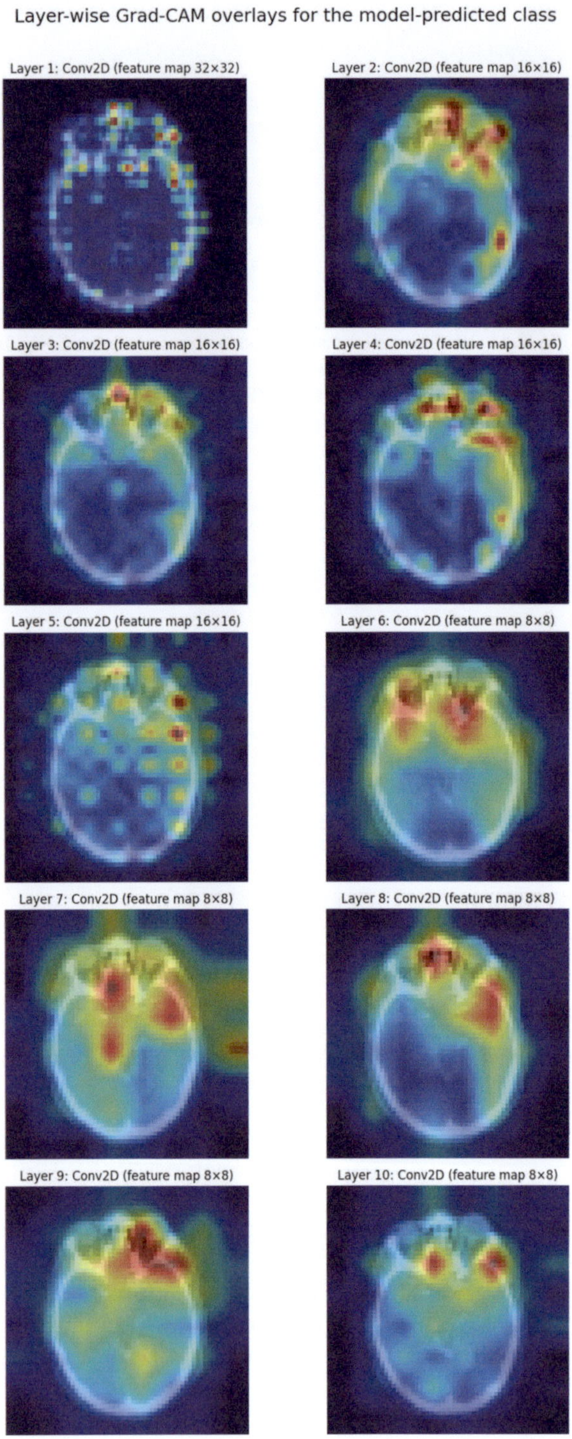

Fig. 1.46 Grad-CAM visualizations from early, intermediate, and deep layers of ResNet18 for HeadCT (class 5) inputs. If the Grad-CAM visualizations show substantial activation in the background and border regions that contain no anatomy, it is often a sign that the model is exploiting padding/cropping or background patterns rather than purely anatomical features. Such issues highlight the importance of extensive data augmentations that break border/background cues such as random crops, patch-based sampling, translation and scaling, random padding, slight rotations, etc. Such visualizations help explain the potential reduction in generalization performance when a Head CT from a different dataset is used. (Background image from Head CT from IRB14-0749)

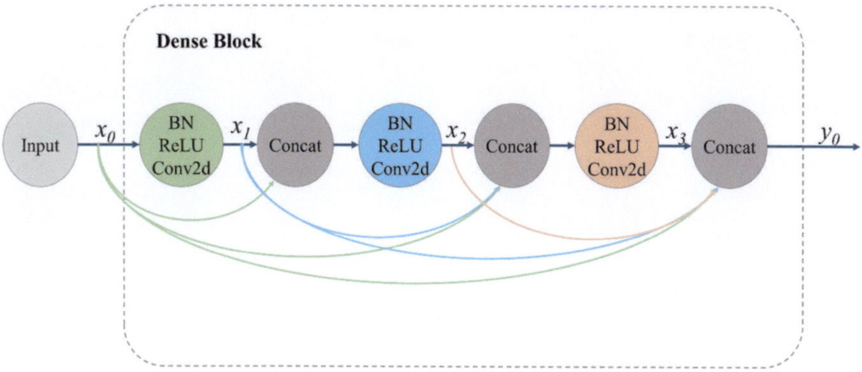

Fig. 1.47 A schematic diagram of a 3-layer dense block used in the DenseNet architecture.

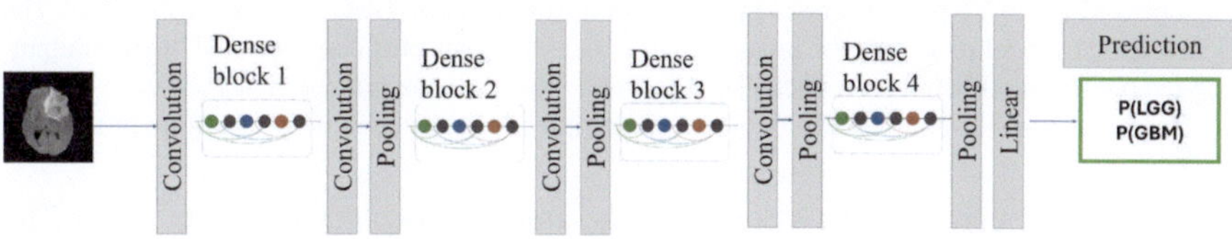

Fig. 1.48 A DenseNet-121 constructed with three 4 dense blocks to perform an LGG/GBM classification task. (Input MRI slice from BraTS-TCGA-GBM, licensed under CC-BY-3.0)

concatenating these dense blocks using a transition layer, usually a 1 × 1 Convolution layer with pooling, as shown in Fig. 1.48.

DenseNet architectures are commonly denoted in practice using the number of trainable layers as a suffix. For example, DenseNet-121, -169, -201, and -264 contain 121, 169, 201, and 264 layers, respectively. Deeper variants use a "BC" design (Bottleneck+Compression) with 1 × 1 bottleneck convolutions and compressed transitions to further reduce parameters.

Since each layer has a short path to the loss via concatenation, gradients flow directly to earlier layers within the block, which improves training convergence. DenseNet's implicit "deep supervision" (every layer has a short path to the loss) acts as a regularizer. Studies observe that DenseNets tend to overfit less on small training sets. Additionally, by concatenating outputs from all preceding layers, DenseNets inherently aggregate multiscale features (from low-level edges to high-level abstractions or semantics) in every subsequent layer. By exploiting features from all layers, DenseNets can capture multiscale information in scans. This has enabled improved automated diagnosis (e.g., brain tumor identification, Alzheimer's detection) in research studies.

For example, let's take the previous use-case from Sect. 2 where we trained a classifier to differentiate GBM from LGG using radiomic features. However, since in this section we are exploring CNNs, let's directly use the MRI images as input instead of the extracted radiomics. The task is illustrated in Fig. 1.49 below.

After training and validation steps are complete, the DenseNet predictions can be explained using Occlusion Sensitivity. In this method, the change in model's

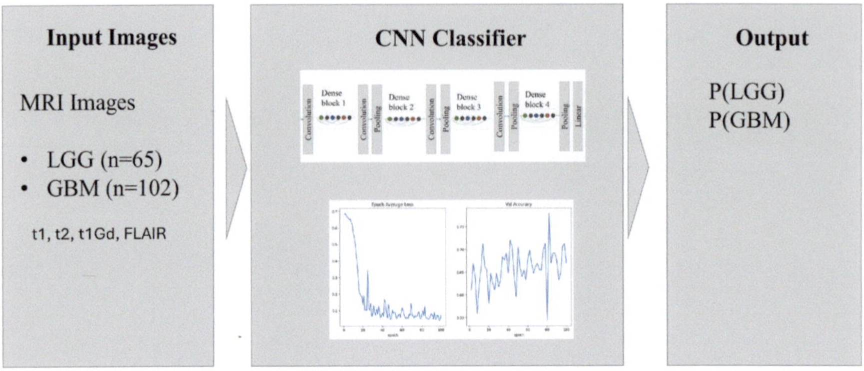

Fig. 1.49 Workflow of a DenseNet121-based classification pipeline for differentiating low-grade glioma (LGG) and glioblastoma (GBM) using multi-sequence MRI. Input data comprise four MRI sequences (T1, T2, T1 post-contrast [T1Gd], and FLAIR) from 65 LGG and 102 GBM cases. The DenseNet121 model processes the images through densely connected convolutional blocks, outputting the predicted probability for each class. Training progress is monitored via epoch-wise average loss and validation accuracy curves. (Code: conv_03_glioma_classification_densenet.ipynb)

predictions is recorded when a portion of the image is "occluded" or set to zero. The model's predictions are expected to change drastically when the occluded patch contains an important region of interest that plays a major role in the final prediction. This is especially useful to ensure that the model is learning to classify using the right features and regions of interest. For this reason, we compare the occlusion sensitivity map to the ground-truth annotations carried out by experienced radiologists (Fig. 1.50).

When the lesion and its enhancing core is occluded (upper-left quadrant of the tumor), the predicted GBM probability drops most dramatically as shown by the red region. In other words, that area is positive evidence for GBM since removing it confuses the network and makes it less confident that it's seeing a high-grade tumor. By contrast, occluding the surrounding normal brain (the blue spots outside the lesion) doesn't affect the prediction by as much, implying that the model treats other areas as negative evidence for GBM (i.e., the model has learnt that these features are more characteristic of LGG or healthy tissue).

Taken together, this spatial map tells us that the DenseNet is keying in on the lesion's central heterogeneity and irregular margins, which are typically characteristics of aggressive, high-grade glioblastoma, while giving far less weight to peritumoral edema or normal parenchyma. The occlusion sensitivity thus provides a post-hoc explanation that aligns with the radiologic features we use clinically to distinguish GBM from LGG.

Encoder-Decoder (U-Shaped)

Encoder-decoder CNNs consist of two symmetric paths: a contracting encoder designed to capture context by progressively downsampling feature maps and an expanding decoder designed to enable precise localization by progressively

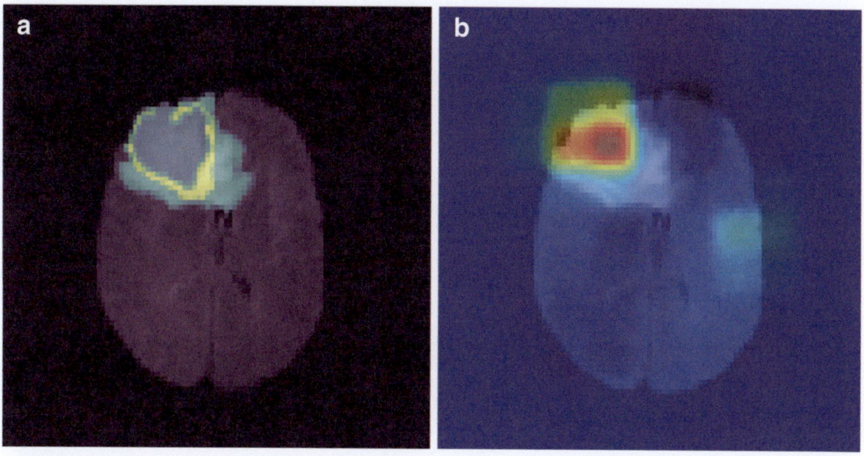

Fig. 1.50 Comparison of expert segmentation and model-derived importance map. The left panel (**a**) shows the ground truth tumor segmentation (here a FLAIR sequence from BraTS-TCGA-GBM, licensed under CC-BY-3.0) annotated by experienced radiologists. The right panel (**b**) displays the occlusion sensitivity heatmap generated from a DenseNet-based classification model, where warmer colors (red/yellow) indicate regions whose occlusion results in a greater drop in the predicted probability, highlighting areas most influential for the model's decision. Such visualizations help carry out qualitative validation to ensure that the model is learning the relevant anatomy and not the data source (center confounding). (Code: conv_03_glioma_classification_densenet.ipynb)

upsampling the downsampled feature maps back to their original dimensions. The encoder is composed of sequentially placed convolutional blocks composed of convolutional, activation and pooling layers. The decoder is composed of transposed convolutions or upsampling + convolution to recover spatial detail (Fig. 1.51). These layers are connected by using skip connections that concatenate the output from each stage of the encoder with the corresponding stage within the decoder module. These skip connections allow high-resolution features to flow directly into the decoder and mitigate information loss.

Encoder-decoder architectures, such as the U-Net, excel at pixel-wise or voxel-wise segmentation tasks for medical imaging, where the neural network is trained to identify lesion vs. healthy tissue pixels. The use of skip connections enables these networks to deliver precise boundary delineation and integrate global anatomical context with local texture patterns. The two-dimensional convolutional kernels can be replaced with three-dimensional kernels natively supporting voxel-based segmentation Fig. 1.52. These architectures also work well with three-dimensional medical images with appropriate isotropic resampling and multi-slice information to address variations in slice thickness and pixel spacing.

In the attached Grad-CAM image, the earliest encoder layers (1–4) light up generic edges and coarse tumor location; the decoder layers (5–8) progressively sharpen that focus, filtering out background as the feature maps go deeper; and the

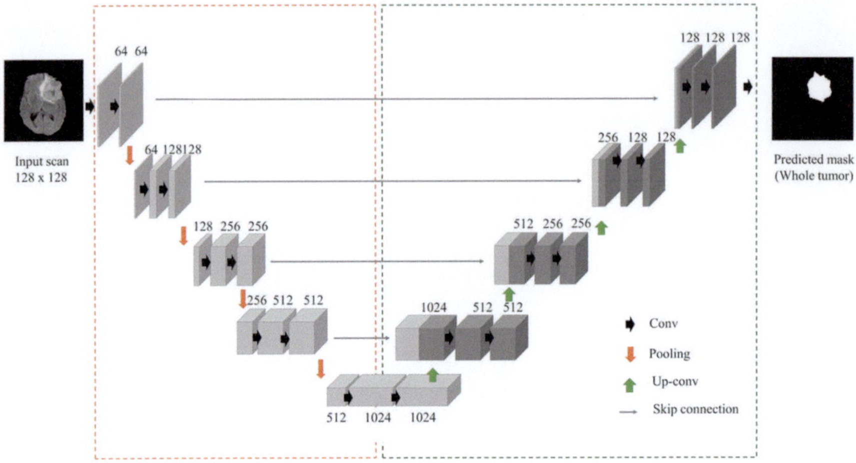

Fig. 1.51 Schematic representation of the U-Net architecture for medical image segmentation. The encoder path (left, orange arrows) progressively reduces spatial resolution through convolutional blocks and pooling, capturing increasingly abstract features. The decoder path (right, green arrows) restores spatial resolution using up-convolutions, while skip connections (gray arrows) transfer high-resolution features from the encoder to the decoder, preserving fine structural details. The final output is a segmentation mask (here, delineating the whole tumor) generated at the original image resolution. Input image from BraTS-TCGA-GBM, licensed under CC-BY-3.0

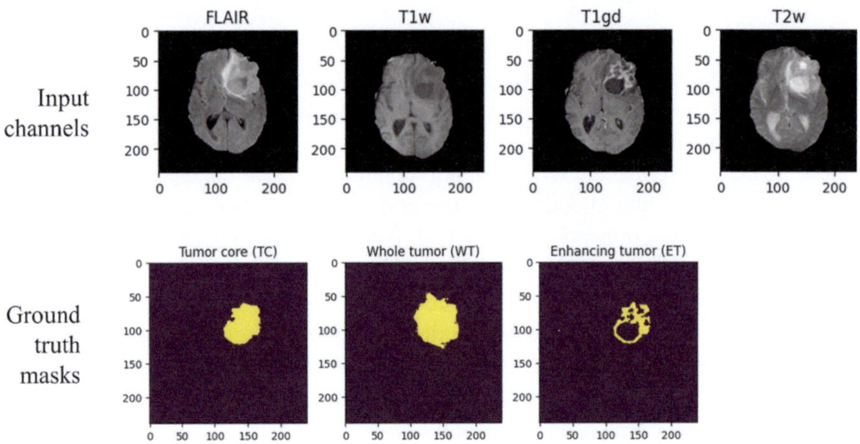

Fig. 1.52 Example case from the BraTS dataset illustrating multi-sequence MRI inputs and corresponding ground truth tumor segmentation labels. *(Top row)* Four MRI sequences: FLAIR, T1-weighted (T1w), contrast-enhanced T1-weighted (T1Gd), and T2-weighted (T2w). *(Bottom row)* Ground truth binary masks for tumor subregions: tumor core (TC), whole tumor (WT), and enhancing tumor (ET), used as segmentation targets for model training and evaluation. Images were generated using a modified version of the MONAI BRATS segmentation tutorial with an input image from BraTS-TCGA-GBM, licensed under CC-BY-3.0

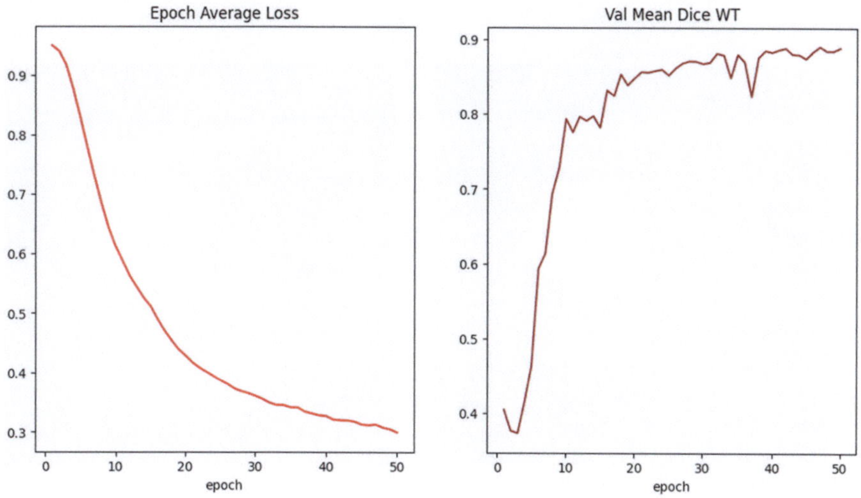

Fig. 1.53 Training performance of a tumor segmentation model on the BraTS dataset. *(Left)* Epoch-wise average loss curve showing a steady decrease, indicating effective model optimization. *(Right)* Validation mean Dice score for the whole tumor (WT) class, demonstrating progressive improvement and convergence toward high segmentation accuracy over 50 epochs. (Code: conv_04_brats_segmentation_unet.ipynb)

final decoder merge (9) shows how up-sampled context and skip connections fuse to delineate the whole-tumor boundary Fig. 1.53. This mirrors the U-Net intuition: a contracting path extracts multi-scale context, skip connections shuttle high-resolution detail forward, and an expanding path combines both to reconstruct a precise segmentation mask.

Although these heat maps give us a useful insight into what each stage is attending to, it is important to understand that we are looking at one 2D slice of a 3D network, with low-resolution feature maps up-sampled and overlaid via a chosen colormap Figs. 1.54 and 1.55. Additionally, only positive gradients for the "whole-tumor" class are shown (negative evidence is typically discarded since we use a ReLU activation function), and spatial alignment can shift slightly due to padding or interpolation. These visualizations reflect correlated activations, not strict causality. The heatmaps in this included image represent only one example, but patterns may vary across cases.

Attention-Augmented CNN

CNNs excel at capturing local patterns, but traditional CNNs lack global context, which can limit generalization in neuroradiology. Attention mechanisms address this challenge by adaptively re-weighting features that allow CNNs to "focus" on parts of the image that are most important in carrying out the task instead of giving equal importance to all areas of the image.

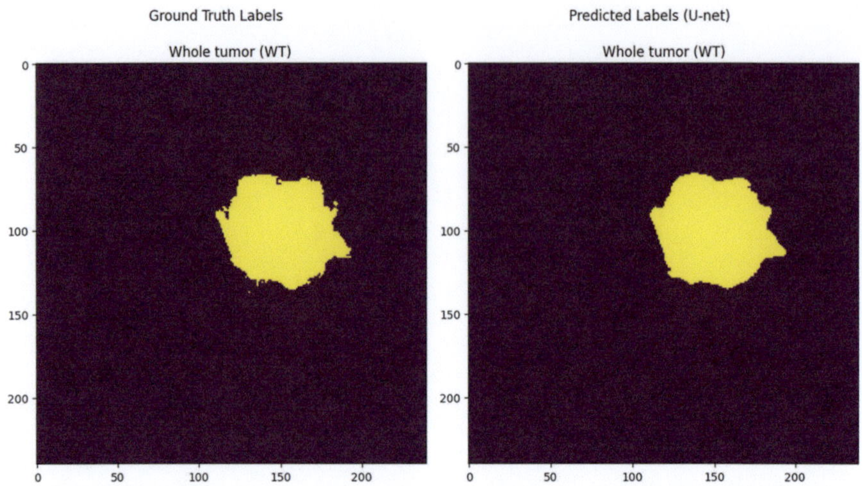

Fig. 1.54 Example of whole tumor (WT) segmentation results on the BraTS dataset. *(Left)* Ground truth label showing the manually annotated tumor region. *(Right)* Predicted label generated by the U-Net model, demonstrating close spatial correspondence with the ground truth annotation. (Tumor mask from BraTS-TCGA-GBM, licensed under CC-BY-3.0)

In practice, the attention models compute weights across spatial locations, channels, or both. *Channel-wise attention methods*, such as Squeeze-and-Excitation, compute a weight for each feature channel to prioritize more important feature maps. *Spatial-attention methods*, such as Convolutional Block Attention Module (CBAM), highlight the most important regions within the feature map, irrespective of the channel. These spatial models are highly effective in suppressing background and concentrating on lesions or anatomical structures. In segmentation tasks, spatial attention modules have been used to adaptively gate skip-connections (as in Attention U-Net) so that the decoder receives only relevant spatial features, improving boundary delineation. *Self-attention methods* help capture long-range dependencies by computing responses at each position within the feature map by relating it to all other positions. Self-attention methods are well-suited to capture global context, which is useful when lesions span large areas or when distant anatomy provides context. Hybrid and multi-scale attention methods combine channel and spatial attention mechanisms. For example, CBAM applies channel attention followed by spatial attention on the same feature map. Attention gates, as used in Attention U-net, can be thought of as a spatial hybrid module that learns to weight features before merging encoder and decoder information.

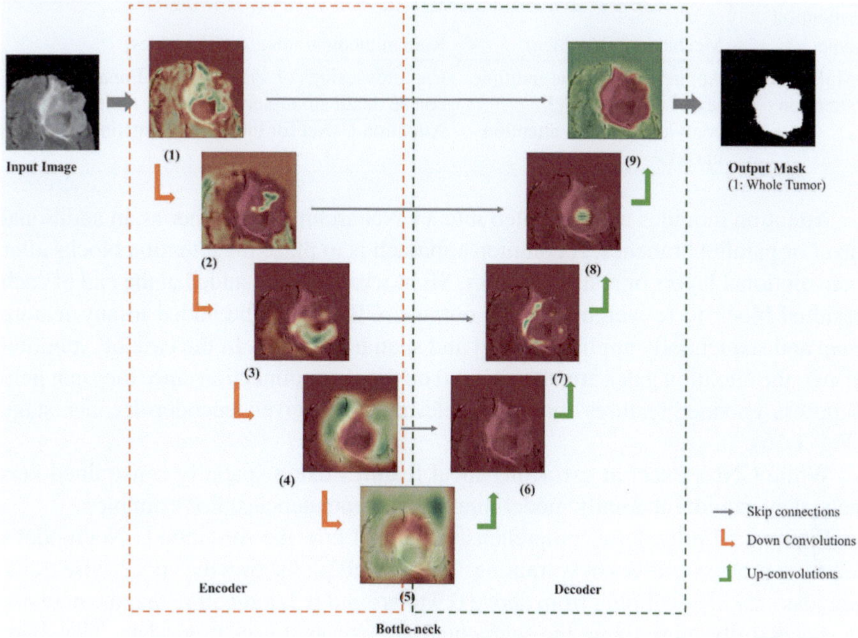

Fig. 1.55 U-Net architecture illustration using an example case (rotated and cropped to illustrate the tumor ROI) from the BraTS dataset for whole tumor (WT) segmentation. The network consists of an **encoder** path (left) with successive down-convolutions to capture contextual features, a **bottleneck** layer (center) for deep feature representation, and a **decoder** path (right) with up-convolutions to restore spatial resolution. Skip connections (gray arrows) transfer feature maps from encoder to decoder at corresponding levels, enabling precise localization. The input multi-sequence MRI slice is progressively transformed through encoding and decoding stages to produce the final binary segmentation mask of the whole tumor. (Code: conv_04_brats_segmentation_unet.ipynb) Input slice from BraTS-TCGA-GBM CC-BY-3.0

Attention type	Mechanism (key idea)	Role in medical imaging (examples)
Channel-wise	Learns a weight for each feature channel (e.g., SE block with global pooling)	Emphasizes important features (e.g., tumor texture, tissue contrasts). Used in classification/segmentation to highlight lesion-related feature maps.
Spatial	Learns a spatial mask over each feature map (e.g. convolutional attention map)	Focuses on salient regions (e.g., tumors, organs). Improves localization (e.g., Attention U-Net gates).
Self-attention (non-local)	Computes pairwise interactions across the image (global attention, multi-head)	Captures long-range context. Useful for large/irregular lesions (e.g., tumor boundaries) and integrating contextual cues from distant anatomy.
Hybrid (channel + spatial)	Combines channel and spatial re-weighting (e.g., CBAM)	Leverages both "what" and "where." For example, combined attention may improve brain tumor classification by focusing on the most informative channels and locations.

Attention type	Mechanism (key idea)	Role in medical imaging (examples)
Multi-scale attention	Applies attention at multiple scales (e.g., parallel conv-kernels with attention masks)	Captures lesions of varying sizes. Enhances fine/coarse detail simultaneously (e.g., multi-scale Attention U-Net for tumor segmentation).

Attention modules are integrated into a CNN architecture either as an additional layer or parallel branches. A common approach is to place the attention blocks after convolutional layers or residual blocks. SE blocks are often added at the end of each residual block to re-weight channel outputs. CBAM can be added to any feature map and sequentially applies channel and spatial attention. In the case of Attention U-net, the attention gates are often placed on the skip connection since they can help suppress encoder features that are irrelevant for a given encoder-decoder stage (Fig. 1.56).

While CNNs excel at extracting local features using spatially constrained kernels, they cannot inherently model long-range dependencies. For example,

Figure 1.57 provides a comprehensive view of how the Attention U-Net model's learning process evolves over training. The top-left plot shows the epoch-wise training loss steadily declining from above 0.9 to around 0.2, indicating that the network is successfully minimizing the segmentation error as it sees more data. The sharp drop in the early epochs suggests that the model quickly captures the most salient spatial patterns, with later epochs focusing on fine-tuning.

The top-right plot tracks the overall validation mean Dice score across all tumor-related classes. It rises rapidly within the first 10 epochs, from roughly 0.25 to over 0.65, before plateauing around 0.72, signaling that the model has reached a stable level of generalization performance. The **bottom row** breaks this down for each

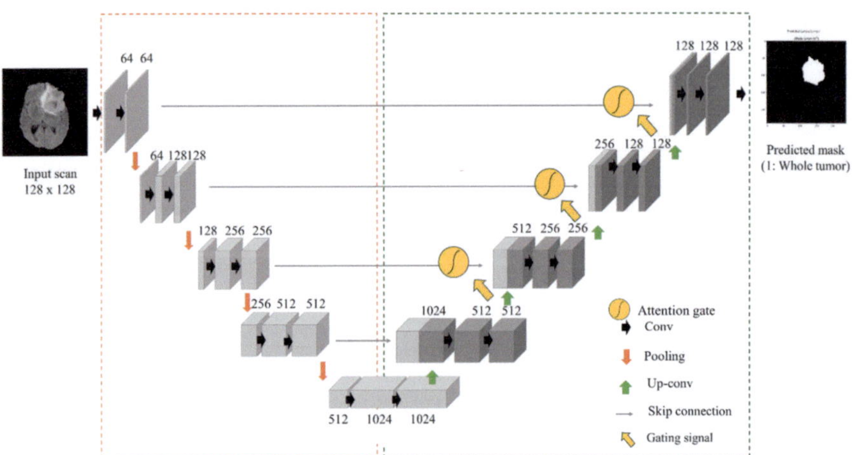

Fig. 1.56 Schematic of Attention U-net. (Input image from BraTS-TCGA-GBM, licensed under CC-BY-3.0)

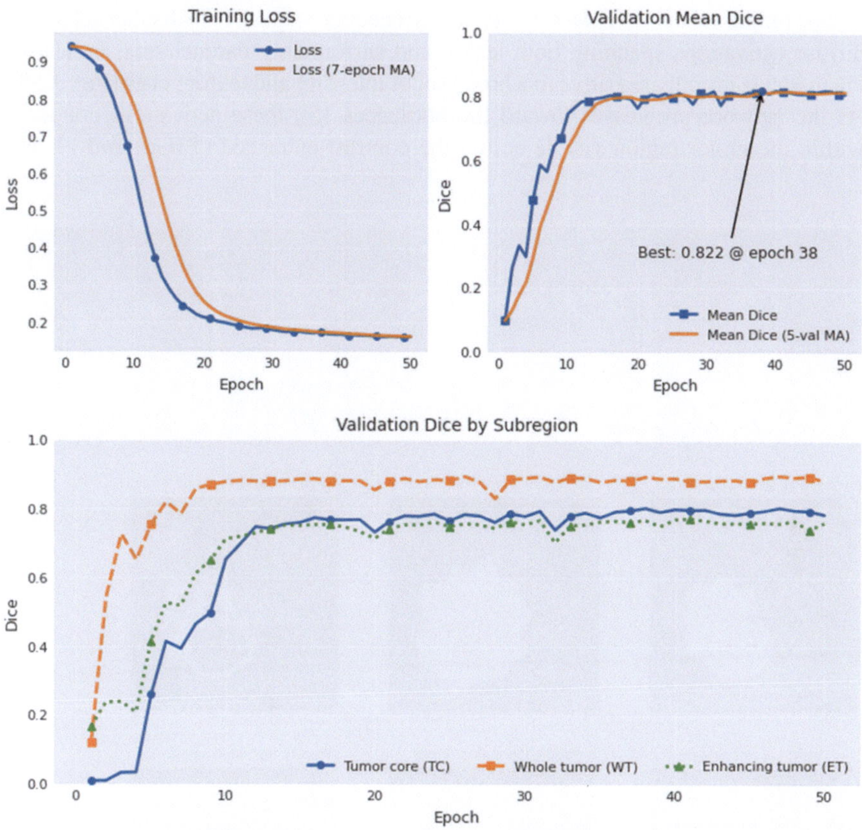

Fig. 1.57 Training and validation performance of the Attention U-Net model for brain tumor segmentation on the BraTS dataset. *(Top left)* Epoch-wise average training loss, showing a steady decrease indicating effective model optimization. *(Top right)* Overall validation mean Dice score across all tumor subregions. *(Bottom row)* Validation mean Dice scores for individual tumor regions: tumor core (TC), whole tumor (WT), and enhancing tumor (ET), demonstrating rapid improvement during early epochs and stable convergence in later stages

target region type, revealing interesting differences in learnability. **Tumor Core (TC)** achieves a Dice of about 0.8, suggesting the model reliably segments this region once trained. **Whole Tumor (WT)** reaches the highest performance (around 0.88–0.90), likely because it has the largest and most spatially coherent target area, making it easier to detect and segment accurately. **Enhancing Tumor (ET)** lags behind, plateauing near 0.53, reflecting the challenge of accurately segmenting smaller, less distinct regions.

Taken together, these curves highlight both the effectiveness of the Attention U-Net in capturing coarse-to-fine spatial features and the inherent difficulty imbalance between different segmentation targets. They also make it clear where further architectural tuning or loss weighting might yield the greatest gains, particularly for smaller, harder-to-segment regions.

For output label *"0: Tumor Core,"* early encoder stages (1-3) display relatively diffuse activations spanning both lesion and surrounding parenchyma, indicating the model is initially sensitive to a broad set of intensity and texture cues (Fig. 1.58). As the network progresses toward the bottleneck (5), these activations condense within the tumor region visible across the contrast-enhanced (T1Gd) and FLAIR

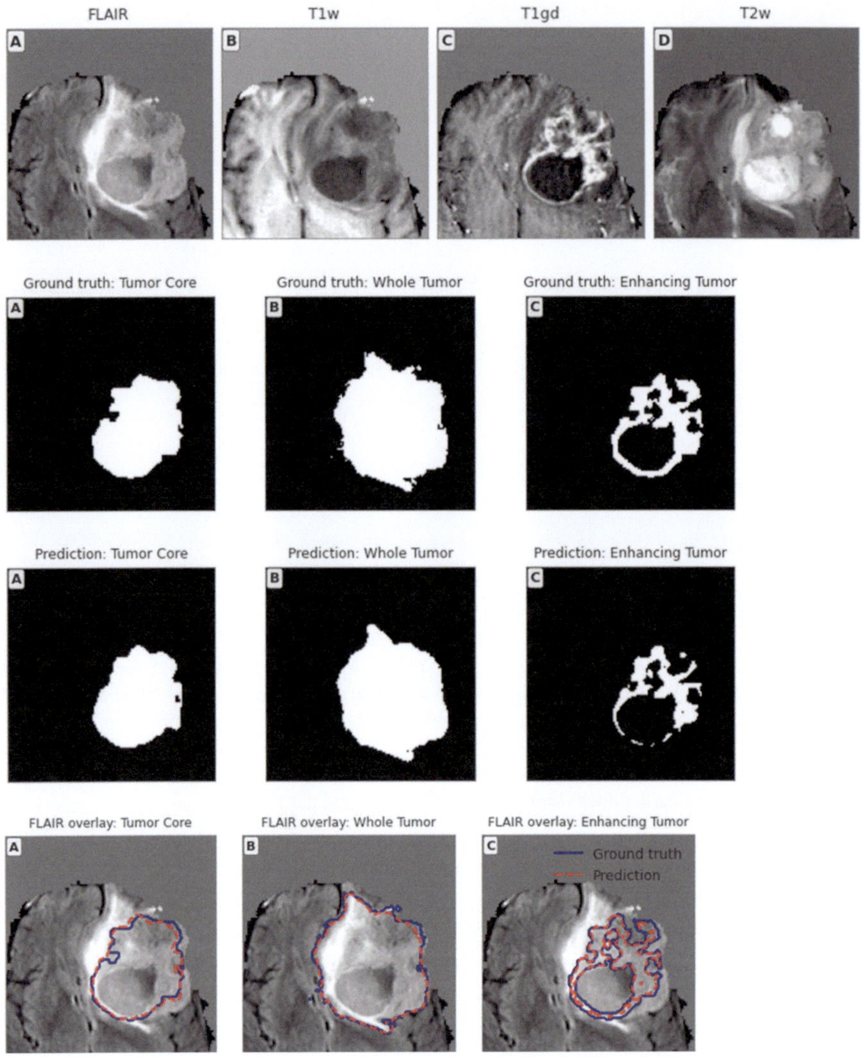

Fig. 1.58 Multi-parametric MRI inputs and tumor segmentation (example case). Top row: four MRI sequences, FLAIR, T1w, T1Gd, and T2w, used as inputs. Middle row: ground-truth masks for (left to right) tumor core (TC), whole tumor (WT), and enhancing tumor (ET), where WT = ET + TC + edema and TC = ET + non-enhancing/necrotic core. Bottom two rows: Attention U-Net predictions for the same three regions. (Example from the BraTS-TCGA-GBM dataset, licensed under CC-BY-3.0)

inputs. The attention gates (A1–A4) clearly suppress peripheral activations and channel skip connection information toward the lesion interior, producing decoder-stage maps (7–9) that align tightly with the tumor's anatomical core in the predicted mask (Fig. 1.59)

For output label *"1: Whole Tumor,"* Grad-CAM reveals a different strategy where the mid-encoder layers already show a more spatially expansive activation pattern that follows peritumoral hyperintensity seen on FLAIR and T2w sequences. Attention gates here act to preserve these wider boundaries rather than overly constrain them, enabling the decoder to reconstruct a contiguous activation map encompassing both core and edema. By the final decoder stage, the attention-weighted focus encompasses the entire tumor extent, matching the whole tumor mask and excluding non-pathological hyperintense regions (Fig. 1.60).

For the output label *"2: Enhancing Tumor,"* the activation pathway is far more selective. Initial encoder layers activate on multiple high-contrast foci within the lesion, but by the bottleneck, the response narrows dramatically to the

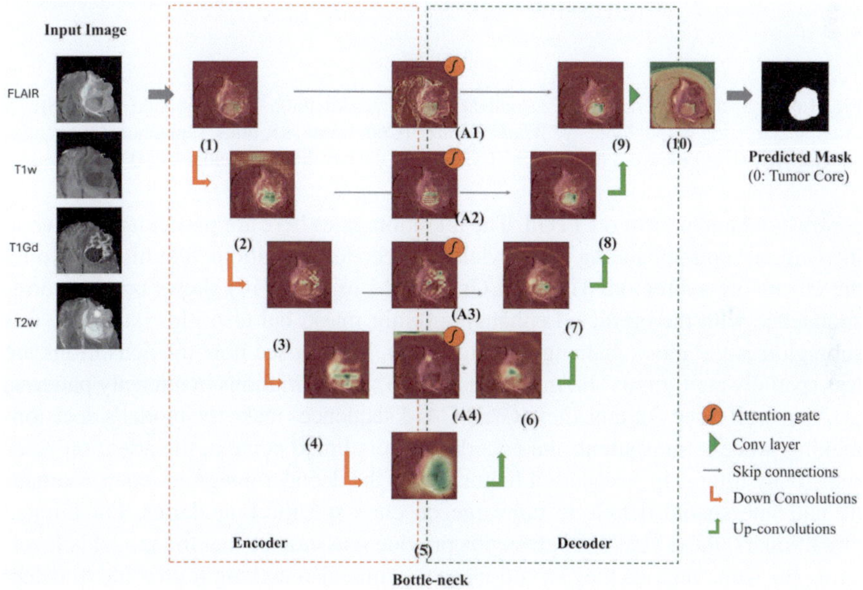

Fig. 1.59 Layer-wise Grad-CAM visualizations for an Attention U-Net applied to an example image from BraTS, targeting output label *"0: Tumor Core."* The model processes four multi-parametric MRI sequences (FLAIR, T1w, T1Gd, and T2w) as input channels. The encoder path (left) performs successive down-convolutions to capture hierarchical features, while the decoder path (right) reconstructs spatial detail via up-convolutions and skip connections. Attention gates (orange icons) modulate skip connection features to enhance focus on tumor-relevant regions. Grad-CAM maps at each selected layer illustrate the network's evolving spatial attention from coarse, global structures in early encoding stages to localized, high-salience tumor regions in the final decoding layers, culminating in the predicted tumor core segmentation mask. (Code: conv_05_brats_segmentation_attentionunet.ipynb) (Example from the BraTS-TCGA-GBM dataset, licensed under CC-BY-3.0)

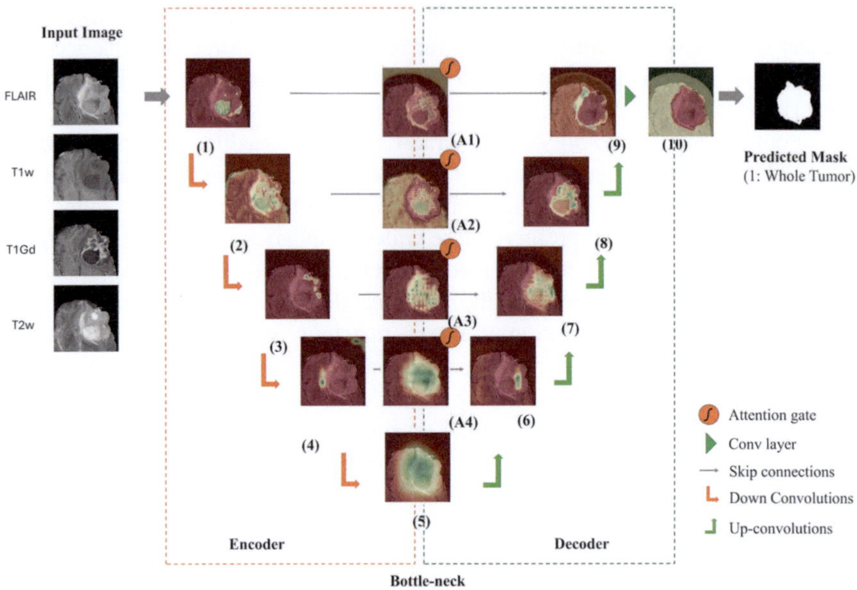

Fig. 1.60 Layer-wise Grad-CAM visualizations for an Attention U-Net applied to the BraTS example, targeting output label *"1: Whole Tumor."* (Code: conv_05_brats_segmentation_attentionunet.ipynb) (Example from the BraTS-TCGA-GBM dataset, licensed under CC-BY-3.0)

contrast-enhancing rim on T1Gd. The attention gates here are particularly active in filtering out non-enhancing areas, yielding decoder activations that highlight only the enhancing subregion. The final Grad-CAM in stage (10) shows precise correspondence with the predicted enhancing tumor mask, but also illustrates why this subregion is the most challenging (Fig. 1.61). We can see how the activations are less spatially contiguous and more sensitive to small variations in intensity patterns.

Across all three outputs, these Grad-CAM sequences make the model's decision-making process transparent: the encoder gathers broad context, the attention gates selectively filter skip connection features, and the decoder integrates coarse semantic and fine spatial details to converge on class-specific boundaries. For clinical practitioners, these visual progressions provide reassurance that the model is leveraging the same regions they would inspect, while also making it possible to detect when the network's attention deviates from expected anatomical correlates. This class-specific, layer-by-layer interpretability is critical for validating model behavior and building trust in its outputs.

Dilated (Atrous) CNN

Dilated convolutions, also known as atrous convolutions, are another method to help CNNS capture multi-scale context. In this operation, the standard convolution is modified by inserting "holes" (usually zeros) between kernel elements. When the

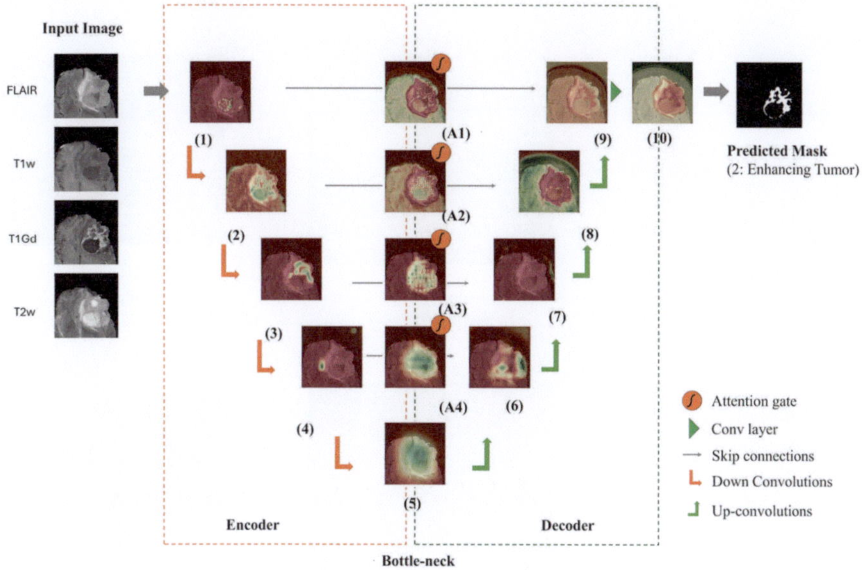

Fig. 1.61 Layer-wise Grad-CAM visualizations for an Attention U-Net applied to the BraTS example, targeting output label *"2: Enhancing Tumor."* (Code: conv_05_brats_segmentation_attentionunet.ipynb)

convolution operation is carried out with this "dilated" kernel, the receptive field is expanded without increasing parameter count or reducing spatial resolution. In contrast, traditional down-sampling operations using strided convolutions tend to reduce the feature map size, which may discard fine-grained details critical for delineating small lesions. The spacing inserted between the kernel elements is controlled using the Dilation rate hyperparameter. A rate or r injects r-1 zeroes between taps, yielding an effective kernel size of $k + (k\text{-}1)(r\text{-}1)$. High dilation rates can cause checkerboard patterns, which can be mitigated by including mixed rates, smoothed dilated convolutions or cascading small rates.

While atrous convolutions can be incorporated into traditional convolutional neural network (CNN) architectures, their uniqueness, or usefulness, lies in enabling flexible control over feature resolution and context aggregation. The DeepLab family (v1, v2, v3, and v3+) of semantic segmentation models leverages this property through a module known as **Atrous Spatial Pyramid Pooling (ASPP)**. ASPP applies multiple parallel atrous convolutions with distinct dilation rates to a shared input feature map (Fig. 1.62). By doing so, it captures contextual information at various spatial scales, enabling the model to recognize both fine details and broader structures in an image. This ability to aggregate multi-scale context is particularly advantageous in semantic segmentation tasks, where objects of interest may vary significantly in size and shape. The resulting features are then concatenated and passed to the classification head, leading to improved localization and boundary delineation in the final segmentation output (Fig. 1.63).

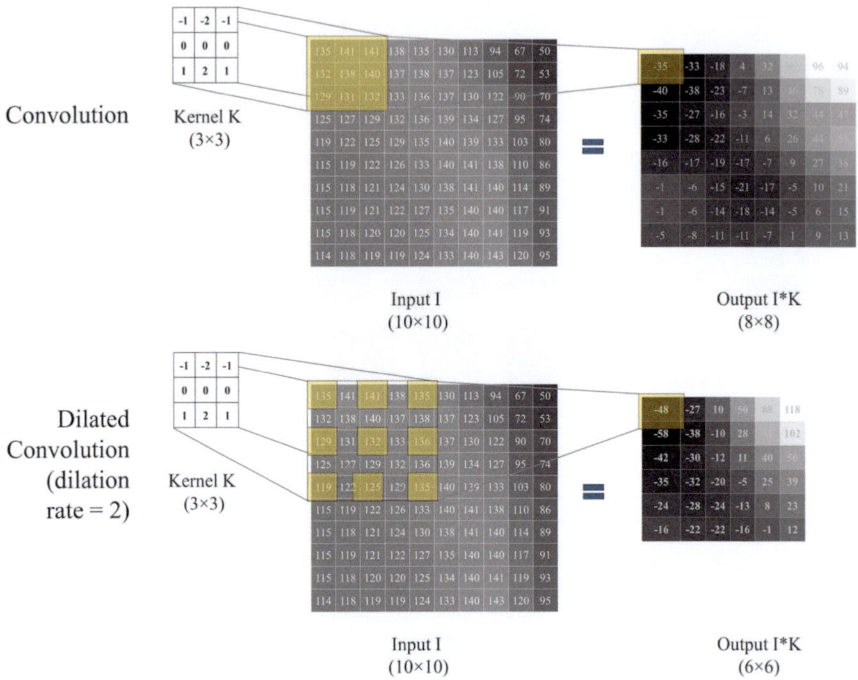

Fig. 1.62 Standard vs. dilated (atrous) convolution. A 3 × 3 kernel is applied to a toy image containing a vertical edge (values 10 → 0) using cross-correlation, stride = 1, padding = 0. In the standard convolution (top), the kernel straddling the edge yields an activation of 30 (sum over three rows). In the dilated case (bottom) with rate r = 2, the kernel samples input locations with gaps, increasing the effective receptive field to k_{eff} = 5 without adding parameters; the output map becomes smaller while producing the same edge response where applicable.

Multi-branch (Multi-stream) CNN

The core innovation in this CNN approach is to pass the inputs through several parallel pathways, often with different input configurations or layer settings, which allows the CNN to learn a more diverse and richer set of features (Fig. 1.64). The different branches can use different kernel sizes or layer types, which can capture a wider array of patterns. Additionally, branches can also process the input at different resolutions, which helps the CNN learn both fine details and high-level contextual information. In tasks involving multi-modal data processing, each branch or stream can also be tailored to a specific modality, where each stream's features are fused later.

Multibranch CNNs can be categorized based on how their information is combined or fused. Early fusion architectures combine information from different streams earlier in the network, for example, near the input. On the other hand, late fusion algorithms process data independently through most of each stream and only combine the outputs near the end. Intermediate fusion architectures can fuse information at one or more points within the network. For example, in the Inception CNN, each "inception"

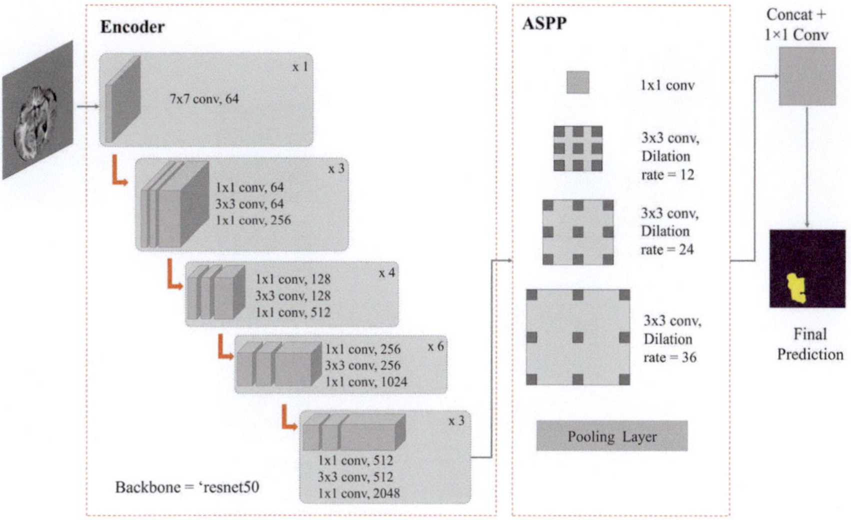

Fig. 1.63 DeepLabv3 architecture for semantic segmentation. A ResNet-50 backbone with atrous (dilated) convolutions forms the encoder (left), maintaining spatial resolution by controlling the output stride. The final encoder feature map feeds the Atrous Spatial Pyramid Pooling (ASPP) module (center), comprising a 1×1 branch, three parallel 3×3 atrous branches with dilation rates 12, 24, and 36 (as depicted for OS = 8), and an image-level (global average) pooling branch. ASPP dilation rates depend on output stride (OS) of the encoder: OS = 16 → {6, 12, 18}; OS = 8 → {12, 24, 36}. Outputs from all branches are concatenated and passed through a 1×1 projection (right) to produce class logits, which are then upsampled to the input resolution for the final prediction. (Example image from Medical Segmentation Decathlon, licensed under CC-BY-SA)

block within the CNN achieves multi-scale processing, and the feature fusion happens at the end of each inception module. Multi-stream architectures such as DeepMedic often use completely parallel pathways with different convolution kernel sizes and layers, and feature fusion happens only close to the end of the CNN.

In neuroradiology, multi-branch CNNs are well-suited for use-cases that require fusion of multi-modal data, such as imaging and clinical data, or even different imaging sequences, such as T1w, T2w, FLAIR, DWI. Each modality highlights different tissue characteristics, and multi-branch architectures allow each branch to process a specific modality independently. The features, which typically provide complementary information, from each data type can be fused at a later stage and used by the model to make a more accurate decision. Interestingly, this mimics how radiologists often mentally synthesize findings from different data sources or sequences. Additionally, brain lesions and anatomical structures can vary significantly in size, shape, and subtlety. Multi-branch CNNs can be designed with different receptive field sizes or down-sampling techniques in each branch. This allows the CNN to learn not only the fine-grained details, such as the texture of a small lesion, but also the broader contextual information, such as the location of the lesion relative to larger brain structures.

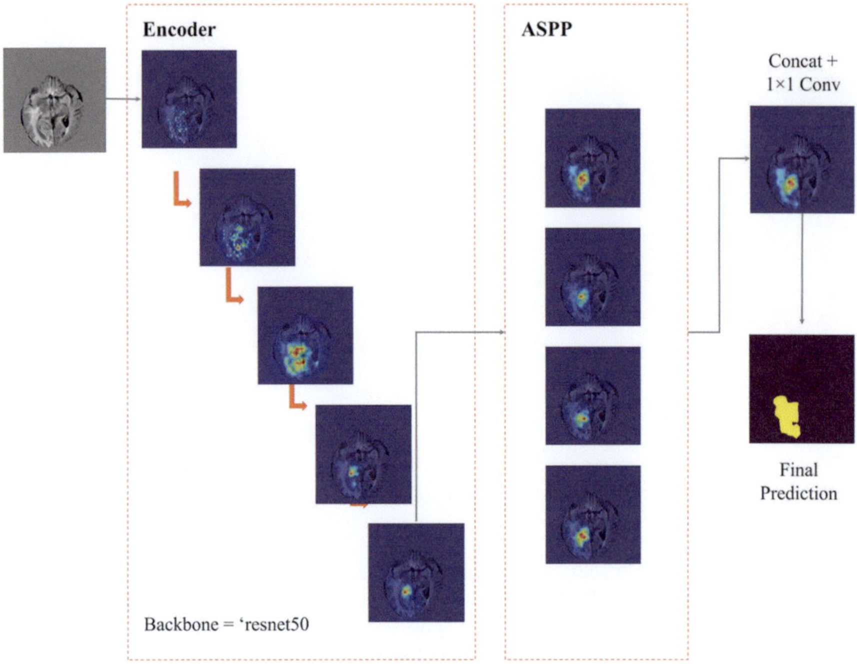

Fig. 1.64 DeepLabv3 with Grad-CAM overlays. Grad-CAM heatmaps are shown at representative encoder bottlenecks (left) and ASPP branches (right) for a ResNet-50 backbone. The encoder maps become progressively more class-specific and spatially coherent from early to late stages, while the ASPP branches show complementary multi-scale responses (1 × 1 and three 3 × 3 atrous paths plus image-level pooling). After concatenation and a 1 × 1 projection, the final classifier produces the per-pixel prediction shown at bottom right. Heatmaps indicate gradient-weighted feature contributions to the target class logit (not probabilities) and are upsampled to input resolution. (Code: conv_06_brats_segmentation_deeplab.ipynb) (Example image from Medical Segmentation Decathlon, licensed under CC-BY-SA)

The DeepMedic architecture proposed by Kamnitsas et al. employs a dual-pathway (multi-scale) approach that simultaneously processes inputs at two different resolutions. In this architecture, the normal resolution pathway operates on images at their original resolution, allowing the network to learn fine-grained and local features from the input data. The downsampled pathway processes image segments extracted from a downsampled (by a factor of 3 along each dimension) version of the input image, allowing the CNN to capture broader contextual information. The feature maps generated by these two parallel pathways are then concatenated at a later stage in the network, typically before the final classification layers.

Efficient Networks

While CNNs have demonstrated increasing accuracy and performance in various neuroradiology tasks, their high performance often comes with a high computation cost. Deeper CNN architectures often contain millions of trainable parameters, sometimes constraining development in resource-limited research settings. Additionally, computationally expensive networks typically take longer during inference, which may be an issue in critical care situations when the time to inference needs to be within an upper limit to be practically viable in clinical practice.

One of the salient features of efficient networks is that they are designed to address the challenge of high computational requirements without compromising performance or accuracy. This is achieved by using several strategies, such as factorized convolutions, squeeze-and-excitation (SE) modules, bottleneck layers, neural architecture search (NAS), compound scaling, etc.

The core concept behind Depthwise separable convolutions is that they split the standard convolution operation, which processes spatial and channel information simultaneously, into two steps: (1) a depthwise convolution and (2) a pointwise convolution. The depthwise convolution operation breaks down the overall feature map into individual feature maps that are separate for each channel. Then it applies a single filter per input channel, thereby capturing spatial features independently for each channel. The pointwise convolution operation uses a 1×1 convolution to combine the outputs of the depthwise convolution across channels. This factorization into two steps is critical since it reduces the number of parameters and computations compared to standard convolutions. It is important to recognize that while carrying out depthwise convolutions, the 3-dimensional contextual information is not lost since the inputs are separated only along the channel direction, which typically contains features that are independent of each other, and the spatial information is still preserved. Depth-wise separable convolutions are used extensively in MobileNets, which are designed for mobile and embedded vision applications.

Bottle-neck layers reduce computational complexity by using 1×1 convolutions to reduce the number of channels before the convolution operations are carried out. The output feature maps are then expanded back to the original number of channels. It is important to recognize that bottleneck layers are not specific to efficient networks. They are used within ResNets and other architectures where the architectures become so deep or large that computation constraints need to be addressed. Squeeze-and-excitation (SE) blocks are used to improve the representational power of a neural network by enabling it to perform dynamic channel-wise feature recalibration. In this approach, each channel is "squeezed" into a single numeric value, typically using pooling. This is followed by an "expand" layer, which is typically a mix of 1×1 and 3×3 convolutions that "excites" or scales the channels based on the squeezed value.

The neural architecture search (NAS) and compound scaling method provide a structured way to scale up models for better accuracy while maintaining high efficiency. Models such as Efficient Net (B0–B7) scale all three dimensions (depth, width, and resolution) using a fixed set of scaling coefficients. The core intuition behind compound scaling is that if the input image is bigger, then the network needs to be deeper to increase the receptive field with more channels to capture more fine-grained features on the bigger image.

In neuroradiology, efficient networks have been crucial in implementing CNN-based algorithms into clinical workflow, where rapid analysis of 3D images is important. For example EfficientNet-B0 to B4 have been used for Alzheimer's disease classification, where the pre-trained EfficientNet models (B0–B4) were used as feature extractors and fine-tuned for classifying Alzheimer's disease (AD), Mild Cognitive Impairment (MCI), and Cognitively Normal (CN) subjects from 2D slices of 3D brain MRI scans. EfficientNets have also been used for segmentation tasks such as for brain tumor segmentation. For example, Preetha et al. implemented a single multi-scale attention U-Net with EfficientNetB4 used as the encoder backbone for segmenting brain tumors from MRI images (BraTS dataset). This aimed to reduce parameters and improve efficiency compared to standard U-Net encoders.

Conclusion

A strong correlation exists between the choice of CNN architecture and the clinical task it is designed to solve. The field is maturing beyond a "one-size-fits-all" mentality, where researchers would apply the newest model to any given problem. Instead, there is a clear pattern of deliberate, informed architectural selection based on the specific demands of the neuroradiological challenge. For instance, segmentation tasks employ a U-Net variant, an architecture whose design is fundamentally optimized for precise spatial localization. Conversely, complex classification and prediction tasks leverage a variety of deep architectures like ResNet, DenseNet, and Multi-Branch CNNs, which are specifically designed to learn the deep, hierarchical feature representations necessary to distinguish subtle pathological patterns. In the case of automated radiology reporting, CNNs are combined with a sequential model, such as the LSTM model, to work with text data. This "architecture-task fit" is not coincidental; it reflects a sophisticated understanding of how the underlying mechanics of these models align with the clinical and imaging-based requirements of the problem at hand. In many respects, generalist architectures like the U-Net deliver robust baseline performance across a variety of neuroradiological tasks. However, when we deliberately adopt specialist designs that tailor the network's structure to the unique, inherently complex patterns and nuances of a given clinical problem, the model accuracy often improves substantially.

Capsule Networks

One of the challenges in traditional CNNs is that the feature map output by a neuron is typically a scalar activation. Scalar activations typically contain information about only the presence of a feature, such as an edge or curve, at a particular location. When passed through the subsequent pooling layers, scalar activations also tend to discard positional information. Additionally, traditional CNNs, with their stacked convolution and pooling layers, are not designed to capture the hierarchical nature of features explicitly.

Capsule networks (CapsNets) address these challenges of traditional CNNs by grouping neurons into "capsules" that output vector activations instead of scalar activations. The intuition behind using a vector activation is that the output vector's length can encode information on the probability that a particular feature, such as a tumor edge or texture, exists, and its direction can encode information on its instantiation parameters, such as orientation, size, and pose. This is implemented by passing the input through convolutional layers as in a traditional CNN. The output feature maps from the convolutional layers are then reshaped to get a set of vectors, which are then squashed to ensure their length is between zero and one. For example, suppose the convolutional layers output an array containing 18 feature maps; these feature maps can be reshaped into two vectors of nine dimensions each for every location, or three vectors of six dimensions each. Since the vector length is used to represent the probability of whether the feature exists, the last step is to ensure that each vector is not longer than one. This is done using a squashing function which preserves the vector's orientation, but squashes it to ensure the length is between zero and one.

Capsule networks use an iterative "routing-by-agreement" method where the lower-level "child" capsules predict outputs for higher-level "parent" capsules using a learned transformation (weight) matrix. These predictions are updated iteratively through a "routing-by-agreement" method. In each iteration, child capsules compute a "prediction vector" for each parent capsule. The predictions are then combined using a weighted sum approach to form the parent's output. The weights, also known as coupling coefficients, are finally updated based on the extent to which predictions align. After multiple iterations, the coupling coefficients grow stronger for child-parent pairs that agree most, effectively "routing" information to the appropriate higher-level capsule and suppressing irrelevant signals.

In neuroradiology, capsule networks have been shown to perform well for both classification and segmentation tasks. In practice, this has been implemented by modifying the latter half of the CapsNet architecture. For example, if the task is to carry out classification, as in the implementation of brain tumor classification, the final layers of the architecture typically include a Capsule layer where each capsule is dedicated to representing one of the classes to be predicted (e.g. one capsule for "glioma," one for "meningioma," one for "pituitary," and one for "no tumor"). These inputs are then processed through a softmax layer which takes the vector lengths and converts them into a probability distribution.

If the task is to carry out segmentation, CapsNets utilize a similar decoder path as used in U-nets, where the condensed feature representations from the capsule layers (encoder path) are progressively upsampled using deconvolutional capsule layers until the full spatial resolution image is reconstructed. For brain structure segmentation (specifically the third ventricle, thalamus, and hippocampus), a 3D Capsule Network achieved Dice scores (92–95%) comparable to UNet architectures. Additionally, the capsule network performed 30% better (Dice score) on images not well-represented in the training data and was significantly more efficient, requiring only 1/10th of the computational memory and being over 25% faster to train than UNets.

Capsule networks are well-suited for neuroradiology tasks since they perform well with limited annotated data. They are robust to anatomical variability and preserve complex spatial hierarchies, which are common challenges in neuroradiology.

Autoencoders

Autoencoders are a class of neural networks that learn by reconstructing their own input. The architecture of an autoencoder is designed in such a way that it forces the network to learn data representations that help reconstruct the image. The core intuition underlying the architecture design of autoencoders is establishing an information "bottleneck" that pushes the network to learn a compressed but meaningful representation of the input data. This bottleneck layer captures the most important features necessary to reconstruct the original input. They are typically used for unsupervised learning tasks, where they can directly learn from the data without requiring specialized annotations. For example, in neuroradiology, autoencoders are well-suited to perform the task of unsupervised anomaly detection, where they are first trained to reconstruct normal brain scans. During this training process, they learn feature representations that characterize a normal brain scan. So, if, during inference, an abnormal scan is provided, the autoencoder performs poorly and has high reconstruction errors. Scans with high reconstruction errors are flagged as potentially containing abnormalities like lesions, with the specific areas that have high reconstruction error highlighted as abnormal areas.

The core components of an autoencoder network are the *Encoder, the Latent space, and the Decoder*. The *encoder* compresses the high-dimensional input data into a lower-dimensional latent space. The encoder typically contains several layers of neurons, where each successive layer progressively reduces the dimensionality of the data. The *latent space* represents the layer where the input data is distilled into its most compressed form. It is also referred to as the "bottleneck" layers because its dimensionality is designed to be significantly smaller than that of the input or output layers. The bottleneck layer is one of the most important characteristics of AEs, and it forces the network to learn and retain only the most important features and representations (Fig. 1.65). The *decoder* takes the latent representations from the encoder and reconstructs the original input data.

During training, the difference between the reconstructed output and the original input is computed using a "loss function." For continuous input values such as pixel

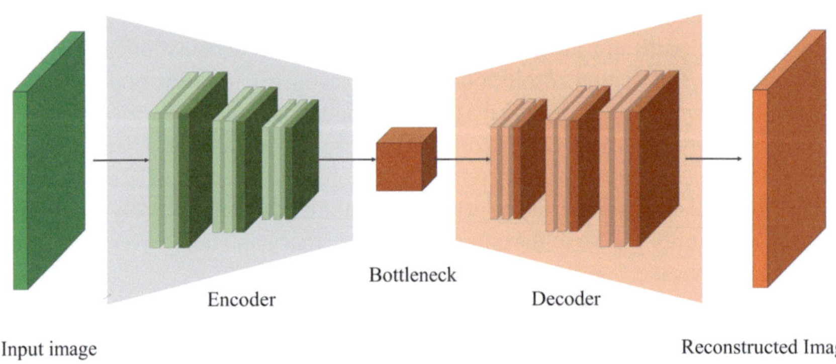

Fig. 1.65 Schematic representation of a Variational Autoencoder (VAE) architecture

intensities in medical images, Mean Squared Error (MSE) is a suitable loss function. In the case of binary input values, Cross-Entropy (CE) loss is more appropriate. The network's parameters (weights and biases of the encoder and decoder structures) are adjusted iteratively (using backpropagation) to identify the optimized set of values that have the lowest reconstruction error.

For example, let's take a **T2-weighted axial MRI slice of a healthy brain** as our input image. We want to train an autoencoder to detect anomalies (like tumors or lesions). Here's how the learning mechanism works specifically for this healthy brain MRI slice.

Step 1: Define Input and Target

Input (x): Our T2-weighted axial MRI slice of a healthy brain is fed into the autoencoder. This image is essentially a grid of numbers, where each number represents the intensity of a pixel (or voxel if it's 3D). For instance, cerebrospinal fluid (CSF) may appear bright (with high pixel values), while white matter may appear darker (with lower pixel values on a T2-weighted image). This entire set of pixel intensity values is x.

Target (x'): The autoencoder processes this input MRI slice x through its encoder (compressing it into a bottleneck) and then its decoder (attempting to reconstruct it). The output x' is a newly generated MRI slice that the autoencoder *thinks* is a faithful copy of the original healthy input x. The goal is for x' to be virtually identical to x.

Step 2: Assign Loss Function

For our MRI slice, MSE is a very suitable loss function. Let's say our input MRI slice x has a specific pixel in the frontal lobe with an intensity value of 150 (on a normalized scale, this might be 0.6). After the autoencoder processes it, the corresponding pixel in the reconstructed output x' might have an intensity of 145 (or 0.58). The squared difference for this pixel is (150–145)2 = 52 = 25. MSE calculates this squared difference for *every single pixel* in the original MRI slice x compared to its corresponding pixel in the reconstructed slice x'. It then averages all these squared differences. So,

$$L(x,x') = \frac{1}{N}\sum_{i=1}^{N}\left(x_i - x_i'\right)^2$$

where N is the total number of pixels, x_i is the intensity of the i-th pixel in the original healthy brain MRI, and x_i' is the intensity of the corresponding i-th pixel in the reconstructed MRI. A lower MSE means the reconstruction is very similar to the original healthy brain scan.

Step 3: Data Preparation

Before our T2-weighted axial MRI slice is fed into the network, its pixel intensity values (which might range from 0 to, say, 2048 depending on the scanner and image format) are **normalized**. This means they are scaled to a standard range, like 0 to 1 or −1 to 1. For example, a pixel value of 1024 in a 0–2048 range would become

0.5 in a 0–1 normalized range. This helps the training process be more stable and efficient.

The entire dataset of healthy brain MRIs would be split: a large portion for **training** (to learn the weights), a smaller **validation** set (to check during training if the model is generalizing well and not just memorizing the training data, helping to decide when to stop training), and a **test** set (completely unseen healthy scans used after training to evaluate final performance).

Step 4: Training Process

Backpropagation: After calculating the MSE for our healthy brain MRI slice, if the error is not zero (meaning the reconstruction isn't perfect), this error value is "blamed" back through the network. For instance, if the ventricles in the reconstructed slice *x'* are blurrier (pixel values are less accurate) than in the original *x*, backpropagation calculates how much each weight and bias in the decoder, and then the encoder, contributed to this specific blurriness. It determines the gradient, i.e., the direction and magnitude of change needed for each weight to reduce that blurriness.

Gradient descent: Using these calculated gradients, an algorithm like Adam (a common choice) updates all the weights and biases in the autoencoder. Suppose a particular weight adjustment is found (via backpropagation) to likely make the reconstructed ventricles sharper (i.e., reduce the MSE for those pixels). In that case, Gradient Descent nudges that weight in the indicated direction. It's like carefully tuning many knobs (the weights) to make the output image (reconstruction) match the input (original healthy MRI) as closely as possible.

Training epochs: This process isn't done with just one healthy brain MRI slice. The autoencoder is shown many different healthy brain MRI slices from the training dataset, perhaps thousands. For each slice, it performs the forward pass (input -> encode -> decode -> output *x'*), calculates the MSE between *x* and *x'*, uses backpropagation to find gradients, and then Gradient Descent to update its weights. An **epoch** is completed when the autoencoder has seen every healthy brain MRI slice in the training set once. Training usually involves many epochs. With each epoch, the autoencoder gets progressively better at reconstructing these *healthy* brain MRIs, meaning the MSE for healthy scans gets lower and lower.

After many epochs of training on various healthy brain MRI slices, the autoencoder becomes an expert at compressing and then accurately reconstructing the patterns, textures, and shapes found in *normal* brain anatomy. The bottleneck forces it to learn the most salient features of "healthiness."

Now, imagine we feed it a *new* T2-weighted MRI slice, but this one contains an abnormal T2 hyperintensity representing a tumor that was *not* in its training data. Because the autoencoder has been optimized to reconstruct *healthy* tissue patterns, it will try to reconstruct the tumor region based on the features of healthy tissue it has learned. Since the tumor's appearance (in terms of pixel intensities, texture, and shape) differs from that of healthy tissue, the autoencoder will most likely struggle to reconstruct it accurately. The resulting reconstructed tumor area in *x'* will likely be blurry, misshapen, or look more like an attempt to "fill in" the space with what it considers normal. Consequently, the MSE calculated between this new anomalous input x and its reconstruction x' will be significantly higher, especially in the tumor region, than the MSE for a typical healthy scan. This high error acts as a red flag, highlighting a potential anomaly.

Vanilla Autoencoder

The Vanilla Autoencoder is the simplest form, featuring an encoder that compresses the input into a lower-dimensional "bottleneck" layer and a decoder that reconstructs the input from this compressed representation. Its defining characteristic is this basic encode-decode structure for learning efficient data coding. It's suited for initial exploratory data analysis in neuroradiology, such as reducing the dimensionality of extracted features from brain MRI scans (e.g., volumetric or texture features) to visualize patient clusters or identify principal modes of variation in a dataset.

For example, autoencoders can help reduce the dimensionality of a large set of handcrafted radiomic features extracted from brain tumor MRIs to identify a smaller subset of the most informative features that differentiate tumor grades. It is well known that radiomic features often exceed the number of patients in a dataset. The autoencoder would be trained on the high-dimensional feature vectors. The encoder part learns to map these features to a lower-dimensional latent space, and the decoder tries to reconstruct the original feature set. The activations in the bottleneck layer then represent the compressed, salient features.

Sparse Autoencoder (SAE)

A Sparse Autoencoder introduces a "sparsity constraint" on the hidden layer activations, meaning only a small number of hidden units are activated at any given time. This is often achieved by adding a penalty term (e.g., L1 regularization or KL-divergence) to the loss function. This is valuable in neuroradiology for learning more interpretable features or for identifying subtle, localized biomarkers because the sparsity encourages the network to learn specific, disjoint features rather than dense, distributed representations.

For example, SAEs can help discover genetic subtypes of glioblastoma from MRI scans by learning sparse representations of the image features that correlate with specific genetic markers (as explored by researchers using SAEs on glioblastoma MRI data). The SAE processes MRI features, and the sparsity constraint forces only a few "neurons" in its hidden layer to fire for any given input. These activated neurons might correspond to specific visual patterns or textures in the MRI that are strongly associated with a particular genetic subtype, aiding in unsupervised discovery of these distinctions.

Denoising Autoencoder (DAE)

A Denoising Autoencoder is trained to reconstruct a clean, original input from a version of that input that has been intentionally corrupted with noise (e.g., Gaussian noise or random pixel dropout). Its defining characteristic is learning robust features by forcing it to undo this corruption. DAEs are well-suited for improving the quality of noisy neuroradiological images (like low-field MRI or low-dose CT scans) and can also be used for unsupervised anomaly detection, as they learn to reconstruct "normal" anatomy well but struggle with unexpected pathological regions.

For example, DAEs can help detect hyperintense lesions (e.g., tumors or stroke lesions) in brain MRI. The DAE is trained on a large dataset of healthy brain MRIs that have artificial noise added. It learns to output clean versions of these images. When a new MRI scan (potentially with an unseen lesion) is fed through the trained DAE (after artificial noise addition), regions corresponding to normal brain tissue will be reconstructed accurately, while anomalous regions (like a lesion) will likely have higher reconstruction errors, highlighting them as potential abnormalities.

Convolutional Autoencoder (ConvAE)
A Convolutional Autoencoder utilizes convolutional layers in both the encoder and decoder, making it highly effective for image data. Its defining characteristic is the use of convolutions to learn spatial hierarchies of features, preserving the spatial relationships in the input images. This makes ConvAEs ideal for tasks involving the direct processing of neuroimages like MRI or CT, such as image reconstruction, segmentation pre-training, or learning powerful image features for downstream tasks like disease classification.

For example, ConvAEs can help reconstruct high-quality brain MRI images from compressed representations or learning features for normative modeling. The convolutional encoder uses filters to learn hierarchical features from an input brain MRI (edges, textures, then more complex structures), progressively downsampling it to a compact latent representation. The convolutional decoder then uses upsampling (often transposed convolutions) and convolutional layers to reconstruct the original brain MRI from this latent code, aiming to minimize the difference between the input and output image.

Variational Autoencoder (VAE)
A Variational Autoencoder is a generative model where, instead of mapping an input to a fixed latent vector, the encoder of a VAE maps the input to a probability distribution (typically a Gaussian with a mean and variance) in the latent space. The decoder then draws from this probability distribution to generate the output. VAEs are excellent for generating realistic synthetic neuroimages (e.g., for data augmentation when real annotated data is scarce), modeling the natural variation in brain anatomy, and for unsupervised anomaly detection by identifying inputs that fall outside the learned distribution of normal data.

For example, VAEs can help generate synthetic brain MRI slices with specific characteristics (e.g., different tumor types or stages of atrophy) to augment training datasets for classification models. The VAE's encoder learns the parameters (mean and variance) of a latent distribution that best describes a given input brain MRI. To generate a new image, a point is sampled from this learned distribution and passed to the decoder, which then reconstructs a new, plausible brain MRI. For anomaly detection, images that result in a latent representation far from the typical learned distributions are flagged.

Generative Adversarial Networks

GANs are a class of generative algorithms that learn to create new synthetic data samples from a provided training dataset. The core concept in a GAN is the competitive process between its two core components: the generator and the discriminator. These two neural networks are trained simultaneously, where the generator attempts to create realistic synthetic data that mimics the training dataset, and the discriminator determines whether the generated image is real or fake. During each training iteration, the generator inputs a random input and uses that input to generate a new data sample that resembles the training data provided. The discriminator receives both the generated image and the real data from the training set and outputs whether the generated image is real or fake. As training iterations progress, the generators improve their output and generate more realistic data, and the discriminator improves its output and gets more accurate in detecting fake data (Fig. 1.66). This training process continues until the generator can produce data that is indistinguishable from real data, and the discriminator can no longer reliably differentiate between them.

There are multiple variants of the GAN architecture that are designed to work well for different types of data and problems.

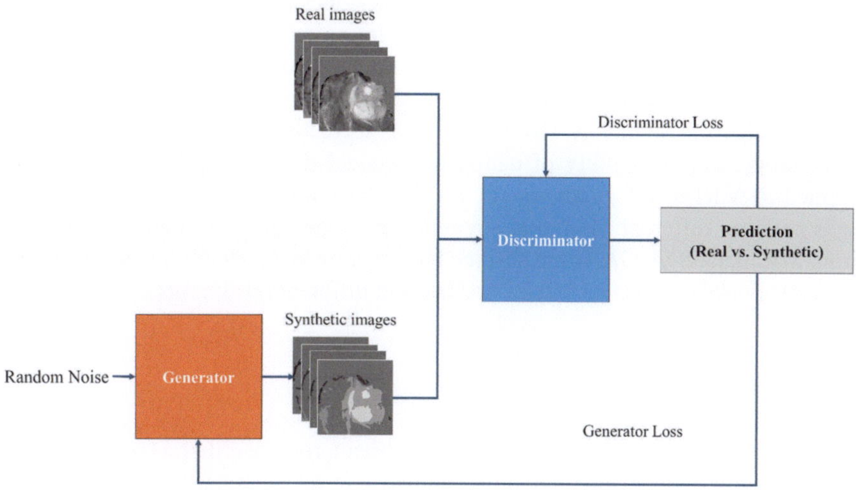

Fig. 1.66 Schematic overview of a Generative Adversarial Network (GAN) architecture. The **generator** G, implemented as a multilayer neural network, transforms a random noise vector into synthetic ("fake") samples. These generated samples, together with **real** samples drawn from the training dataset, are presented to the **discriminator** D, another multilayer neural network trained to distinguish real from fake. During each training iteration, D is updated by backpropagating its classification loss to improve its ability to correctly label inputs, while G is simultaneously updated via backpropagation of the generator's loss, derived from D's feedback, to produce increasingly realistic outputs. The adversarial, minimax objective drives both networks toward an equilibrium in which generated samples become indistinguishable from real data. (Example image from BraTS-TCGA-GBM, licensed under CC-BY-3.0)

The vanilla GAN architecture proposed by Goodfellow et al. uses fully connected neural networks for both the generator and discriminator. While it served as a conceptual application, it needed to be modified to work with different data types.

Deep-convolutional GANs (DCGANs) are a type of GAN that uses convolutional layers for both the generator and discriminator components. They are well-suited for image generation and translation tasks. Conditional GANs (cGAN) improved upon the baseline architectures by allowing for the generation of specific types of images based on conditional inputs. For example, cGANS have been used to generate images of a specific pathology, say a brain scan depicting a glioma, given the label "glioma."

Pix2Pix GAN, a type of cGAN, is used for image-to-image translation tasks where the GAN learns a mapping from an input image to another image type that is aligned to the input image. For example, Pix2Pix GANs have been widely used for synthetic contrast generation of MRI sequences, where the input image is a non-contrast or low-dose contrast image and the GAN is trained to generate a full-dose contrast image from those inputs. Pix2Pix is highly relevant for tasks where paired data can be obtained, such as MRI-to-CT synthesis if co-registered scans are available, medical image enhancement, generating realistic images from segmentation masks, or translating between different contrast-enhanced sequences.

CycleGANs enable unpaired image-to-image translation (e.g., MRI to CT when direct pairs are unavailable), using a cycle-consistency loss. One of the core innovations in CycleGAN is the cycle consistency loss, which ensures that if an image from domain A, say MRI, is translated to another domain B, say CT, and then reverse translated back to domain A, the resulting image should be close to the original one from domain A. CycleGAN helps solve an important challenge in neuroradiology, i.e. availability of paired multimodal data. It has been successfully applied to MRI-to-CT synthesis, T1-to-T2 MRI translation, translating neuroimages between different MRI field strengths, and generating synthetic PET images from MRI data. StyleGANs are designed to generate high-fidelity images with fine-grained control over visual "style" attributes at different resolutions.

Transformer Networks

Transformers are a class of neural network architectures that utilize a "self-attention" mechanism to dynamically weight the influence of all input data points while generating a contextual representation for any single data point. This is an essential aspect since, unlike CNNs and RNNs, transformer networks process the entire data input in parallel instead of sequential processing (RNNs) or using localized receptive fields (CNNs). To offer an analogy, imagine a radiologist reviewing a complex patient report. One way to review the report would be to read each word from start to finish and try to retain all the details in memory. This is akin to how an RNN or, more specifically, LSTM would work, which is quite challenging, especially with long sequences within reports. More realistically, a radiologist would review all the words in a significant section, or even the entire patient report, and subsequently determine how different findings interrelate to form the complete clinical picture. In the case of a neuroradiologist examining an MRI scan, their attention is not uniformly distributed across the image. For example, when interpreting a scan for a suspected glioma, the radiologist's focus is typically drawn to areas of abnormal signal intensity, and they mentally connect these areas with surrounding structures, such as the ventricles or cortical sulci, to assess the mass effect or infiltration. This is akin to how a transformer operates, where the complex, long-range dependencies and global context are captured well.

The foundational step in applying transformer networks to spatial grid-like data in medical imaging is the process of "tokenization." For example, vision transformers begin by partitioning the input images, say an MRI image, into a grid of fixed-size non-overlapping patches. Let's say that an input image with a resolution of 128 × 128 pixels is provided to the tokenizer. This image is typically divided into 64 patches of 16 × 16 pixels. Each of these patches is then flattened into a 1-dimensional vector, which is subsequently passed through a trainable linear projection layer. This linear projection layer learns to map the flattened 1-dimensional vector into a high-dimensional vector space known as the "patch embedding" vectors. Each vector in this sequence now represents a specific spatial region of the original image. This process, where the original image, a grid of pixels, is transformed into a sequence of embedding vectors, opens up the applications toward the development of universal, modality-agnostic architectures.

Before the patch embeddings are fed into the first layer of the transformer, they are incorporated with positional embeddings, which contain information about the position of each patch within the original image grid. This step re-injects the spatial information, such as the structural and anatomical relationships within the neuroimaging data, that was lost during the flattening process.

Query, Key, and Value vectors For each vector in the input patch embedding, the self-attention mechanism calculates an output vector that incorporates context from the entire sequence. First input embedding is multiplied by three separate, trainable weight matrices, W_Q (for the query), W_K (for the key), and W_V (for the value) to result in the Query vector (q), Key vector (k), and the Value vector (v) for every patch in the image sequences. The Query vector can be intuitively thought of as the current patch's "question" or "request for information. It represents what the patch is looking for in other parts of the image. The Key vector acts as a label or identifier for each patch, which signals "this is the information contained." The Value vector contains the actual information or feature representation of the patch that will be passed on if that is something that will be attended to. To determine how much attention a specific patch I should pay to another path j, the model calculates an attention score, which is computed by taking the dot product of the Query vector of the patch i (q_i) and the Key vector of the patch j (k_j). This dot product measures the relevance between the question from patch I and the label of patch j. This calculation is performed between the query patch and every other patch in the sequence, including itself. These scores are then scaled, and a softmax function is applied to the score, converting it into a probability distribution, which is visualized using an attention map. A patch with high weight is considered highly relevant to the query patch—Fig. 1.67. The final step involves the computation of an output (which is typically a weighted sum of Value vectors of all patches in the sequence). The output is a new, context-aware representation for the query patch.

There are some fundamental ways in which the self-attention mechanism processes input patches differently when compared to how a CNN would process them. A neuron in a CNN layer processes information from only a local region of the previous layer, known as the receptive field. The global context in CNNs comes from the stacking of many layers that gradually increase the receptive field through successive convolutional and pooling operations. In contrast, the self-attention mechanism has a global receptive field right from the first layer. In a transformer network, every patch can directly interact with and attend to every other patch, regardless of their spatial distance. This makes transformer networks very effective at modeling the long-range dependencies and distant correlations that are crucial for understanding the complex dynamics in neuroradiology. In CNNs, the filters learnt are static, meaning that once trained, they are applied uniformly across every input image. The "filter" created by self-attention is dynamic and content-dependent and is calculated for each specific input image based on the internal relationship between its component patches. For example, when the input image is an MRI containing a large diffuse tumor, the attention mechanism would typically learn to create an expansive attention maps that link

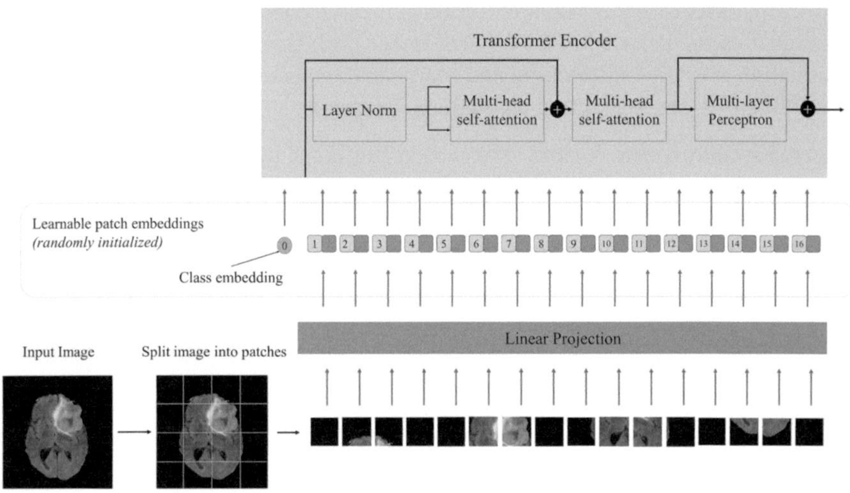

Fig. 1.67 Vision Transformer (ViT) pipeline. An input image is split into fixed-size patches, each flattened and linearly projected to a *D*-dimensional patch embedding. A learnable class token is prepended to the sequence. Learnable absolute positional embeddings are added to all tokens. The resulting sequence is processed by a Transformer encoder block (pre-layer normalization, multi-head self-attention, residual add; then MLP, residual add), repeated *L* times. The final class token is used by a classifier head (not shown). Concepts follow Dosovitskiy et al., *An Image is Worth 16 × 16 Words: Transformers for Image Recognition at Scale*, ICLR 2021. (Example image from BraTS-TCGA-GBM, licensed under CC-BY-3.0)

distant patches containing tumor infiltration. Still, for a small metastatic lesion, it would learn to focus attention on a smaller, more specific region. This adaptability to variations in pathology size, shape, and location is a key factor in the success of Transformer networks in complex neuroradiology tasks, such as segmenting tumors of varying morphologies (Fig. 1.68). These tasks are generally challenging for CNN-based models that are typically constrained by receptive fields.

Encoder-Only Models (e.g., BERT) These architectures are designed to build a deep, bidirectional understanding of an input sequence. They are ideal for discriminative tasks such as classifying clinical text or extracting named entities from a radiology report.

Decoder-Only Models (e.g., GPT) These models are optimized for autoregressive, or generative, tasks. They excel at generating new, coherent text, making them suitable for creating report summaries or impressions.

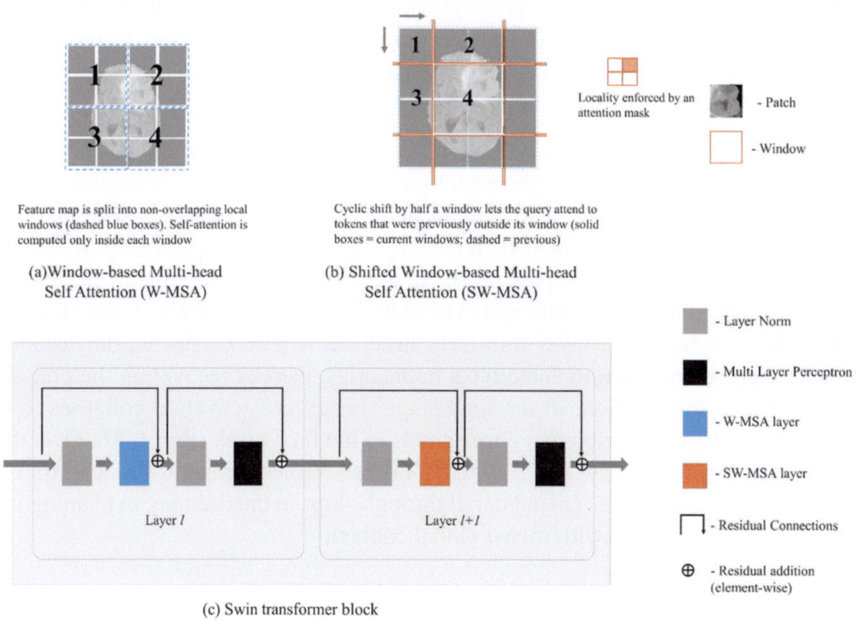

Fig. 1.68 Swin Transformer: Windowed and shifted-window self-attention. (**a**) W-MSA: the feature map is partitioned into fixed non-overlapping M × MM{\times}MM × M windows (dashed blue); self-attention is computed only within each window. (**b**) SW-MSA (cyclic shift): features are shifted by $(\lfloor M/2 \rfloor, \lfloor M/2 \rfloor)$ and attention is computed inside the shifted windows (solid orange); after unshifting, tokens can exchange information across former window boundaries while locality is preserved via an attention mask. (**c**) Two consecutive Transformer blocks within a stage alternate W-MSA and SW-MSA; each block uses pre-layer normalization, a residual add around the attention, then pre-norm, MLP, and another residual add. Concepts follow Liu et al., *Swin Transformer: Hierarchical Vision Transformer using Shifted Windows*, ICCV 2021 (https://arxiv.org/abs/2103.14030). (Example image from BraTS-TCGA-GBM, licensed under CC-BY-3.0)

Vision Transformers (ViT) This variant adapts the transformer for image analysis by dividing an image into a grid of patches and treating them as a sequence. This reframes the imaging task as a sequence-to-sequence problem, allowing the model to apply self-attention across the entire image.

Swin Transformers The Swin (shifted window) addresses the limitations of ViTs in terms of inefficiencies with high-resolution images by using patch merging layers that downscale the feature map by grouping adjacent patches and concatenating their features.

UNETR This architecture (named using a mix of UNET and Transformers) uses a transformer as the encoder network. This process works by dividing the input volume into sequences of patches and embeddings, similar to a ViT. The skip connections pass the feature maps at different layers of the transformer encoder, which captures information at various levels of abstraction, to produce the final detailed voxel-wise segmentation task. The Swin-UNETR replaces the ViT-based encoder with the more efficient and hierarchical Swin Transformer encoder. Hybrid architectures that combine a transformer-based encoder with a CNN-based decoder (e.g., UNETR, Swin UNETR) have become exceptionally powerful for classifying Alzheimer's disease and segmenting stroke lesions (Fig. 1.69).

These CAMs illustrate SwinUNETR's coarse-to-fine reasoning. The early encoder layers demonstrate high-resolution stages react to local contrast and textures (edges, illumination), not yet class-specific—useful for boundary seeding. The deeper encoder/bottleneck layers demonstrate a larger effective context from shifted windows, with responses expanding over the lesion and suppressing the background—capturing what to segment. The skip fusion in the decoder is the stage at which the skip features convey mid-level structure. After each fusion, the decoder CAMs sharpen and align to anatomical boundaries, thereby recovering the precise shape of the segmentation. In the final stage (head), the activation collapses to a compact, contiguous region that corresponds to the final mask (Fig. 1.70). Overall, the maps support the view that SwinUNETR establishes semantics in deep transformer stages and restores spatial detail through skips in the decoder, explaining its strong boundary fidelity with robust global context.

Diffusion Models

Diffusion models are a class of generative algorithms that, at their core, operate through 2 interconnected steps: a forward diffusion process and a reverse diffusion process. In the "forward process," the input, such as a high-resolution T1-weighted MR image of the brain, is processed through a sequence of steps where a small amount of random noise is added to each step in an incremental manner. The "reverse process" starts with the noise as input and generates a new clean image statistically similar to the original training data distribution. During training, the

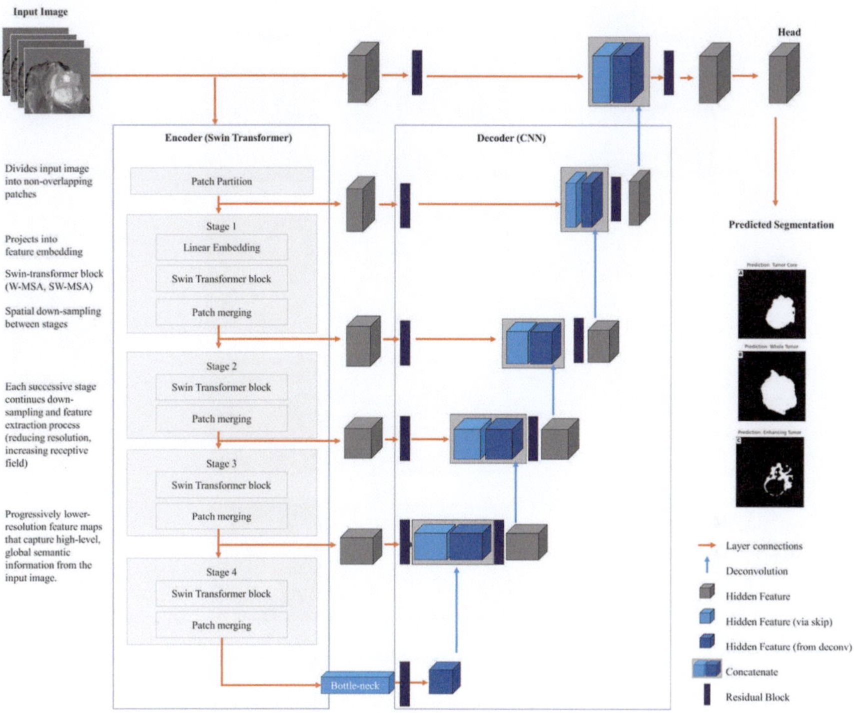

Fig. 1.69 Schematic of the Swin-UNETR architecture. The encoder partitions the input (3D) image into non-overlapping patches and applies a linear embedding, followed by four stages of Swin Transformer blocks using windowed and shifted-window self-attention (W-MSA/SW-MSA). Patch-merging halves the spatial resolution between stages while increasing channel capacity (C, 2C, 4C, 8C). A U-Net-like CNN decoder progressively upsampled features via transposed convolutions and residual blocks, concatenating encoder features at matching resolutions through skip connections. A final $1 \times 1 \times 1$ convolutional head produces the segmentation logits, which are mapped to the predicted label mask. (Hatamizadeh, Ali, et al. "Swin unetr: Swin transformers for semantic segmentation of brain tumors in MRI images." *International MICCAI brainlesion workshop*. Cham: Springer International Publishing, 2021). (Example image from BraTS-TCGA-GBM, licensed under CC-BY-3.0)

neural network learns the transformations necessary to incrementally remove the noise and reconstruct a coherent, new image.

For example, let's take an application in neuroradiology: denoising a brain MRI scan. The objective is to train a diffusion model that can take a noisy brain MRI (e.g., a T2 FLAIR image acquired with a fast protocol) and produce a high-quality version as if it were acquired with a much longer protocol. For this task, the first step is to collect the training data. Had this been framed as a supervised learning task, the data collection process would have involved collecting thousands of pairs of noisy and clean images. However, the advantage of using generative AI architectures such as diffusion models is that to become an expert at removing noise from a real MRI, the model doesn't need to see real noisy MRIs during training. Instead, it

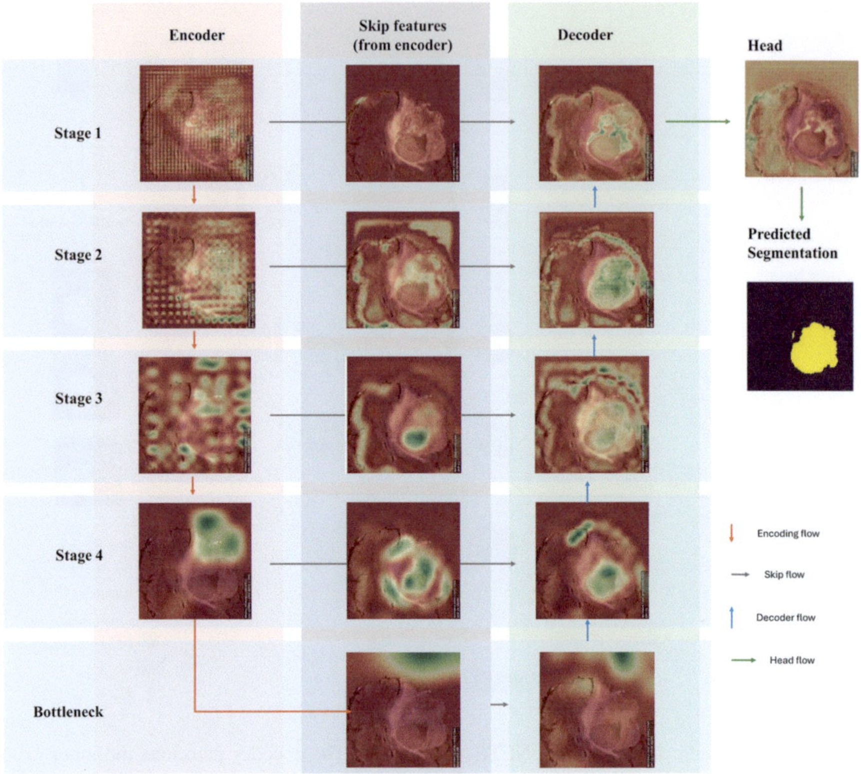

Fig. 1.70 Grad-CAM visualizations across SwinUNETR for class *Tumor Core*. From left to right: encoder stages (1–4), skip features passed to the decoder, decoder stages (1–4), and the final segmentation head. Each row shows the same slice; columns track the forward path and skip fusion. Grid-like patterns at shallow depths reflect windowed self-attention and patching that are typical of Swin blocks. (Code: https://github.com/rbramkumar/Artificial-Intelligence-in-Neuroradiology-A-Practical-Guide/blob/main/Chapter%201/Section%203%20-%20The%20promise%20of%20deep%20learning/transformers_01_brats_swinunetr.ipynb) (Example image from BraTS-TCGA-GBM, licensed under CC-BY-3.0)

can become an expert at practicing on an almost infinite number of artificially noised images. In the case of CNNs, this is usually done using extensive data augmentations, but generative AI algorithms take it one step further. By learning to remove the noise we add artificially, the model develops a fundamental understanding of the difference between the "true" anatomical signal and "random" noise.

Denoising diffusion probabilistic models (DDPMs) are a type of diffusion models that model the forward process and reverse process as a Markov Chain. A Markov Chain represents a sequence of events where the probability of each event depends only on the state of the previous event. In a forward diffusion process, adding noise is a Markov chain where each new slightly noisier image is created based only on the image from the step right before it. Similarly, in the reverse diffusion process, the model learns to create a reverse Markov chain, where each cleaner image is predicted only from the previous noisier image.

Latent diffusion models (LDMs) were developed to address the scalability issue with DDPMs, where the computational burden can increase significantly with higher pixel dimensions of the 3D medical image volumes. LDMs perform the computationally intense diffusion and reversion diffusion processes in a "latent space" where the high-dimensional input images are first compressed into a compact representation with much lower dimensions. For this purpose, the encoder network from an autoencoder is used to compress the input image into a compact latent representation. The diffusion model then operates entirely within this latent space, where the computational burden is significantly reduced. Once the reverse diffusion process generates a denoised latent representation, the decoder part of the autoencoder maps this latent representation back to the full-resolution pixel space to produce the final image.

Vision Language Models

Vision-language models are a class of neural networks designed to process and correlate information from both visual and textual inputs simultaneously. Unlike traditional neural networks, such as computer vision algorithms (typically CNN-based or transformer-based), and large-language models (typically transformer-based), vision-language models create a "shared embedding space" where visual and textual data can be jointly represented.

VLM is typically composed of three components that work together to form an AI system capable of taking an image and a text prompt as input and generating a relevant textual output.

1. Vision Encoder: The vision encoder's responsibility is to process the input image and generate features or patches that can be transformed into a set of numerical representations, known as embeddings. These embeddings capture important visual features from the input image, such as shapes, textures, and spatial relationships. This is typically constructed using a computer vision algorithm, such as a CNN or a Vision Transformer (ViT). This model is pre-trained on millions of image-text pairs, which enables it to correlate images and text.
2. Language Model: At the other end of the VLM, the language model's responsibility is to generate the contextually relevant text. This component is typically a pre-trained LLM (e.g., GPT or LLaMa families) that is based on the transformer architecture. These are pre-trained algorithms that excel at understanding text, grammar, context, and high-level abstractions and semantic relationships.
3. Fusion mechanism: This part of the network connects the vision encoder and language model, and its design is a key area of active research. In simpler architectures, this could be constructed using a simple linear projection layer ("the projector") that maps the visual embeddings from the vision encoder to the same dimensional space used by the LLM. In more complex architectures, this part can be constructed using complex adapter modules or cross-attention mechanisms that enable the visual and textual embeddings to interact more deeply. For example, a "Querying transformer" can learn to extract the most relevant visual features from the image based on the context provided by the text prompt.

The powerful capabilities of VLMs come from a sophisticated learning process centered around the concept of a *"shared representation space."* In this high-dimensional space, all concepts, whether they originate from pixels in images or words in a sentence, are represented using numerical vectors. Intuitively, this space can be understood as a vast, intelligently organized library of concepts. In a traditional library, an MRI image of a brain hemorrhage would be in the "Medical Imaging" section, while a neurology report describing the hemorrhage would be in the "Medical Texts" section. In the VLM's shared embedding space, the vector representing the image of the hemorrhage and the vector representing the text "acute non-traumatic intraparenchymal hemorrhage in the left temporal lobe" would be mapped very close to each other in the same conceptual "neighborhood." This co-location of related visual and text information is the key to the model's power. This conceptual library is built through a training process, typically called ***"Contrastive Language-Image Pre-training (CLIP)***, on large datasets, often comprising billions of image-text pairs available from public sources.

However, since these pre-trained encoders and language models are typically trained using image-text pairs from the internet, which contain natural images and everyday language, they need to be adapted to specialized images and text within the neuroradiology space. This is because medical imaging possesses a different statistical distribution from natural images. For example, medical images are characterized by subtle grayscale textures and specific anatomical features that are fundamentally different from natural images (e.g., photos of landscapes, cats, and cars). Similarly, medical reports use a dense, precise vocabulary with complex, non-intuitive semantic relationships that are quite different from natural text. Without specialized training using radiology images and reports, there exists a critical mismatch between the concepts learned during the pre-training and the specialized knowledge needed for neuroradiological inference.

To address these domain gaps, several foundational steps have been developed, such as the creation of in-domain medical datasets. For example, datasets such as ***MIMIC-CXR***, which contain a publicly available set of 227,835 imaging studies from 65,379 patients, where the medical images are paired with their corresponding radiology reports. Another dataset called ***Radiology Objects in Context (ROCO)*** contains over 81K radiology images from several imaging modalities such as CT, Ultrasound, X-Ray, Fluoroscopy, PET, Mammography, MRI, and Angiography, with their corresponding captions, keywords, Unified Medical Language Systems Concept Unique Identifiers, and Semantic Type. More recently, datasets such as ***PMC-15M*** have been proposed that include 15 million biomedical image-text pairs collected from 4.4 million scientific articles from PubMed Central. Models such as the ***BiomedCLIP*** model, which was fine-tuned using the PMC-15M dataset, demonstrate improved performance on biomedical tasks over their generalist predecessors. Another dataset is the ***BrainMD*** dataset, which contains 3d MRI scans with corresponding radiology reports and EHR data.

After the model is pre-trained using medical domain datasets, it is further refined using a dataset of specific instructions, typically formatted as medical questions and answers. This step, referred to as instruction tuning, teaches the model to follow clinical commands and perform specific tasks such as Visual question answering, report generation, etc. Additionally, the architecture of VLMs is modified to suit the domain better. For example, the generalized vision encoders are sometimes replaced with other architectural model designs:

(a) *Cross-modal align embedding*: This shows a dual-encoder architecture. The image and the medical report are passed through separate encoders (an Image Encoder and a Text Encoder). The model is trained to align the output embeddings (In and Tn) in a shared space.
(b) *Cross-attention module*: This architecture uses a cross-attention mechanism to allow the image and text representations to influence each other. After initial encoding, the model has specific layers where information from the image modality can focus on relevant parts of the text modality, and vice versa. This enables a more granular fusion of information than simply aligning the final embedding.
(c) *Joint input:* This depicts a fusion-encoder architecture. Here, the image and text data are combined (concatenated) at an early stage and fed as a joint input into a single Transformer Encoder. This forces the model to learn combined image-text features from the very beginning.
(d) *Condition prompt layer*: In this method, the text report is first encoded into an embedding that acts as a "condition" or "prompt." This prompt is then fed into the layers of a generative network that directs the image generation or reconstruction process.

Performance Evaluation

Introduction to ML Tasks

> A computer program is said to learn from experience E to some task T and some performance measure P, if its performance on T, as measured by P, improves with experience E (Thomas Mitchell 1997).

A crucial step in any machine learning project is the precise definition of the task. This is important since it sets the expectation of what the ML algorithm is supposed to do. Conversely, this also means that the ML algorithm is not expected to perform any other tasks beyond this task definition. In medical imaging, ML has been shown to perform multiple tasks with remarkable accuracy. Segmentation is the task of delineating anatomical structures or lesions on scans. Classification tasks involve assigning diagnostic labels. Regression tasks involve predicting continuous variables, such as tumor volume reduction and treatment response. In image reconstruction tasks, the primary goal is typically to enhance image quality or reduce acquisition time. In image registration, the task can be defined as aligning images from different modalities or at different points in time. While this is not exhaustive, it serves to highlight that the ML task is typically closely aligned with the clinical application or problem it is intended to address.

> If I had an hour to solve a problem, I'd spend 55 minutes thinking about the problem and five minutes thinking about solutions. (Albert Einstein)

The definition of the ML task directly dictates the subsequent steps in a typical algorithm training pipeline. This typically includes data collection, data pre-processing, model selection, development, validation, and testing. For example, a segmentation task requires pixel-wise annotations, which are more labor-intensive to obtain than image-level labels needed for classification. The choice of evaluation metrics, such as Dice coefficient for segmentation or area under the receiver operating characteristic curve (AUC-ROC) for classification, must align with the clinical goals of the task. In multi-modal imaging, tasks may include the fusion of information from MRI, CT, and PET, requiring sophisticated data integration techniques.

Depending on the complexity of the clinical task at hand, a singular task definition may not be sufficient. The task may need to contain multiple subtasks that are part of larger workflows. For example, let's assume we are building an AI system to input MRI/CT images of the neck, and its task is to provide a response on whether the patient's lymph nodes are benign or metastatic. Depending on the clinical application of this AI system, we can either approach this as a Classification problem or a combination of Segmentation and Classification problems. For example, we can define the goal of the ML algorithm as providing a classification score directly from the input MRI/CT image. This is quite beneficial in clinical situations, such as workflow prioritization, in which the presence/absence of metastatic lymph nodes is the only concern. In this setting, the data collection would involve only labeling whether the acquired sequence contains Lymph node metastasis. These labels are relatively easy to acquire and not very time-consuming. However, this approach also needs a lot of data samples to train since this algorithm is expected to learn features that distinguish metastatic lymph nodes from benign lymph nodes entirely from the data. On the other hand, if the clinical application of this AI system is to supplement the current diagnostic toolkit using radiomics, the ML overall task needs to be broken down into three sub-tasks. In this case, the first sub-task would be to develop an ML algorithm that can carry out auto-segmentation of lymph nodes, the second sub-task would be to generate radiomic features of the segmented lymph node, and the third sub-task would be to predict using the radiomic features whether or not the lymph node is metastatic. In recent works involving deep learning, it is possible to combine the latter two steps into one by using both hand-crafted and deep learning-generated radiomic features.

As we explore the AI algorithms, it is important to think of the different algorithms and paradigms as a toolbox for the practitioner (Fig. 1.71). Each paradigm offers distinct capabilities and is well-suited to address specific problems. Supervised learning excels when high-quality labeled data is available and the task is well-defined, such as disease classification or lesion segmentation. Unsupervised learning is invaluable for exploratory analysis, pattern discovery, and feature extraction, especially in the early stages of research or when labels are unavailable. Semi-supervised learning algorithms provide a pragmatic solution when labeled data is scarce but unlabeled data is abundant, as is often the case in large hospital data

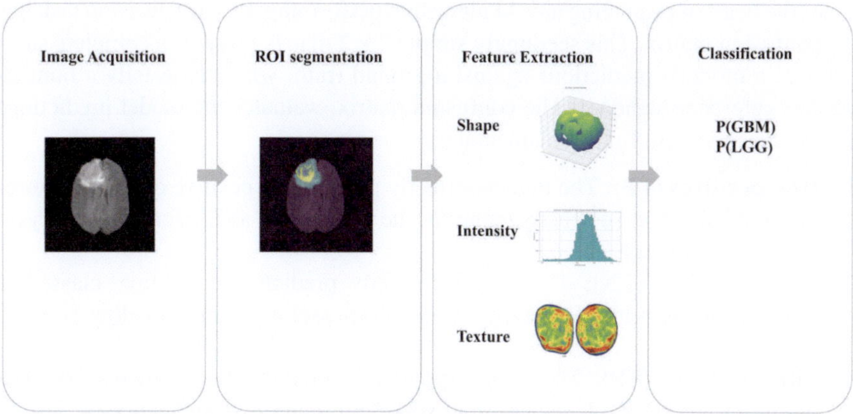

Fig. 1.71 Illustration of a multi-step machine learning pipeline in medical imaging. The process begins with image acquisition, followed by region-of-interest (ROI) segmentation, which uses segmentation algorithms to delineate anatomical structures or lesions. The segmented regions are then subjected to radiomic feature extraction, capturing quantitative descriptors such as shape, intensity, and texture. These features serve as inputs to a downstream classification model, enabling tasks such as diagnosis or prediction of treatment outcomes. Each sub-task, from segmentation to feature extraction and classification, represents a critical component supporting robust and clinically meaningful AI applications. (Example image from BraTS-TCGA-GBM, licensed under CC-BY-3.0)

management systems. Reinforcement learning is uniquely positioned to address problems involving sequential decisions, adaptive protocols, or real-time control.

The clarity with which the task is defined determines the success of the entire machine learning pipeline. Ambiguities in task definition can lead to inconsistent data collection, suboptimal model selection, and misleading performance evaluations. Additionally, to address the problem of limited data samples, which is often the case with medical imaging datasets, power analysis, which estimates the amount of data (i.e., the number of samples) required to achieve reliable results, is an essential component of task definition.

Task-Specific Evaluation Metrics

Evaluation metrics are used to provide a rigorous performance assessment of the AI algorithms. These metrics highlight the utility of AI algorithms not only from a performance perspective but also to highlight some of the challenges that must be addressed before a model can transition from code to clinic. Additionally, these evaluation metrics must highlight not only the scenarios where the algorithms work well, but also the scenarios where they don't, so that the clinical practitioners can make an informed decision. This section covers some of the foundational principles and metrics that are used in current research works.

At the heart of evaluating any AI algorithm performing a binary decision task lies the confusion matrix. This seemingly simple 2 × 2 matrix presents a complete summary of a model's predictions against a ground truth, which is usually a human-verified reference standard. The confusion matrix evaluates the model predictions and places them into four fundamental categories:

1. **True positives (TP):** The model correctly predicts the positive class. For example, an AI algorithm correctly identifies the presence of an intracranial aneurysm on a CT angiogram
2. **True negatives (TN):** The model correctly predicts the negative class. For example, the algorithm currently identifies a vessel segment as healthy and free of aneurysms.
3. **False positives (FP):** The model incorrectly predicts the positive class. The algorithm incorrectly flags a normal vessel bifurcation as an aneurysm. This is also known as the Type 1 error. Type 1 errors may lead to false alarms.
4. **False negatives (FN):** The model incorrectly predicts the negative class. In this case, the AI fails to detect a present aneurysm, potentially missing a critical diagnosis.

The confusion matrix provides the basis from which nearly all threshold-based classification and overlap-based segmentation metrics are derived. Also, the clinical implications for these errors (False Positives and False Negatives) in neuroradiology are quite asymmetric. For example, false negatives (missing aneurysms) can potentially lead to catastrophic subarachnoid hemorrhages. On the other hand, false positives can trigger unnecessary anxiety and lead to invasive testing. This is important since AI algorithms, similar to diagnostic testing, are rarely 100% accurate. The more we try to reduce the type-1 error, the higher the type-2 errors get. Understanding this trade-off is essential and the choice of evaluation metrics must be closely aligned with the clinical use-case and tolerance for each type of error.

The ultimate test of any AI algorithm's clinical value is its ability to generalize. This means that the algorithm maintains its performance across diverse populations, imaging hardware and clinical settings. The evaluation metrics, as evaluated on a test set (hold-out independent dataset) that is used only once after all the training and hyperparameter tuning steps are complete, can provide an unbiased estimate of the model's performance on unseen data.

Classification Tasks

Classification tasks involve the assignment of a predefined label to an input which can be an list of numerical features (such as numerical values of radiomic features for each patient), image (such as an MRI image or sequence), region of interest (patches or bounding boxes within an image), text-based report (radiology reports) or multi-modal data (combination of the above). The metrics that are used to evaluate these tasks can be broadly divided into 2 categories: those that assess model performance at a single, fixed decision threshold, and those that evaluate the model's overall discriminative ability across all possible thresholds.

Threshold-Dependent Metrics
These metrics are calculated from the confusion matrix at a specific operating point, which is determined by a chosen probability threshold.

Accuracy Accuracy is one of the most intuitive metrics, representing the proportion of all predictions that were correct.

$$Accuracy = \frac{TP + TN}{TP + TN + FP + FN}$$

Accuracy as an evaluation metric can provide a sense of the overall correctness of the model in a simple and widely understood manner. However, it is a notoriously misleading metric in the presence of class imbalance, which is a common scenario in neuroradiology where pathological findings are rare. For example, in a dataset where only 1% of brain MRIs show a specific rare tumor, a model that classifies every scan as "normal" would achieve 99% accuracy, despite being clinically useless, as it fails to identify any positive cases. Therefore, while simple to understand, accuracy is almost never reported in a stand-alone manner without further evaluation metrics as below.

Precision (Positive Predictive Value—PPV) Precision quantifies the reliability of positive predictions. One can think of precision as an answer to the question "if the AI algorithm identifies a positive finding, what is the probability that the finding is truly present?" The higher the precision, the lower the false positives. Higher precision is required in scenarios where a false positive can lead to significant harm or cost (such as an invasive brain biopsy for a suspected tumor). ML algorithms with low precision may potentially generated many false alarms, eroding trust in the clinical setting and unnecessary, potentially harmful follow-up procedures. Precision is calculated as the proportion of predictions in the positive class that were actually correct:

$$Precision = \frac{TP}{TP + FP}$$

Recall (Sensitivity or True Positive Rate—TPR) Recall, also known as sensitivity, measures the model's ability to identify all actual positive cases. One can think of precision as an answer to the question "of all the patients who actually have a specific condition, what fraction did the AI model correctly detect?" The higher the recall, lower the False negatives. High recall is required in scenarios where a false negative could potentially lead to significant negative consequences (a missed aneurysm could lead to hemorrhage). It is represented as the proportion of true positive instances that were correctly classified by the model.

$$Recall = \frac{TP}{TP + FN}$$

Specificity (True Negative Rate—TNR) Specificity measures the model's ability to correctly identify all actual negative cases. Specificity quantifies how well a model can rule out a disease. The higher the specificity, the lower the false positives. Specificity is required in large-scale screening programs, where a highly specific test would correctly identify most healthy individuals, preventing widespread patient anxiety and costs of unnecessary follow-up imaging for those without the disease. It is represented as:

$$Specificity = \frac{TN}{TN + FP}$$

F1-score F1-score provides a single, balanced measure of a model's performance by combining precision and recall into a single measure of effectiveness. Unlike accuracy, it does not include true negatives in its calculation, focusing only on the correct prediction of the positive class, making it more robust for class imbalance.

It is calculated as the harmonic mean of precision and recall:

$$F1 - score = \frac{2}{\frac{1}{Precision} + \frac{1}{Recall}} = 2 \times \frac{Precision \times Recall}{Precision + Recall}$$

Mathews Correlation Coefficient (MCC) Matthews Correlation Coefficient is a more complex but highly robust metric that computes the correlation between the actual and predicted binary classifications, and is calculated as

$$MCC = \frac{TN \times TP - FN \times FP}{\sqrt{(TP + FP)(TP + FN)(TN + FP)(TN + FN)}}$$

Unlike F1-score, which ignores true negative values, the MCC takes into account all four values (TP, FP, TN, FN). Higher values of MCC indicate better performance on both the positive and negative classes. The MCC is 0 when the model performance is no better than random guessing, and the MCC is −1 when the actual and predicted values show total disagreement.

Threshold-Independent Metrics

While threshold-dependent metrics are crucial for evaluating a model at a specific clinical operating point, threshold-independent metrics provide a more holistic view of a model's discriminative capability across its entire range of decision thresholds.

AUROC (ROC-AUC) The Receiver Operating Characteristic (ROC) curve is a graphical plot of the True Positive Rate (Recall/Sensitivity) on the y-axis against the False Positive Rate (1-Specificity) on the x-axis for every possible classification threshold (Table 1.5). The Area under the ROC Curve (AUROC) is a single scalar value derived from the ROC curve that represents the probability that the model will rank a randomly chosen positive instance higher than a randomly chosen negative one Fig. 1.72. The higher the value of AUROC (close to 1.0), the better the model's ability to distinguish pathology from normal. For example in Fig. 1.72 below, the binary classifier demonstrates strong discriminative capability, achieving an Area Under the Curve (AUC) of 0.860. This value signifies an 86% probability that the model will correctly rank a random positive sample higher than a random negative one. The curve illustrates the performance trade-off at various decision thresholds, where an optimal threshold could be selected at the point closest to the top-left corner (e.g., an FPR of approximately 0.2 and a TPR of 0.8), as this point represents a favorable balance between high sensitivity and a low false positive rate.

AUPRC (PR-AUC)
Precision-Recall (PR) curve plots precision (PPV) on the y-axis against recall (TPR) on the x-axis for every possible classification threshold. The Area Under the PR Curve (AUPRC) summarizes this relationship into a single value. The PR curve is a more specialized and often more informative metric than the ROC curve, particularly for tasks with significant class imbalance. The reason for this is that the calculation of the False Positive Rate in an ROC curve includes the number of true negatives (FPR = FP/(FP + TN)). In a highly imbalanced dataset where the number of true negatives is vast (e.g., millions of healthy voxels for every few lesion voxels), a large increase in the number of false positives may result in only a minuscule change in the FPR, making the ROC curve appear deceptively optimistic. The PR curve, by contrast, does not use true negatives in its calculation (Precision = TP/(TP + FP)). It therefore directly illustrates the trade-off between correctly identifying positive cases (recall) and the reliability of those positive predictions (precision), providing a much clearer picture of performance on the minority (positive) class.

The Precision-Recall (PR) curve in Fig. 1.73 illustrates the model's performance on the validation set, achieving a high Area Under the PR Curve (AUPRC) of 0.865. This score, being significantly above the baseline for an imbalanced dataset, indicates a strong ability to identify positive instances correctly while minimizing false positive predictions. The curve demonstrates the inherent trade-off between precision and recall, showing that the model can maintain high precision (e.g., >0.85) while correctly identifying up to 90% of all positive cases (recall of 0.9). An optimal classification threshold would be selected from this curve based on the specific application's priority: prioritizing high precision for tasks where false alarms are costly, or prioritizing high recall for tasks where missing a positive case is unacceptable.

The relationship between ROC and PR spaces was formalized by Davis and Goadrich (2006), who proved that for a fixed dataset, one curve dominates in ROC space if and only if it also dominates in PR space. PR plots are often more informative for imbalanced problems. For example, a screening tool for unruptured

Table 1.5 Consolidated summary of threshold-dependent classification metrics

Metric	Formula	Clinical Question Answered	Key Limitation
Accuracy	$\frac{TP+TN}{TP+TN+FP+FN}$	What fraction of all predictions were correct?	Highly misleading on imbalanced datasets.
Precision (PPV)	$\frac{TP}{TP+FP}$	If the model predicts positive, how likely is it to be correct?	Does not account for false negatives (missed cases).
Recall (Sensitivity)	$\frac{TP}{TP+FN}$	Of all actual positive cases, what fraction did the model find?	Does not account for false positives (false alarms).
Specificity	$\frac{TN}{TN+FP}$	Of all actual negative cases, what fraction did the model correctly rule out?	Does not provide information on the positive class.
F1-Score	$2\times\frac{Precision\times Recall}{Precision+Recall}$	What is the balanced performance between precision and recall?	Ignores true negatives, which can be important in some contexts.
MCC	$\frac{TN\times TP-FN\times FP}{\sqrt{(TP+FP)(TP+FN)(TN+FP)(TN+FN)}}$	How well do the predictions correlate with the ground truth overall?	Less intuitive to interpret than other metrics.

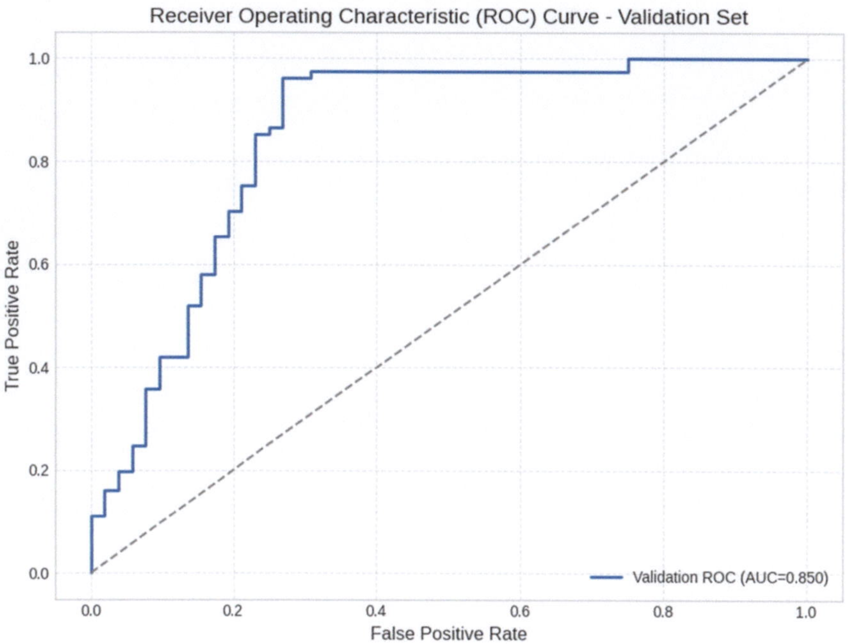

Fig. 1.72 An example of an ROC curve that is generated for a binary classification task to differentiate GBM (positive class) from LGG (negative class) using an SVM classifier trained on the TCGA-GBM and TCGA-LGG data. (Codes: https://colab.research.google.com/drive/1pN2HjHY3qaloCb7Oppj6jKXIydq9MoDT#scrollTo=3VuJvVrzTJAf)

aneurysms must operate at very high recall to minimize catastrophic misses; a high overall AUROC does not guarantee good performance at that operating point, so evaluation should match the clinical question.

Segmentation Tasks

Image segmentation tasks involve partitioning a digital image into multiple segments or sets of pixels (or voxels in 3D), often to delineate anatomical structures (e.g., gray matter, white matter, ventricles) or pathological regions (e.g., tumors, ischemic strokes, white matter hyperintensities). Architectures like the U-Net are frequently employed for this purpose. Metrics for segmentation evaluation can be broadly categorized into those that measure volumetric overlap and those that measure boundary or surface distance.

Dice Similarity Coefficient (DSC)
The Dice Similarity Coefficient (DSC) is a statistic used to gauge the similarity of two samples. For two sets of voxels, A (predicted) and B (ground truth), it is defined as the size of their overlap doubled, divided by the sum of their sizes:

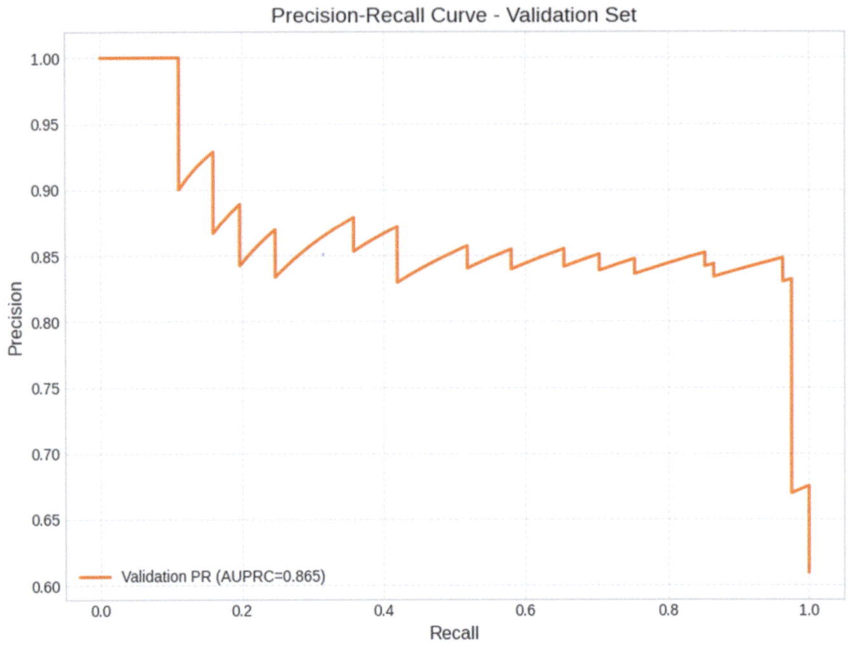

Fig. 1.73 An example of a Precision-Recall curve that is generated for a binary classification task to differentiate GBM (positive class) from LGG (negative class) using an SVM classifier trained on the TCGA-GBM and TCGA-LGG data. (Codes: https://colab.research.google.com/drive/1pN2HjHY3qaloCb7Oppj6jKXIydq9MoDT#scrollTo=3VuJvVrzTJAf)

$$DSC(A,B) = \frac{2 \times (A \cap B)}{(A \cup B)}$$

The DSC is the most widely used and standard metric for evaluating segmentation performance in medical imaging. This is because the DSC is relatively insensitive to class imbalance (i.e., the size of the foreground object relative to the image background), making it more reliable than per-pixel accuracy. Its value ranges from 0 (no overlap) to 1 (perfect overlap).

Let's refer back to our example where we trained a U-net algorithm in Sect. 3.2.3.4. and visualize the predicted segmentations based on how well they align with the ground truth. Figure 1.74 below provides a detailed, multi-faceted evaluation of the brain tumor segmentation model. The Dice Similarity Coefficient (DSC) for each class can be calculated directly from the provided pixel areas/volumes for the intersection, false positives, and false negatives. In this case, since we resample all our input images to a voxel size of 1 mm × 1 mm × 1 mm, each pixel/voxel in the images corresponds to 1 mm width. While the visualization below shows Dice scores calculated for a specific slice, it is important to note that this is done only for visualization and explanation purposes. Typically, for such 3D segmentation tasks, the Dice score is calculated for the overall volume.

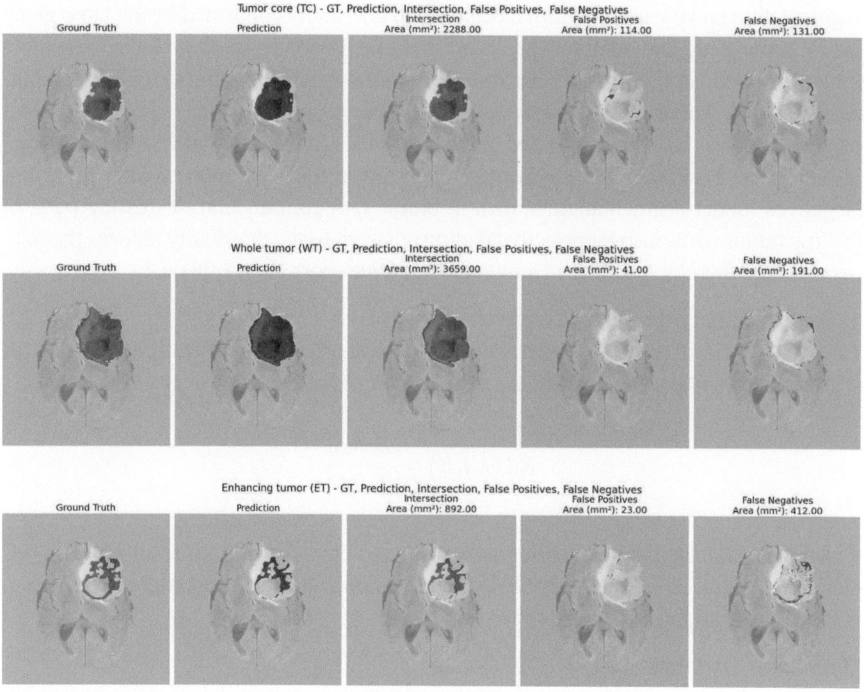

Fig. 1.74 Example comparison of automatic and reference tumor segmentations on an axial brain MR image. Panels are organized by row and column. Rows show the three BraTS sub-regions: tumor core (TC), whole tumor (WT), and enhancing tumor (ET). Columns show, left-to-right: Intersection (true positives), False Positives, and False Negatives. The segmentation overlays are displayed on the grayscale MR slice (green = intersection/TP; red = FP; blue = FN). The area of each overlay is reported in mm^2 at the top of every panel. This layout highlights where the model agrees with the reference mask and where it over- or under-segments each sub-region. Codes for this visualization are available at: conv_04_brats_segmentation_unet.ipynb. (Example image from BraTS-TCGA-GBM, licensed under CC-BY-3.0)

For the Tumor Core (TC), with an intersection of 2250 mm^2 (or pixels), false positives of 213 mm^2 (or pixels), and false negatives of 169 mm^2 (or pixels), yielding a DSC of approximately 0.92. Similarly, the Whole Tumor (WT) class, with an intersection of 3789 mm^2 (or pixels), false positives of 179 mm^2 (or pixels), and false negatives of 61 mm^2 (or pixels), results in a high DSC of approximately 0.97. Finally, the process demonstrates how the large error volumes for the Enhancing Tumor (ET), an intersection of only 1076 mm^2 (or pixels), against false positives of 1280 mm^2 (or pixels), and false negatives of 39 mm^2 (or pixels), translate into a significantly lower DSC of approximately 0.62. Note how the dice calculations are confined to the union of predicted and ground truth segmentations and don't include the rest of the areas/volumes in the scan.

The model performs exceptionally well for the Whole Tumor (WT) and Tumor Core (TC) regions, achieving high Dice scores of 0.97 and 0.92, respectively. These scores approaching 1.0 indicate a very strong spatial overlap between the predicted segmentation and the ground truth labels, which is visually confirmed by the large green intersection areas and minimal presence of False Positives (red) or False Negatives (blue). In contrast, the model's performance on the Enhancing Tumor (ET) is significantly poorer, with a Dice score of only 0.62. The visualization panels provide a clear diagnosis for this low score. The dedicated error maps for ET reveal substantial volumes of both False Positives (over-segmentation, shown in red) and minor volumes of False Negatives (under-segmentation, shown in blue). This combination of missing parts of the true tumor while also incorrectly labeling adjacent tissue drastically reduces the relative overlap, thereby resulting in a much lower Dice score (Fig. 1.74).

Jaccard Index (Intersection over Union—IoU)
Another metric that measures the overlap between the ground truth and predicted segmentations is the Jaccard Index, also known as Intersection over Union (IoU).

$$IoU(A,B) = \frac{|A \cap B|}{|A \cup B|}$$

IoU is a standard metric for segmentation and conceptually quite similar to DSC (Jaccard = Dice/(2 − Dice)), but IoU penalizes misclassifications more heavily and is therefore a slightly stricter metric of overlap.

Hausdorff Distance (HD)
While overlap-based metrics are useful for assessing overall volumetric agreement, they can be insensitive to errors in the boundary delineation of the segmented object. Distance-based metrics address this by directly measuring the distance between the surfaces of the predicted and ground truth segmentations. The Hausdorff Distance (HD) for segmentations A and B is represented as:

$$HD(A,B) = \left(d(a,b), d(a,b)\right)$$

where *d(a,b)* is the Euclidean distance between points *a* and *b*. Intuitively, we can understand that the function for HD identifies the point on the predicted boundary that is farthest from any point on the boundary of ground truth.

In neuroradiology studies, HD is almost always reported along with Dice as a critical evaluation metric when the clinical applications involve precise boundary delineation. This is especially important when a high DSC score could mask a large HD, where a small "spike" or deviation in the predicted boundary extends into critical structures. For example, in radiotherapy where high doses of radiation are delivered, it is essential to identify and avoid surrounding healthy tissues. In such scenarios, HD is a much more clinically relevant evaluation metric to measure the quality of segmentation.

For example, in Fig. 1.75 the predicted TC closely overlaps the reference except for a small "spike" where the boundary deviates outward. A Dice score would remain high because the overall volumes still largely agree, yet the HD of 8.49 mm reveals a substantial local error, exactly the kind of deviation that matters when a

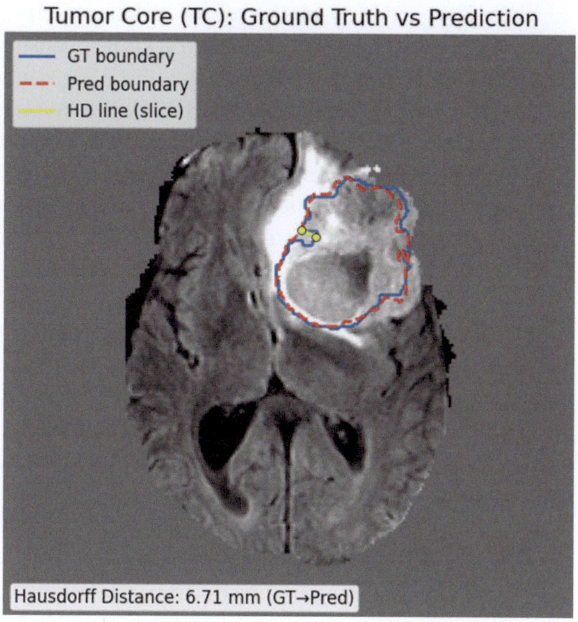

Fig. 1.75 Example of a boundary-based evaluation using the Hausdorff distance (HD) on an axial brain MR slice. The tumor-core (TC) reference contour (blue) and the model prediction (red) are overlaid. Although most of the outlines coincide, a localized protrusion in the predicted boundary produces a worst-case surface-to-surface separation (yellow line) of 6.71 mm in physical units. (Code: conv_04_brats_segmentation_unet.ipynb). (Example image from BraTS-TCGA-GBM, licensed under CC-BY-3.0)

contour approaches dose-limiting organs or eloquent tissue. Reporting HD (or the robust variant HD95, the 95th-percentile surface distance) alongside Dice provides complementary information: Dice summarizes volumetric agreement, while HD quantifies the largest boundary discrepancy clinicians must account for. In practice, distances should always be computed in physical space using image spacing, since anisotropic voxels can otherwise distort the measured HD.

95th Percentile Hausdorff Distance (HD95)
The primary limitation of the standard HD is its extreme sensitivity to outliers; a single misclassified voxel far from the true boundary can dramatically increase the HD score. To mitigate the sensitivity of the standard HD to outliers, the 95th percentile Hausdorff Distance (HD95) is often used. Instead of taking the maximum distance, it calculates the 95th percentile of the distances between the boundary points. HD95 is a more robust and practical metric for boundary evaluation.

Average Symmetric Surface Distance (ASSD)
The Average Symmetric Surface Distance (ASSD) averages the distances between the boundaries of predicted and ground truth segmentations. Unlike HD and Hd95, which provide worst-case segmentation errors, the ASSD provides a global measure of the average boundary error. ASSD averages the distances from every point on the surface set A to the closest point on the surface of set B (and vice versa). It is represented as:

$$ASSD(A,B) = \frac{1}{|S(A)| + |S(B)|}\left(\sum_{s_A \in S(A)} d\left(s_A, S(B)\right) + \sum_{s_B \in S(B)} d\left(s_B, S(A)\right)\right)$$

where *S(A)* and *S(B)* are the sets of surface voxels.

As with any average metric, the ASSD is less sensitive to single outliers than HD but more sensitive to the overall shape of the segmentation than DSC, and is typically reported alongside the HD (or HD95). It is helpful in evaluating the segmentation of complex or branching structures such as the cerebral vessels.

Table 1.6 presents a summary of key segmentation metrics. It is worthwhile to point out that in segmentation use-cases, the overlap metrics and boundary metrics convey complementary information that clinical practitioners can use to assess the model's performance. A segmentation can achieve a DSC score greater than 0.9, suggesting excellent performance while simultaneously having a large and clinically unacceptable HD. For example, this can happen when large parts of a tumor are segmented correctly, but a small portion of its boundary significantly extends into surrounding normal tissues. Therefore, for a comprehensive and clinically meaningful evaluation, it is essential to report both overlap-based and distance-based metrics. More recent works have explored metrics that better correlate with clinical utility. The Surface Dice Similarity Coefficient (Surface DSC), which at tolerance measures how much of two surfaces lie within a specified tolerance (a pre-defined distance e.g., 1 mm, 2 mm, 3 mm and so on) of each other.

Generative Tasks

Evaluating generation AI algorithms within neuroradiology presents a unique challenge, since these algorithms don't produce a single correct output but rather a distribution of potentially correct outputs. For example, Generative AI algorithms

Table 1.6 Summary of key segmentation metrics

Metric	Definition / How computed (short)	What it measures (intuition)	Strengths / Why use it	Limitations / Pitfalls
Dice Similarity Coefficient (DSC)	$\frac{2\times(A\cap B)}{(A\cup B)}$	Overlap between predicted and ground-truth masks	Most common; intuitive 0 to 1 scale	Insensitive to small structures; volume-dependent
Intersection-over-Union (IoU/ Jaccard)	$\frac{\lvert A\cap B\rvert}{\lvert A\cup B\rvert}$	Overlap (stricter than DSC)	Widely used; comparable to natural-image literature	Harder to interpret clinically
Hausdorff Distance (HD) / HD95	Max (or 95th pct) surface-to-surface distance	Worst-case boundary error	Captures outlier boundary errors	Max HD sensitive to noise; prefer HD95
Average (Symmetric) Surface Distance (ASD/ASSD)	Average bidirectional surface distance	Typical boundary error	Less sensitive to outliers than HD	Requires accurate surface extraction

could be used to synthesize contrast-enhanced MRI sequences from non-contrast or low-contrast sequences, or generate a descriptive radiology report (text) from an input sequence. Image generation algorithms, which are used for tasks such as synthetic-MRI or CT images, super-resolution, and denoising, require different evaluation strategies from text generation algorithms, which are used for tasks such as generating radiology reports from images. The evaluation of these tasks is a rapidly evolving field, and while these algorithms are still mainly assessed using metrics adapted from other domains, they are getting more clinically-grounded in their assessments.

The evaluation metrics for image generation algorithms can be broadly divided based on whether a ground truth or input image exists (reference-based metrics) or the images are purely synthetic (distribution-based).

For reference-based tasks, the intuition behind evaluation metrics is to compare how similar the generated image is to the reference image.

Structural similarity index (SSIM) measures the perceptual similarity between a generated image and a reference image. Perceptual similarity is typically evaluated along three characteristics: luminance, contrast, and structure. SSIM can range from −1 to 1, where values closer to 1 indicate that the AI-generated image is very similar to the real image. SSIM is widely used to evaluate super-resolution or image-to-image translation tasks in neuroradiology. For example, an algorithm trained to generate synthetic contrast-enhanced MRI images from non-contrast or low-dose contrast images can be evaluated using SSIM. However, low SSIM values don't necessarily translate to low clinical utility since even slightly blurry images can have lower SSIM even if clinically acceptable.

Peak Signal-to-Noise Ratio (PSNR)

PSNR is another reference-based metric that quantifies the ratio of the maximum possible signal and reconstruction noise. The higher the PSNR value, the closer the generated image is to the original (less error). PSNR is based on the Mean Squared Error (MSE), which represents the cumulative squared error between the reference and generated image. The PSNR is expressed in decibels (dB) and is calculated using the Mean Squared Error (MSE):

$$PSNR = 10\left(\frac{MAX^2}{MSE}\right)$$

where MSE is the average of squared differences between the corresponding pixels in the reference and generated images and MAX is the maximum possible pixel value of the image. The MSE for two images I and K of dimensions m and n are given by

$$MSE = \frac{1}{mn}\sum_{i=0}^{m-1}\sum_{j=0}^{n-1}\left[I(i,j) - K(i,j)\right]^2$$

When developing or testing algorithms to remove noise from neuroimaging, PSNR can be used to quantitatively prove their effectiveness. By comparing a denoised image to an original image with noise, a higher PSNR shows that the algorithm successfully reduced the noise while preserving the original image's signal. While PSNR is an objective metric, it doesn't always perfectly align with human perception. In neuroradiology, it needs to be paired with subjective clinical assessments from radiologists to ensure that algorithms performing well on PSNR also produce images of diagnostic quality.

For unpaired generative tasks that involve creating synthetic images without one-to-one ground truth, the intuition behind evaluation metrics is to compare the distribution of generated images with that of real images. Many evaluation metrics, such as the Fréchet Inception Distance (FID), Inception Scores (IS), that are well-defined for natural image tasks, are not adapted to medical imaging or neuroradiology. The InceptionV3 network was trained on ImageNet, a dataset of natural images (e.g., cats, dogs, cars). The features it has learned to extract may not be relevant or optimal for capturing the subtle tissue contrasts, textures, and anatomical structures present in medical images like MRIs or CTs. An image could have a low FID score by matching the low-level statistical properties of real MRIs but contain anatomically impossible features, rendering it clinically useless. An intuitive solution to the domain gap is to replace the ImageNet-trained feature extractor with one trained on a large corpus of medical images, such as RadImageNet. This could potentially be a domain-specific adaptation of the FID metric. Due to the limitations of automated metrics, qualitative evaluation by domain experts remains the gold standard for assessing generative models. "Visual Turing Test" (VTT) is often employed: radiologists or experts are asked to distinguish AI-generated images from real images in a mixed set. If experts cannot reliably tell the difference, the generative model is considered successful in realism.

For text generation tasks such as automated radiology report generation from images or summarizing findings, the evaluation metrics are drawn from natural language processing with adaptations made for clinical relevance.

Bilingual evaluation understudy (BLEU) measures n-gram overlap between the generated text and reference text. Higher BLEU scores correspond to closer language overlap between the reference text and generated text. For example, a BLEU-4 score (4-gram matches) of 0.25 would be reported when there is a 25% overlap on four-word sequences. Additionally, to prevent models from achieving a high score by generating very short, precise sentences, BLEU applies a penalty if the candidate text is shorter than the reference text.

BLEU only measures word-level overlap and cannot assess whether the generated report captures the same meaning as the reference. Also, this metric is not designed to capture the nuance of clinical language, such as assertions of certainty (for example, "suspicious for malignancy" vs "consistent with malignancy").

Recall-oriented understudy for gisting evaluation (ROUGE) looks at the longest common subsequence between the generated and reference text and gauges how many of the essential findings in the reference text were accurately captured within the generated text. Higher ROUGE scores indicate that the model captured more essential findings and did not omit key information.

The **metric for evaluation of translation with explicit ordering (METEOR)** includes synonym matches and the weighted harmonic mean of precision and recall. METEOR considers both how much of the generated text is correct (precision) and how much of the reference text is covered (recall), with a heavier emphasis on recall. Unlike simpler metrics that only count exact word matches, METEOR also accounts for stemming, which includes matching words with the same root (e.g., "imaging" and "imaged") and synonyms, which involve matching words with similar meanings (e.g., "scan" and "imaging"). For example, when comparing a radiology report generated by an AI algorithm with a radiologist's reference report, METEOR is helpful to determine if the generated report captured all critical findings and relevant details, even if the report used different phrasing. The word-order penalty also encourages the algorithm to logically structure the output into a fluent, readable, and structured report.

Let's take an example of a Human reference report and an AI-generated report and intuitively evaluate their scores.

- **Human reference report:** "Findings are consistent with an acute to subacute infarct in the right middle cerebral artery territory. There is no evidence of intracranial hemorrhage or mass effect. Mild chronic microvascular ischemic changes are also noted."
- **AI-generated report:** "Acute stroke in the right MCA distribution. No hemorrhage is seen. Chronic small vessel ischemic disease is present."

The BLEU score for this example would be relatively low since BLEU focuses strictly on exact n-gram overlap. While both reports qualitatively describe the same clinical findings, they use different words and phrases. For example, the 1-gram (single word) overlap would identify some words such as "acute," "in," "the," "right," "no," "hemorrhage," and "chronic." However, the 2-gram (two-word) and higher overlap is very low. For example, phrases such as "middle cerebral artery territory" and "MCA distribution" share no overlap even though they mean the same thing. This evaluation metric doesn't consider the fact that "stroke" is a synonym for "infarct" and "MCA" is an abbreviation for "middle cerebral artery."

However, the ROUGE score would be high. This is because ROUGE is designed to measure if the essential findings from reference text (such as "acute/subacute infarct," "located in the right MCA territory,", "no hemorrhage," "no mass effect," and "chronic microvascular changes") are successfully captured in the generated text. We can analyze the generated report and identify that most of the essential findings were captured, except "no mass effect."

The METEOR score of this report would also be high since this metric would identify the synonyms and stemming (in this context, "infarct" and "stroke" are synonyms). Also, the "middle cerebral artery territory" and "MCA distribution" are semantically identical. This metric would consider the high precision (the generated report did not add incorrect information), and also the high recall was only lowered because of the omission of "mass effect." The sentences are fluent and logically structured, so it is unlikely to incur a word-order penalty.

Synthesis and Future Directions

The evaluation of AI algorithms in neuroradiology is a complex process that requires a nuanced understanding of not only technical metrics but also their clinical implications. It is very important to note that no single metric is sufficient and that a robust evaluation requires a suite of complementary metrics tailored to assess the model's performance for the specific clinical task. Choosing the most appropriate evaluation metrics is fundamental to producing meaningful and reproducible research. Table 1.7 provides a comprehensive summary of recommended evaluation metrics. While this table can serve as a quick-reference guide for researchers and clinicians, it is important to select appropriate metrics that align with the specific research question and clinical goals.

Validation Frameworks

Validation frameworks establish clear benchmarks for quality, transparency, and reproducibility, which build trust among clinicians, patients, and regulatory bodies. These frameworks provide evidence-based, consensus-driven checklists and recommendations and offer a clear roadmap for researchers to ensure their research is reported with the necessary completeness and clarity. Since AI models can be complex with opaque decision-making processes, these frameworks establish clear benchmarks for quality, transparency, and reproducibility. Some of the key frameworks for AI in neuroradiology are:

Table 1.7 Summary of recommended evaluation metrics

AI task category	Specific task example	Typical/standard metrics	Recommended specialized/advanced metrics
Image classification	Tumor grading from MRI; Stroke detection from CT	Accuracy, Area Under the ROC Curve (AUC)	Area Under the Precision-Recall Curve (AUPRC), Matthews Correlation Coefficient (MCC), F1-Score
Text classification	Triage of reports for urgent findings	Accuracy, F1-Score	Macro- and Micro-averaged F1-Scores (for multi-class tasks), Precision/Recall at specific operating points
Image segmentation	Delineation of brain tumors or white matter lesions	Dice Similarity Coefficient (DSC), Intersection over Union (IoU)	95th Percentile Hausdorff Distance (HD95), Average Symmetric Surface Distance (ASSD), Surface DSC
Image generation	MRI contrast synthesis; Data augmentation	Fréchet Inception Distance (FID)	Domain-Specific FID, Qualitative Visual Turing Test (VTT) by Radiologists
Text generation	Automated radiology report generation	BLEU, ROUGE, METEOR	F1-Score on extracted clinical facts (F1RadGraph)

- **Checklist for artificial intelligence in medical imaging (CLAIM) and minimum information about clinical artificial intelligence modeling (MI-CLAIM)**
  CLAIM is a reporting guideline that provides a checklist of essential items for authors and reviewers aimed at improving the clarity, transparency, and reporting clarity of AI in medical imaging. MI-CLAIM is a comprehensive checklist aimed at providing transparent, reproducible reporting guidelines for clinical AI modeling studies, and is structured into six essential components (Study, design, Data partitioning, Model optimization and selection, Performance evaluation, Model examination, Reproducible Pipeline). These guidelines acknowledge the practical realities of medical AI research, such as the protection of commercial intellectual property and safeguarding patient privacy, and propose a tiered system for transparency, where the highest tier is complete open sharing of code, while lower tiers involve releasing executable files without revealing underlying source code.
- **Transparent reporting of a multivariable prediction model for individual prognosis or diagnosis (TRIPOD)**
  The TRIPOD statement aims to improve the transparent reporting of studies that develop, validate, or update multivariable prediction models for either diagnostic or prognostic purposes. TRIPOD provides a 22-item checklist that is designed to be relevant to any type of multivariable model, from traditional statistical methods such as logistic regression to more complex ML algorithms. Additionally, TRIPOD strongly recommends validation of the prediction model on an external test set, typically from a different time period or a different hospital.
- **Minimum information for medical AI reporting (MINIMAR)**
  MINIMAR proposes a minimum set of reporting standards to ensure that intended predictions, target populations, hidden biases, and the model's generalizability can be clearly understood and evaluated.
- **Radiomics quality score (RQS)**
  RQS provides a 16-item checklist that is designed to evaluate and improve the quality of radiomics studies. These results (scores) range from −8 to +36 to quantify study rigor and reproducibility. Higher RQS scores include steps that ensure feature stability and calibration, analyzing imaging at multiple time points, correlating radiomic features with biological correlates, and making the source code and data publicly available.
- **Consolidated standards of reporting trials—artificial intelligence (CONSORT-AI)**
  CONSORT-AI aims to provide specific reporting guidelines for randomized controlled trials (RCTs) that evaluate a health intervention with an AI component to ensure transparency and allow for critical appraisal. This includes a 14-item checklist that includes recommendations such as providing clear descriptions of the AI intervention and its various versions, integration into clinical settings, handling of data, analysis of errors, and code/data accessibility.
- **FUTURE-AI: International consensus guideline for trustworthy and deployable artificial intelligence in healthcare**
  Future AI is a holistic international consensus guideline that provides a framework of principles and best practices to guide the development and deployment

of trustworthy AI tools. Table 1.8. Unlike frameworks that focus on retrospectively reporting a completed study, FUTURE-AI provides a proactive roadmap around six core guiding principles—Future, Universality, Traceability, Usability, Robustness, and Explainability.

The frameworks analyzed in this section are not static endpoints but are part of an ongoing, dynamic process of community-wide learning and improvement. As AI technology continues to evolve, so too will the standards required to govern it. The neuroradiology community, comprising clinicians, researchers, data scientists, and industry partners, must remain actively engaged in the use, critique, and refinement of these guidelines. By collectively committing to a culture of transparency, rigor, and ethical responsibility, the field can navigate the challenges ahead and build a future where artificial intelligence serves as a trustworthy, indispensable, and equitable partner in advancing neurological patient care.

Common Pitfalls and Mitigations

Researchers and AI practitioners may face several challenges during the development and implementation of AI algorithms, which can compromise their clinical utility and reliability. As summarized in Table 1.9, these challenges can either be data-related, model-related, training-related, or around Implementation & Trust. While these are not an exhaustive list of challenges, they capture several common challenges and practical mitigation strategies.

Table 1.8 Consolidated summary of selected validation frameworks

Framework	Primary goal	Scope	Stage of AI lifecycle	Key deliverable
CLAIM	Transparent reporting of AI studies	Medical Imaging	Reporting	44-item checklist
MI-CLAIM	Transparent reporting of AI models	General Clinical AI	Development & Reporting	6-part guideline
TRIPOD	Transparent reporting of prediction models	Diagnosis & Prognosis	Development & Validation	22-item checklist
CONSORT-AI	Transparent reporting of clinical trials	AI Interventions (RCTs)	Clinical Evaluation	14-item extension
RQS	Methodological quality assessment	Radiomics Research	Development & Validation	16-item scoring system
MINIMAR	Minimum information for reporting to assess bias	General Medical AI	Reporting	4-part standard
FUTURE-AI	Guidance for trustworthy AI	Healthcare AI Lifecycle	Full Lifecycle	6 principles, 30 practices

Table 1.9 Common pitfalls and mitigation strategies

Pitfall category	Pitfall description	Mitigation strategies
Data-related	Insufficient or Poorly Curated Data: Small, noisy, or poorly annotated datasets limit model performance.	Data Augmentation: Artificially expand the dataset (e.g., rotations, scaling). Transfer Learning: Fine-tune models pre-trained on large datasets. Federated Learning: Train across institutions without sharing private data.
Model-related	Overfitting & Poor Generalization: The model performs well on the training data but fails on new, unseen data from different sources (domain shift).	Rigorous External Validation: Test on completely independent datasets. Regularization: Use techniques like Dropout to prevent memorization. Cross-Validation: Systematically split data to get a robust performance estimate.
Training-related	Mode-collapse, Vanishing/Exploding gradients	Hyperparameter tuning Usage of appropriate task-specific loss functions Architectures with better gradient propagation
Implementation & trust	The "Black Box" Problem: The model's decision-making process is opaque, hindering clinical trust and adoption.	Explainable AI (XAI): Use methods like saliency maps (heatmaps) to visualize the model's focus and reasoning.
	Inherent Algorithmic Bias: The model learns and amplifies demographic or systemic biases present in the training data, leading to health disparities.	Data Auditing & Fairness Metrics: Analyze data for balance and test for equitable performance across subgroups. Bias-Aware Training: Use algorithms designed to reduce bias. Curate Diverse Datasets: Actively collect representative data.

Clinical Translation Benchmarks

While evaluation metrics around model performance, such as accuracy, AUROC, precision, and recall, are essential for model development, they do not reliably estimate the model's real-world clinical utility. Clinical translation benchmarks are designed to assess a model's readiness for deployment by evaluating its performance on tasks that directly impact patient care and clinical workflow. As summarized in Table 1.10, clinical translation benchmarks help ensure that the AI algorithms are not only technically robust but also safe, effective and beneficial for patients.

Table 1.10 Clinical translation benchmarks

Benchmark area	Objective	Common evaluation methods
Robustness & generalizability	To ensure the model performs reliably across different scanners, hospitals, and patient populations.	External validation on datasets from unseen institutions. Testing across different scanner models and protocols.
Efficiency & workflow integration	To confirm the model is fast and integrates smoothly into existing clinical systems (like PACS).	Measure model inference time. Compare AI-assisted workflow time vs. manual time. Assess ease of integration with PACS.
Interpretability & trust	To ensure clinicians can understand the basis for the model's predictions, fostering trust.	Use Explainable AI (XAI) methods like saliency maps. Conduct qualitative reviews with clinical experts.
Clinical impact	To measure the model's tangible benefit to diagnostic accuracy and patient outcomes.	Conduct reader studies comparing clinician performance with and without AI assistance. Evaluate improvements in diagnostic accuracy or reductions in inter-reader variability.

Beyond Neural Networks: ML in Practice

> Those of us in machine learning are really good at doing well on a test set, but unfortunately deploying a system takes more than doing well on a test set. All of AI…has a proof-of-concept-to-production gap. (Andrew Ng from "Andrew Ng X-Rays the AI Hype" (May 2021))

Machine learning (ML) in neuroradiology extends beyond the technical sophistication of neural networks, demanding careful attention to clinical integration, interpretability, fairness, and reliability. While deep learning architectures have driven remarkable advances, their adoption in real-world practice hinges on addressing challenges unique to healthcare settings. This section reviews three critical domains-explainability, bias mitigation, and uncertainty quantification-that underpin responsible and effective deployment of ML in clinical neuroradiology.

The potential of these deep learning applications is immense. They promise to reduce diagnostic turnaround times, particularly in emergency settings; decrease physician error by providing a consistent "second reader"; and enable the analysis of impracticably large datasets for research and population health studies. Commercially available algorithms are already being implemented in clinical practice to flag time-sensitive findings like ICH, demonstrating a tangible impact on patient care pathways.

However, the path from promising research to widespread, robust clinical implementation is fraught with challenges. A recurring theme in the literature is the critical need for greater research standardization, model generalizability, and external validation. Many high-performing models are developed and tested on private institutional datasets or curated public challenge datasets, and their performance often degrades when applied to "in-the-wild" clinical data from different scanners, patient populations, and imaging protocols. Furthermore, the "black box" nature of many deep learning models, where the internal reasoning is not transparent, poses a significant barrier to clinical trust and adoption. Addressing these hurdles of validation, generalization, and interpretability is the central focus of the ongoing effort to translate deep learning research into routine neuroradiological practice.

Explainable AI for Clinical Trust

A persistent barrier to clinical adoption of AI is the "black box" nature of many models, especially deep neural networks. Clinicians require transparency to verify that algorithmic decisions align with established radiological knowledge and to identify potential model failures. Explainable AI (XAI) methods provide this transparency, enabling users to interpret and trust model outputs.

Saliency maps and related visualization techniques, such as Grad-CAM, highlight image regions most influential to a model's prediction. These tools allow radiologists to confirm that the AI is focusing on clinically relevant features, such as a lesion or abnormality, rather than spurious artifacts. SHAP (SHapley Additive exPlanations) and LIME (Local Interpretable Model-agnostic Explanations) offer quantitative explanations by attributing importance scores to input features, making it possible to assess not only where the model is looking but also why it made a particular decision.

SHAP

The SHAP technique uses Shapley values from game theory to attribute the contribution of each feature in the model to the final prediction. SHAP visualizations are a method for explaining the output of a machine learning model (Fig. 1.76).

Each dot represents a patient; the position on the x-axis indicates that patient's SHAP value (feature contribution), which indicates how much the feature contributed to the model's output (to the right) or detracted from it (to the left). Features are ordered by mean |SHAP|, so those at the top have the most considerable overall impact. Dot color encodes the raw feature value (blue = low, pink = high). Clinically, larger enhancing-tumor burden (e.g., VOLUME_ET, VOLUME_ET_OVER_BRAIN, VOLUME_ET_OVER_WT) consistently drives higher predicted risk/probability (rightward shift), which aligns with domain knowledge and helps clinicians trust that the model is using sensible signals. Texture features show mixed, patient-specific effects, and the vertical spread at each row reveals heterogeneity across cases, supporting case-level auditability. Together, SHAP offers both global importance and per-patient attributions, enabling transparent, clinician-interpretable validation of model behavior.

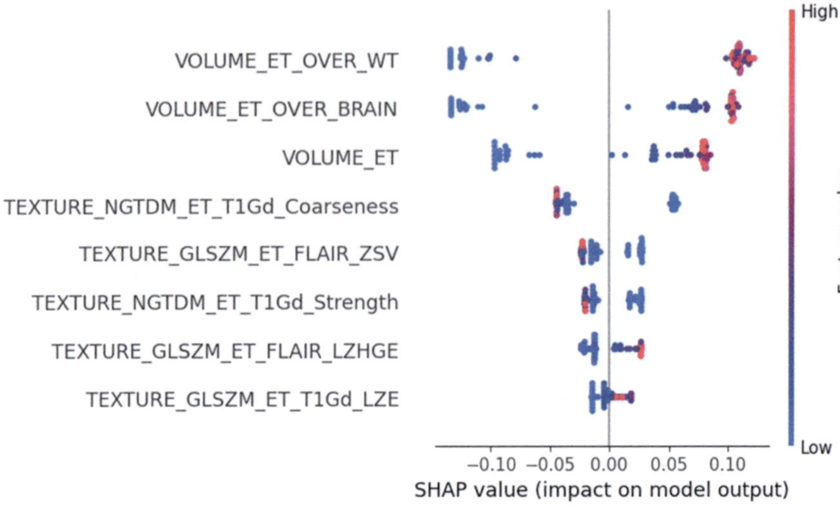

Fig. 1.76 Illustrative SHAP summary ("beeswarm") plot explaining a radiomics model trained on TCGA-GBM and TCGA-LGG. (Code to reproduce this figure: shap_visualization.py.py)

Grad-CAM

Explainable AI (XAI) techniques

, such as the attention visualizations shown here, play an important role in bridging the gap between algorithmic decision-making and clinical trust. By revealing which image regions the model prioritizes at each stage of processing, clinicians can verify whether the network's focus aligns with clinically relevant structures. This transparency helps in identifying potential failure cases, such as attention drifting to irrelevant anatomy, and supports informed decision-making when integrating AI into workflow. In neuroradiology, where diagnostic decisions carry significant consequences, such interpretable outputs enable more rigorous validation, facilitate multidisciplinary review, and foster clinician confidence in model-assisted assessments. Over time, systematic use of XAI methods can help build a reproducible evidence base for safe, accountable AI adoption in clinical practice.

While integrating XAI tools into clinical workflows increases radiologists' confidence and facilitates error detection, these methods are not without limitations. Saliency maps can be inconsistent, and different XAI techniques may yield divergent explanations for the same prediction. Therefore, validation of XAI methods on clinically relevant tasks and datasets remains essential.

Figure 1.77 demonstrates how the Attention U-Net model's spatial focus aligns with its segmentation outputs across three target categories. The top row shows Grad-CAM heatmaps from the final convolutional layer, highlighting the areas that contributed most to the model's predictions. For each category, tumor core, whole tumor, and enhancing tumor, the regions highlighted

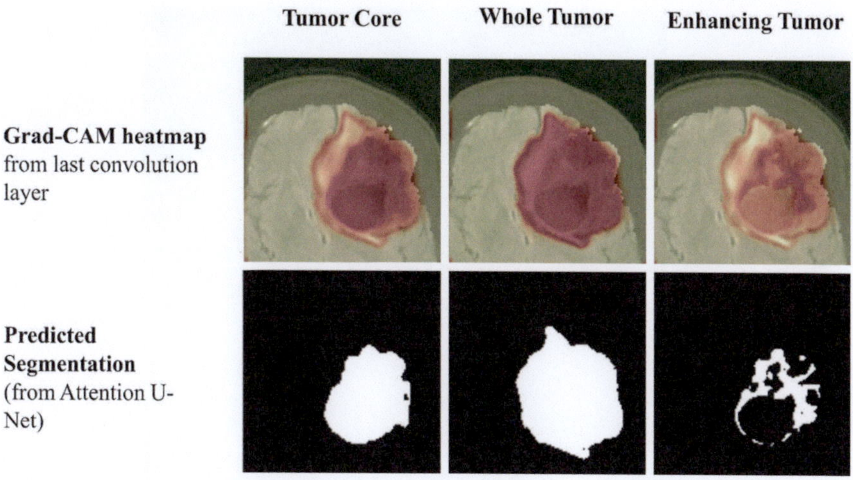

Fig. 1.77 Illustrative Grad-CAM visualizations and predicted segmentations from an Attention U-Net for brain tumor subregion segmentation using the BraTS dataset. (Code: conv_05_brats_segmentation_attentionunet.ipynb) (Example image from BraTS-TCGA-GBM, licensed under CC-BY-3.0)

in red indicate where the network allocated the most attention during inference. These maps provide a visualization of the model's internal decision-making, revealing how its focus regions differ depending on the target class being predicted.

The bottom row presents the corresponding binary segmentation masks predicted by the Attention U-Net. When we compare these masks with the Grad-CAM heatmaps, we can observe the relationship between high-attention regions and predicted positive areas. Larger, more spatially coherent structures (e.g., whole tumor) show a close match between heatmap coverage and segmentation, while smaller, more complex structures (e.g., enhancing tumor) display more fragmented attention patterns, Fig. 1.77, reflecting the increased difficulty of the task.

Overall, this pairing of attention heatmaps and predicted masks provides an interpretable link between feature activation and output, enabling researchers to assess whether the network's focus is semantically consistent with the intended segmentation target.

Occlusion Sensitivity

Occlusion Sensitivity measures the resulting changes in the model's output when parts of the inputs are systematically masked or "occluded. A significant drop in the predicted probability when a specific region is occluded indicates that the occluded region is more important for the model's prediction decision (Fig. 1.78).

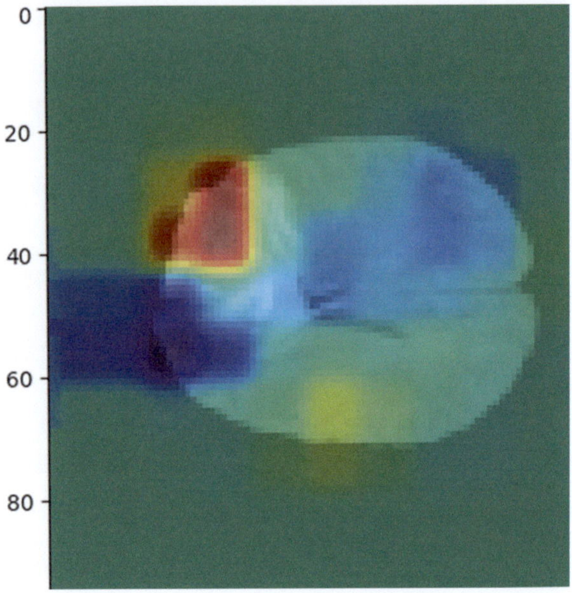

Fig. 1.78 Occlusion sensitivity map for a glioblastoma (GBM) classification model. Warmer regions (red/yellow) indicate areas where occluding the input image most strongly reduces the model's confidence in the GBM class, highlighting spatial zones most critical for the decision. Cooler regions (blue) have minimal or opposite influence, illustrating the model's localized dependence on specific high-importance features. (Code: conv_03_glioma_classification_densenet.ipynb) (Example image from BraTS-TCGA-GBM, licensed under CC-BY-3.0)

Transfer Learning

Transfer learning in neuroradiology involves adapting a model pre-trained on a large dataset, often ImageNet or, when available, a large medical imaging corpus, to perform a specific neuroradiological task such as classification, detection, or segmentation. Two common strategies are feature extraction, where the pre-trained layers are kept frozen and only a new task-specific head is trained, and fine-tuning, where some or all layers are further trained on the target dataset. This approach helps address the scarcity of labeled neuroradiology data, reduces training time, and can improve generalization. However, performance gains depend on the similarity between the pre-training and target domains, the fine-tuning strategy, and the size of the available dataset.

Data Augmentation

Augmentation category	Technique & description	Clinical rationale/purpose
Geometric transformations	Rotation, Scaling, Flipping: Applying affine transformations to alter image orientation.	Simulates variations in patient positioning and anatomy; teaches the model key invariances.
	Elastic Deformations: Applying non-linear, local warping to the image.	Mimics natural anatomical variability and soft-tissue differences between patients.
Intensity & pixel-level	Brightness & Contrast Jitter: Randomly adjusting the intensity range of the image.	Improves robustness to different scanner protocols, vendors, and acquisition settings.
	Gaussian Noise: Adding random noise from a normal distribution to pixel values.	Makes the model more resilient to inherent noise in MRI and CT images.
Generative	Generative Adversarial Networks (GANs): Using a generator-discriminator framework to create new, synthetic images.	Creates novel, realistic training samples, especially useful for augmenting data for rare diseases.
	Style Transfer: Adapting an image to match the textural style of another image set.	Addresses domain shift by making data from one scanner appear as if it came from another.

Predictive Uncertainty for Decision Support

Integration of AI algorithms into clinical practice depends on how much clinicians trust and interpret the predictions from these complex algorithms. For classification tasks, the AI algorithm's output typically consists of a single prediction, for example, "aneurysm present" with 95% probability. However, such point estimates do not convey the full picture of the model's confidence in its own prediction. Predictive uncertainty addresses this limitation by providing estimates on how reliable the model's output is for specific samples.

The practical importance of uncertainty is recognized in clinical medicine, where differential diagnoses and alternate impressions are standard practice. An AI model that can express when it is "uncertain" mimics this crucial aspect of clinical reasoning. For neuroradiologists, an uncertainty estimate can be the key to distinguishing between a confident, reliable AI finding and a speculative one that requires closer scrutiny. This is not merely an academic exercise; it has direct implications for patient safety and clinical workflow. For instance, if a model predicts an "aneurysm present" with high probability but this prediction is accompanied by high uncertainty, a notification can automatically be triggered for an expert radiologist's review, ensuring that ambiguous or unusual cases receive the necessary attention.

In the context of deep learning, predictive uncertainty is generally decomposed into two main types: aleatoric and epistemic uncertainty. Understanding the distinction is vital for interpreting an AI's output in a clinical scenario.

1. **Aleatoric uncertainty**: This type of uncertainty is inherent in the data itself and cannot be reduced by collecting more data. It stems from intrinsic randomness or noise. In neuroradiology, this could be due to factors such as low-resolution images, imaging artifacts resulting from patient motion, or the inherent ambiguity in distinguishing certain tissue types, even for experienced experts.
2. **Epistemic uncertainty**: This uncertainty relates to the model itself and its parameters. It reflects the model's lack of knowledge about the optimal parameters to describe the data, often because it has been trained on a limited or non-comprehensive dataset. Epistemic uncertainty is reducible; it can be decreased by training the model on more diverse data. Such uncertainties are significant in the AI domain since there are cases when the model may encounter a rare pathological condition or an image from a scanner model it was not trained on. The AI model would provide its prediction, but the prediction would have a high epistemic uncertainty. This indicates that the output for that patient or study is unreliable because the model is operating outside its domain of expertise. This is a crucial safety mechanism that prevents the model from making overconfident errors on "out-of-distribution" data.

Domain Shift and Label Shift

Domain shift, also known as covariate shift, occurs when the distribution of the input data changes while the relationship between the input data and output labels remains the same. These changes are typically due to different scanner manufacturers, acquisition protocols, reconstruction software, patient positioning, and other factors. For example, imagine an AI algorithm trained to segment brain metastases on 3T MRI scans from a single vendor (e.g., Siemens). The "domain" in this task is 3T Siemens MRI scans. When this algorithm is deployed in a hospital where 1.5T and 3T scans are routinely acquired using different vendors (e.g., GE or Philips), this model is said to encounter a domain shift. It is important to note that the underlying pathology (i.e., metastasis) is still the same, but the images in the new setting may have different characteristics, such as signal-to-noise ratio, contrast settings, imaging resolution, and slice thickness. Mitigating domain shift involves careful validation, continuous monitoring, and strategic adaptation to the target clinical environment. Domain Adaptation techniques, such as transfer learning, aim to align the distribution from the target domain with the source domain. In this method, the model trained in the source setting would typically fine-tune the model on a smaller, labeled dataset from the target hospital. Another method to mitigate domain shift is the use of extensive data augmentation. Data augmentations are applied to the input data right at the time of training to simulate variations in brightness, contrast, and various noise conditions. Another time-tested method to build a generalizable algorithm that is robust to domain shift is the use of diverse multi-center datasets from multiple scanners, vendors, and hospitals.

Label shift is a distributional shift where the relative frequency of labels differs between the training data and the real-world deployment data. These models can become unreliable, leading to poor performance in real-world scenarios where the target distributions often differ from the training distribution. For example, let's take the case of an AI algorithm trained to classify brain tumor types that is trained on a dataset from a tertiary academic neuro-oncology center. Due to referral bias, this center might have a high prevalence of more aggressive forms, such as glioblastomas, and a lower prevalence of lymphomas. If this algorithm is then deployed at a community hospital, where the distribution of tumor types will likely be different, the change in prior probability may lead to situations where the algorithm overdiagnoses glioblastomas simply because it was trained on a dataset with a high proportion of glioblastomas. To address label shift, the developed AI algorithms need to be tested on a target, labeled dataset to estimate the local disease prevalence and subsequently calibrate the model's output probabilities to reflect the target patient population better. Post deployment, the model's predictions need to be regularly monitored against confirmed diagnoses to assess if the model's decision thresholds need intervention or recalibration.

Low-Code/No-Code

Low-code and no-code tools are increasingly used in neuroradiology to speed up AI model development with minimal coding. Research-focused frameworks (Table 1.11), such as nnU-Net, SAM, and Auto3Dseg, automate preprocessing, architecture selection, and training for segmentation-Table 1.11. These platforms are designed to simplify or automate the complex aspects of training an AI algorithm, including pre-processing, model selection, training, and deployment. Such platforms are designed for accessibility and speed, but they often lack flexibility, control, and customization.

General ML suites, such as PyCaret and Scikit-learn, enable rapid experimentation with imaging-derived features and radiomics. Cloud-based AutoML (e.g., GCP) offers scalable model training and deployment without local infrastructure. Commercial solutions, such as Aidoc and Qure.ai, provide regulatory-cleared AI tools for specific neuroradiology tasks. While these platforms lower technical barriers, robust validation and domain-specific tuning remain essential for reliable clinical use (Table 1.12).

These are not exhaustive and capture only a slice of representative platforms/tools. These lists are intended to serve as a quick reference for AI researchers and developers to plan/evaluate their AI Algorithm pipelines for applicability.

Table 1.11 A summary of low-code solutions for commonly used neuroradiology tasks

Category	Platform/tool	Primary function	Neuroradiology applicability
Automated segmentation frameworks	nnU-Net	A self-configuring framework that automates the entire workflow for semantic segmentation. Applicability:	State-of-the-art brain tumor segmentation (e.g., BraTS challenge) and segmentation of various brain structures.
	MONAI Label	An AI-assisted annotation tool that integrates into viewers like 3D Slicer. It accelerates dataset creation using active learning.	Rapidly creating high-quality labeled datasets for brain tumors, stroke lesions, or anatomical regions.
	TotalSegmentator	A pre-trained model capable of segmenting over 100 different anatomical structures in CT scans with a single command.	Segmenting cranial structures for surgical planning or analysis without manual annotation.
	Auto3dSeg	An automated self-configuring framework for preprocessing and semantic segmentation	Automated training process for segmenting specific structure/ROI
General & cloud AutoML platforms	Google Cloud Vertex AI	A managed cloud platform for building, training, and deploying ML models with a graphical interface (AutoML) or custom code.	Training custom classifiers on brain MRI/CT without managing infrastructure.
	NVIDIA MONAI Deploy	A framework for packaging and deploying medical AI models into clinical environments using standardized application formats (MAPs).	Bridging the gap between a trained segmentation/classification model and its use in a hospital's PACS system.
	PyCaret	An open-source, low-code ML library that automates workflows for tasks like classification and regression.	Building predictive models from radiomics features extracted from brain scans
	Hugging Face	A platform for accessing thousands of pre-trained models and fine-tuning them on custom data with simplified tools.	Fine-tuning pre-trained vision models (like SAM or Swin Transformer) for specific neuroradiology segmentation or classification tasks.

Table 1.12 No-code AI solutions for neuroradiology

Category	Platform/ tool	Primary function	Neuroradiology applicability
AI-Assisted data annotation	3D Slicer	An open-source platform for medical image visualization and analysis with numerous plugins for AI-assisted segmentation.	Manual and semi-automated segmentation of brain structures and pathologies for research and surgical planning.
	V7 / Labelbox	Commercial platforms that provide sophisticated tools for AI-powered data labeling and dataset management.	Managing large-scale annotation projects for neuroradiology datasets with features like automated pre-segmentation.
End-to-end commercial solutions (no-code for clinicians)	Aidoc	An FDA-cleared AI platform that analyzes medical images in real-time to detect acute abnormalities and prioritize workflow.	Automated, real-time detection of intracranial hemorrhage and large vessel occlusion
	Viz.ai	An AI-powered care coordination platform focused on synchronizing stroke care teams.	Automatically detecting large vessel occlusion on CT angiography and alerting the entire stroke care team via a mobile app.
	RapidAI	A suite of tools for cerebrovascular imaging analysis, providing clinicians with actionable insights.	Automated CTP/MRI perfusion maps, ASPECT scoring, and detection of intracranial hemorrhage and vessel occlusions.
	Qure.ai	AI solutions for CT and X-ray interpretation across emergency and acute-care settings.	Triage for intracranial hemorrhage, skull fractures, mass effect, and midline shift.

Developer-focused AI frameworks (Table 1.13) such as PyTorch, Tensorflow, and MONAI Core help AI researchers and developers create novel algorithms by building highly specialized networks from scratch. They typically require strong programming skills, primarily in Python (Fig. 1.79).

Public Datasets for Neuroradiology

Publicly available datasets have been a major driver of AI technologies within the field of neuroradiology. These curated repositories serve as the fundamental building blocks for training, validating, and benchmarking the current and next generation of AI algorithms. In neuroradiology, the principles of Open Science are operationalized through such initiatives that promote data sharing according to FAIR principles—Findable, Accessible, Interoperable, and Reusable. The table

Table 1.13 High-code (developer-focused) AI frameworks for neuroradiology

Category	Framework/ library	Primary function	Neuroradiology applicability
Core deep learning	PyTorch	Flexible, Python-centric deep learning framework widely used in academic research. It provides tensor computation with GPU acceleration	Building, training, and experimenting with novel neural network architectures
	TensorFlow (with Keras)	Comprehensive, scalable deep learning ecosystem developed by Google. Keras serves as its user-friendly high-level API for rapid prototyping	Developing and deploying production-grade models
Specialized medical imaging	MONAI Core	PyTorch-based, open-source framework specifically designed for deep learning in medical imaging. It provides domain-specific building blocks for data handling, transformations, and network architectures.	Accelerating the development of custom medical AI models by providing pre-built, optimized components for 3D/4D data loading, image augmentation
Radiomics & machine learning	PyRadiomics	Open-source library for extracting a wide range of quantitative radiomic features from medical images.	Extracting hundreds of shape, intensity, and texture features from a pre-specified ROI
	Scikit-learn	Python library for classical machine learning (i.e., non-deep learning). It offers a wide array of algorithms for classification, regression, clustering, and dimensionality reduction.	Training models like Support Vector Machines (SVM) or Random Forests on radiomic features or clinical data
Image processing & handling	SimpleITK/ ITK	A foundational, high-performance toolkit for medical image analysis. It is not a deep learning library itself, but is critical for preprocessing and post-processing steps.	Performing essential image manipulation tasks like reading/writing DICOM files, image registration, filtering

below contains a consolidated inventory of major publicly available datasets (Table 1.14). This list is not exhaustive and is intended to serve as a quick-reference guide for researchers to identify and compare datasets based on their primary characteristics.

Specifically for Brain Tumor segmentation tasks, there have been many public challenges that have focused on Glioma segmentation, as summarized in Table 1.15 below.

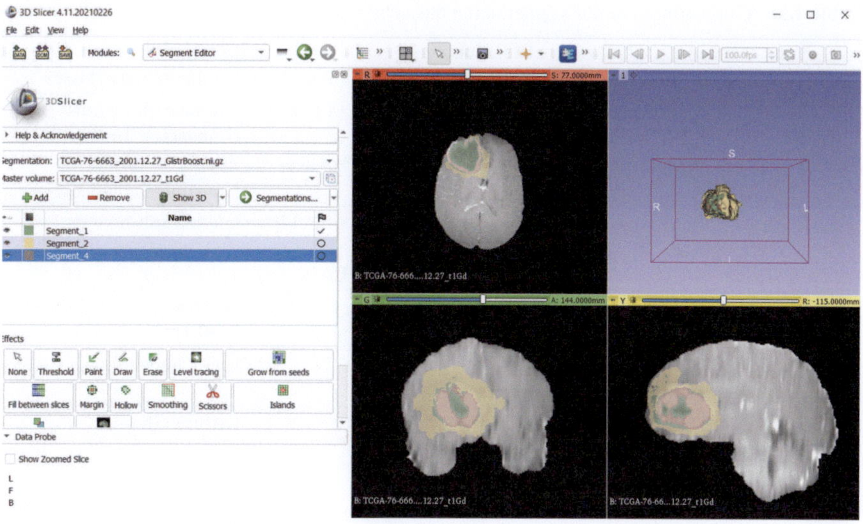

Fig. 1.79 Multi-class glioma segmentation shown in 3D Slicer (v4.11). Axial, coronal, and sagittal post-contrast T1-weighted images from TCGA-GBM case TCGA-76-6663 with color overlays denoting the enhancing tumor core (ET), non-enhancing tumor core (NET), and peritumoral edema (ED). (Data source: BraTS–TCGA-GBM analysis results, licensed under CC-BY-3.0. https://www.cancerimagingarchive.net/analysis-result/brats-tcga-gbm/)

Table 1.14 Public datasets for neuroradiology tasks

Dataset name	# Patients	Modalities	Segmentations/classes
BraTS Intracranial Meningioma (Pre-op Meningioma Dataset)	1344 patients	MRI (T1 pre/post, T2, T2-FLAIR)	Yes, manually annotated tumor sub-compartments
Yale Brain Metastases Longitudinal	1430 patients (11,892 MRI studies)	MRI (T1 pre & post, T2, FLAIR)	No lesion masks (clinical annotations only); all cases have $\geq$1 metastasis
ATLAS (Anatomical Tracings of Lesions After Stroke) v2.0	1271 stroke patients (655 public + 300 hidden test set)	MRI (T1-weighted)	Yes, manual lesion masks for chronic stroke lesions
Acute Stroke MRI Dataset	2888 patients	MRI (Diffusion DWI/ADC; many with FLAIR, T2, T1, SWI, etc.)	Yes, manual acute stroke lesion masks
RSNA Intracranial Hemorrhage (2019 Challenge)	> 25,000 annotated cranial CT exam	CT (non-contrast head CT)	Slice-level hemorrhage subtype labels
HECKTOR (Head & Neck Tumor Segmentation Challenge)	883 cases	PET/CT (FDG-PET with co-registered CT)	Ye, tumor volume and lymph node segmentations
IXI dataset	~600 healthy, normal subjects 2005–2006	MRI (T1, T2 and PD, MRA, DWI)	N/A

Table 1.15 Glioma/brain tumor segmentation datasets

Dataset name	Institution	# Patients/ subjects	Modalities	Segmentations/classes
BraTS (Multiple Years)	U. of Pennsylvania (CBICA), TCIA, others	1251 (BraTS-2021 training)	MRI (T1, T1c, T2, T2-FLAIR)	Glioma sub-regions (Enhancing Tumor, Edema, Necrotic/ Non-Enhancing Core)
BraTS-Africa	TCIA, Lacuna Fund	146	MRI (T1, T1c, T2, T2-FLAIR)	Glioma sub-regions
TCGA-GBM	TCIA / The Cancer Genome Atlas	262	MRI, CT, DX	Glioblastoma Multiforme (GBM)
TCGA-LGG	TCIA / The Cancer Genome Atlas	199	MRI, CT	Low-Grade Glioma (LGG)
UCSF-PDGM	TCIA / UCSF	~500 subjects	MR	Diffuse Glioma
Brain Tumor MRI Dataset (Kaggle)	Kaggle (combination of sources)	7023 images	MRI	4 classes: Glioma, Meningioma, No Tumor, Pituitary

Conclusion

This chapter set out to demystify the complex world of machine learning, framing its role not as a replacement for clinical expertise but as a powerful augmentation. We have explored the technologies that enable a truly symbiotic model of human-machine collaboration, where AI serves to enhance and accelerate the radiologist's capabilities. Starting from the basic principles behind supervised learning to the sophisticated deep learning architectures, we intended to bridge the critical gap between an algorithm's performance and a clinical practitioner's understanding. We discussed Explainable AI (XAI) with practical techniques such as SHAP, Grad-CAM, and saliency maps that are designed to address this gap. These techniques help clinical practitioners to trust the technology better by understanding its reasoning and limitations, thereby transforming the "black box" nature into a transparent and reliable copilot.

The advances discussed in this chapter are driven by the converging trends highlighted at the beginning. AI algorithms are data-hungry and computation-heavy. Such powerful models were trained and refined by the open-source data repositories like TCIA and BraTS, which have not only democratized research but also reliably helped benchmark algorithms. The specialized network architectures adapted to mechanical imaging, such as U-Net, Vision Transformers, are testaments to a community focused on solving real-world medical imaging problems. Hopefully, this chapter has equipped the reader with the conceptual knowledge necessary to appreciate the applications discussed in the subsequent chapters, as well as to critically evaluate them as they are applied in practice.

Ultimately, the path from an algorithm developed in a research lab to clinical impact in physicians and hospitals lies in building robust, interpretable AI systems that enhance accuracy and empower the clinician. As we move forward, the true benchmark of success will not be measured only by standalone algorithmic accuracy, but also by how effectively these tools are integrated into workflows to improve diagnostic confidence, streamline patient care, and ultimately achieve better outcomes. The concepts in this chapter provide the foundational blueprint for understanding, trusting, and effectively wielding the powerful AI technologies that will continue to shape our field.

Suggested Reading

1. Goodfellow I, Bengio Y, Courville A. Deep learning. MIT Press; 2016.
2. Géron A. Hands-on machine learning with Scikit-learn, Keras & TensorFlow: concepts, tools, and techniques to build intelligent systems. 3rd ed. O'Reilly Media; 2022.
3. Aboian M, Bousabarah K, Kazarian E, et al. Clinical implementation of artificial intelligence in neuroradiology with development of a novel workflow-efficient picture archiving and communication system-based automated brain tumor segmentation and radiomic feature extraction. Front Neurosci. 2022;16 https://doi.org/10.3389/fnins.2022.860208.
4. Savage N. Digital assistants aid disease diagnosis. Nature. 2019;573(7775) https://doi.org/10.1038/d41586-019-02870-4.
5. O'Neill TJ, Xi Y, Stehel E, et al. Active reprioritization of the reading worklist using artificial intelligence has a beneficial effect on the turnaround time for interpretation of head CT with intracranial hemorrhage. Radiol Artif Intell. 2020, 3(2):e200024. https://doi.org/10.1148/ryai.2020200024.
6. de Vries BM, Zwezerijnen GJC, Burchell GL, van Velden FHP, van Oordt CWM d H, Boellaard R. Explainable artificial intelligence (XAI) in radiology and nuclear medicine: a literature review. Front Med. 2023;10:1180773. https://doi.org/10.3389/fmed.2023.1180773.
7. Chae A, Yao MS, Sagreiya H, et al. Strategies for implementing machine learning algorithms in the clinical practice of radiology. Radiology. 2024;310(1) https://doi.org/10.1148/radiol.223170.
8. Wagner DT, Tilmans L, Peng KA, et al. Artificial intelligence in neuroradiology: a review of current topics and competition challenges. Diagnostics. 2023;13(16):2670. https://doi.org/10.3390/diagnostics13162670.
9. van Leeuwen KG, de Rooij M, Schalekamp S, van Ginneken B, Rutten M. How does artificial intelligence in radiology improve efficiency and health outcomes? Pediatr Radiol. 2021;52(11):2087. https://doi.org/10.1007/s00247-021-05114-8.
10. Khalighi S, Reddy K, Midya A, Pandav K, Madabhushi A, Abedalthagafi M. Artificial intelligence in neuro-oncology: advances and challenges in brain tumor diagnosis, prognosis, and precision treatment. npj Precis Oncol. 2024;8(1):80. https://doi.org/10.1038/s41698-024-00575-0.
11. Elhalawani H, Mohamed A, White A, et al. Matched computed tomography segmentation and demographic data for oropharyngeal cancer radiomics challenges. Sci Data. 2017;4:170077. https://doi.org/10.1038/sdata.2017.77.
12. Antonelli M, Reinke A, Bakas S, et al. The medical segmentation decathlon. Nat Commun. 2022;13:4128. https://doi.org/10.1038/s41467-022-30695-9.
13. Bakas S, Akbari H, Sotiras A, Bilello M, Rozycki M, Kirby JS, Freymann JB, Farahani K, Davatzikos C. Advancing The Cancer Genome Atlas glioma MRI collections with expert segmentation labels and radiomic features. Sci Data. 2017;4(1):170117. https://doi.org/10.1038/sdata.2017.117.

14. Johnson AEW, Pollard TJ, Berkowitz SJ, et al. MIMIC-CXR, a de-identified publicly available database of chest radiographs with free-text reports. Sci Data. 2019;6:317. https://doi.org/10.1038/s41597-019-0322-0.
15. Zhang S, Xu Y, Usuyama N, Xu H, Bagga J, Tinn R, et al. Biomedclip: a multimodal biomedical foundation model pretrained from fifteen million scientific image-text pairs. 2023. arXiv preprint https://arxiv.org/abs/2303.00915.
16. Ronneberger O, Fischer P, Brox T. U-net: convolutional networks for biomedical image segmentation. In: International conference on medical image computing and computer-assisted intervention. Cham: Springer international publishing; 2015, October. p. 234–41.
17. Dosovitskiy A, Beyer L, Kolesnikov A, Weissenborn D, Zhai X, Unterthiner T, et al. An image is worth 16x16 words: transformers for image recognition at scale. 2020. arXiv preprint https://arxiv.org/abs/2010.11929.
18. Isensee F, Jaeger PF, Kohl SAA, et al. nnU-Net: a self-configuring method for deep learning-based biomedical image segmentation. Nat Methods. 2021;18:203–11. https://doi.org/10.1038/s41592-020-01008-z.
19. Selvaraju RR, Cogswell M, Das A, Vedantam R, Parikh D, Batra D. Grad-cam: visual explanations from deep networks via gradient-based localization. In: Proceedings of the IEEE international conference on computer vision. 2017. pp. 618–26.
20. Ribeiro MT, SinghS., Guestrin C. "Why should i trust you?" Explaining the predictions of any classifier. In: Proceedings of the 22nd ACM SIGKDD international conference on knowledge discovery and data mining. 2016, August. pp. 1135–44).
21. Lundberg SM, Lee SI. A unified approach to interpreting model predictions. In: Advances in neural information processing systems, 30. 2017.
22. Bakas S, Akbari H, Sotiras A, Bilello M, Rozycki M, Kirby J, Freymann J, Farahani K, Davatzikos C. Segmentation labels and Radiomic features for the pre-operative scans of the TCGA-LGG collection [Data set]. The Cancer Imaging Archive. 2017. https://doi.org/10.7937/K9/TCIA.2017.GJQ7R0EF.
23. Bakas S, Akbari H, Sotiras A, Bilello M, Rozycki M, Kirby J, Freymann J, Farahani K, Davatzikos C. Segmentation labels for the pre-operative scans of the TCGA-GBM collection [Data set]. The Cancer Imaging Archive. 2017. https://doi.org/10.7937/K9/TCIA.2017.KLXWJJ1Q.
24. Rückert J, Bloch L, Brüngel R, et al. ROCOv2: radiology objects in COntext version 2, an updated multimodal image dataset. Sci Data. 2024;11(1):688. Published 2024 Jun 26. https://doi.org/10.1038/s41597-024-03496-6.
25. Lu J, Xu W, Chen X, Wang T, Li H. Noninvasive prediction of IDH mutation status in gliomas using preoperative multiparametric MRI radiomics nomogram: a mutlicenter study. Magn Reson Imaging. 2023;104:72–9. https://doi.org/10.1016/j.mri.2023.09.001.
26. Jafari M, Rahmani M, Alibabaie S, et al. Hybrid radiomics and machine learning for brain tumors multi-task classification: an exploratory study on integrating GLCM and curvelet-based features for enhanced accuracy. Health Sci Rep. 2025;8(8):e71195. Published 2025 Aug 20. https://doi.org/10.1002/hsr2.71195.
27. Silva MA, Patel J, Kavouridis V, et al. Machine learning models can detect aneurysm rupture and identify clinical features associated with rupture. World Neurosurg. 2019;131:e46–51. https://doi.org/10.1016/j.wneu.2019.06.231.
28. Xie G, Li T, Ren Y, et al. Radiomics-based infarct features on CT predict hemorrhagic transformation in patients with acute ischemic stroke. Front Neurosci. 2022;16:1002717. Published 2022 Sep 21. https://doi.org/10.3389/fnins.2022.1002717.
29. Xie Y, Jiang B, Gong E, et al. JOURNAL CLUB: use of gradient boosting machine learning to predict patient outcome in acute ischemic stroke on the basis of imaging, demographic, and clinical information. AJR Am J Roentgenol. 2019;212(1):44–51. https://doi.org/10.2214/AJR.18.20260.
30. van Engelen JE, Hoos HH. A survey on semi-supervised learning. Mach Learn. 2020;109:373–440. https://doi.org/10.1007/s10994-019-05855-6.

31. Srivastava N, Hinton G, Krizhevsky A, Sutskever I, Salakhutdinov R. Dropout: a simple way to prevent neural networks from overfitting. J Mach Learn Res. 2014;15(1):1929–58.
32. Plaat A. Deep reinforcement learning. Springer Singapore; 2022. https://doi.org/10.1007/978-981-19-0638-1.
33. Smilkov D, Carter S. TensorFlow playground. n.d. Retrieved September 25, 2025, from https://playground.tensorflow.org
34. Schmidt RM. Recurrent neural networks (RNNs): a gentle introduction and overview. 2019. arXiv preprint https://arxiv.org/abs/1912.05911.
35. Hochreiter S, Schmidhuber J. Long short-term memory. Neural Comput. 1997;9(8):1735–80. https://doi.org/10.1162/neco.1997.9.8.1735.
36. Lee C, Kim Y, Kim YS, Jang J. Automatic disease annotation from radiology reports using artificial intelligence implemented by a recurrent neural network. AJR Am J Roentgenol. 2019;212(4):734–40. https://doi.org/10.2214/AJR.18.19869.
37. Schuster M, Paliwal KK. Bidirectional recurrent neural networks. IEEE Trans Signal Process. 1997;45(11):2673–81. https://doi.org/10.1109/78.650093.
38. Han Y, Yuan Y, Mou L. A dual-view approach to classifying radiology reports by co-training. 2024. arXiv preprint https://arxiv.org/abs/2406.05995.
39. Ng A. Supervised learning [lecture notes]. In: A. Ng, Machine learning. Coursera. n.d. Retrieved from https://www.coursera.org/learn/machine-learning
40. Cardoso, MJ, Li W, Brown R, Ma N, Kerfoot E, Wang Y, Murrey B et al. Monai: an open-source framework for deep learning in healthcare. 2022. arXiv preprint https://arxiv.org/abs/2211.02701.
41. Krizhevsky A, Sutskever I, Hinton GE. ImageNet classification with deep convolutional neural networks. In: Pereira F, Burges CJ, Bottou L, Weinberger KQ, editors. Advances in neural information processing systems, vol. 25. Curran Associates, Inc; 2012.
42. Simonyan K, Zisserman A. Very deep convolutional networks for large-scale image recognition. 2014. arXiv preprint https://arxiv.org/abs/1409.1556
43. Wang X, Peng Y, Lu L, Lu Z, Bagheri M, Summers R. ChestX-ray8: hospital-scale chest X-ray database and benchmarks on weakly-supervised classification and localization of common thorax diseases. In: IEEE CVPR. 2017. pp. 3462–71.
44. Halabi SS, Prevedello LM, Kalpathy-Cramer J, et al. The RSNA pediatric bone age machine learning challenge. Radiology. 2019;290(2):498–503. https://doi.org/10.1148/radiol.2018180736.
45. He K, Zhang X, Ren S, Sun J. Deep residual learning for image recognition. In: Proceedings of the IEEE conference on computer vision and pattern recognition. 2016. pp. 770–8.
46. Huang G, Liu Z, Van Der Maaten L, Weinberger KQ. Densely connected convolutional networks. In: Proceedings of the IEEE conference on computer vision and pattern recognition. 2017. pp. 4700–8.
47. Oktay O, Schlemper J, Folgoc LL, Lee M, Heinrich M, Misawa K, et al. Attention u-net: Learning where to look for the pancreas. 2018. arXiv preprint https://arxiv.org/abs/1804.03999.
48. Niu Z, Zhong G, Yu H. A review on the attention mechanism of deep learning. Neurocomputing. 2021;452:48–62. https://doi.org/10.1016/j.neucom.2021.03.091.
49. Chen LC, Zhu Y, Papandreou G, Schroff F, Adam H.. Encoder-decoder with atrous separable convolution for semantic image segmentation. In: Proceedings of the European conference on computer vision (ECCV). 2018. pp. 801–18.
50. Kamnitsas K, Ledig C, Newcombe VFJ, et al. Efficient multi-scale 3D CNN with fully connected CRF for accurate brain lesion segmentation. Med Image Anal. 2017;36:61–78. https://doi.org/10.1016/j.media.2016.10.004.
51. Tan M, Le Q. Efficientnet: rethinking model scaling for convolutional neural networks. In: International conference on machine learning. PMLR; 2019, May. p. 6105–14.
52. Agarwal D, Berbís MÁ, Luna A, Lipari V, Ballester JB, Díez I d l T. Automated medical diagnosis of Alzheimer's disease using an efficient net convolutional neural network. J Med Syst. 2023;47(1):57. https://doi.org/10.1007/s10916-023-01941-4.

53. Preetha R, Jasmine Pemeena Priyadarsini M, Nisha JS. Brain tumor segmentation using multi-scale attention U-Net with EfficientNetB4 encoder for enhanced MRI analysis. Sci Rep. 2025;15(1) https://doi.org/10.1038/s41598-025-94267-9.
54. Mensah KP, Adekoya FA, Ayidzoe AM, Edward BY. Capsule networks—a survey. J King Saud Univ Comput Inf Sci. 2022;34(1):1295–310. https://doi.org/10.1016/j.jksuci.2019.09.014.
55. Berahmand K, Daneshfar F, Salehi ES, et al. Autoencoders and their applications in machine learning: a survey. Artif Intell Rev. 2024;57:28. https://doi.org/10.1007/s10462-023-10662-6.
56. Solanki A, Naved M. GANs for data augmentation in healthcare. Cham: Springer; 2023. https://doi.org/10.1007/978-3-031-43205-7.
57. Hatamizadeh A, Nath V, Tang Y, Yang D, Roth HR, Xu D. Swin unetr: Swin transformers for semantic segmentation of brain tumors in mri images. In: International MICCAI brainlesion workshop. Cham: Springer International Publishing; 2021, September. p. 272–84.
58. Devlin J, Chang MW, Lee K, Toutanova K. Bert: pre-training of deep bidirectional transformers for language understanding. In: Proceedings of the 2019 conference of the North American chapter of the Association for Computational Linguistics: human language technologies, volume 1 (long and short papers). 2019, June. pp. 4171–86.
59. Radford A, Narasimhan K, Salimans T, Sutskever I. Improving language understanding by generative pre-training [preprint]. OpenAI. Published 2018. Accessed 25 Sept 2025.
60. Yang L, Zhang Z, Song Y, Hong S, Xu R, Zhao Y, et al. Diffusion models: a comprehensive survey of methods and applications. ACM Comput Surv. 2023;56(4):1–39.
61. Wang Y, Peng J, Dai Y, et al. Enhancing vision-language models for medical imaging: bridging the 3D gap with innovative slice selection. In: Proceedings of the 38th conference on neural information processing systems (NeurIPS 2024), datasets & benchmarks track. 2024. Accessed 25 Sept 2025.
62. Radford A, Kim JW, Hallacy C, Ramesh A, Goh G, Agarwal S, Sastry G, et al. Learning transferable visual models from natural language supervision. In: International conference on machine learning. PmLR; 2021. p. 8748–63.
63. Tang Y, Yuan Y, Tao F, Tang M. Cross-modal augmented transformer for automated medical report generation. IEEE J Transl Eng Health Med. 2025;13:33–48. Published 2025 Jan 29. https://doi.org/10.1109/JTEHM.2025.3536441.
64. Chicco D, Jurman G. The advantages of the Matthews correlation coefficient (MCC) over F1 score and accuracy in binary classification evaluation. BMC Genomics. 2020;21:6. https://doi.org/10.1186/s12864-019-6413-7.
65. Bradley AP. The use of the area under the ROC curve in the evaluation of machine learning algorithm performance. Pattern Recogn. 1997;30(7):1145–59. https://doi.org/10.1016/S0031-3203(96)00142-2.
66. Davis J, Goadrich M. The relationship between Precision-Recall and ROC curves. In: Proceedings of the 23rd international conference on machine learning (ICML '06). New York: Association for Computing Machinery; 2006. p. 233–40. https://doi.org/10.1145/1143844.1143874.
67. Zou KH, Warfield SK, Bharatha A, et al. Statistical validation of image segmentation quality based on a spatial overlap index. Acad Radiol. 2004;11(2):178–89. https://doi.org/10.1016/s1076-6332(03)00671-8.
68. Hicks SA, Strümke I, Thambawita V, et al. On evaluation metrics for medical applications of artificial intelligence. Sci Rep. 2022;12(1):5979. Published 2022 Apr 8. https://doi.org/10.1038/s41598-022-09954-8.

69. Huttenlocher DP, Klanderman GA, Rucklidge WJ. Comparing images using the Hausdorff distance. IEEE Trans Pattern Anal Mach Intell. 1993;15(9):850–63. https://doi.org/10.1109/34.232073.
70. Yeghiazaryan V, Voiculescu I. Family of boundary overlap metrics for the evaluation of medical image segmentation. J Med Imaging (Bellingham) 2018;5(1):015006. doi:https://doi.org/10.1117/1.JMI.5.1.015006.
71. Zhang L, Wang M, Liu M, Zhang D. A survey on deep learning for neuroimaging-based brain disorder analysis. Front Neurosci. 2020;14:779. Published 2020 Oct 8. https://doi.org/10.3389/fnins.2020.00779.
72. Celaya A, Rivière BM, Fuentes DT. A generalized surface loss for reducing the Hausdorff distance in medical imaging segmentation. 2023.
73. Lin C-Y. ROUGE: a package for automatic evaluation of summaries. In: Proceedings of the workshop on text summarization branches out, post-conference workshop of ACL 2004, July 25–26, 2004, Barcelona, Spain.
74. Papineni K, Roukos S, Ward T, Zhu W-J. BLEU: a method for automatic evaluation of machine translation. In: Proceedings of the 40th annual meeting of the Association for Computational Linguistics (ACL), July 2002, Philadelphia, PA. pp. 311–318.
75. Banerjee S, Lavie A. METEOR: an automatic metric for MT evaluation with improved correlation with human judgments. In: Goldstein J, Lavie A, Lin C-Y, Voss C, editors. Proceedings of the ACL workshop on intrinsic and extrinsic evaluation measures for machine translation and/or summarization; June 2005. Ann Arbor: Association for Computational Linguistics; 2005. p. 65–72. Available from: https://aclanthology.org/W05-0909/.
76. Horé A, Ziou, D. Image quality metrics: PSNR vs. SSIM. In: 2010 20th international conference on pattern recognition, Istanbul, Turkey, 2010, pp. 2366–9. https://doi.org/10.1109/ICPR.2010.579.
77. Tejani AS, Klontzas ME, Gatti AA, et al. Checklist for artificial intelligence in medical imaging (CLAIM): 2024 update. Radiol Artif Intell. 2024;6(4):e240300. https://doi.org/10.1148/ryai.240300.
78. Collins GS, Moons KGM, Dhiman P, et al. TRIPOD+AI statement: updated guidance for reporting clinical prediction models that use regression or machine learning methods. BMJ. 2024;385:e078378. Published 2024 Apr 16. https://doi.org/10.1136/bmj-2023-078378.
79. Hernandez-Boussard T, Bozkurt S, Ioannidis JPA, Shah NH. MINIMAR (MINimum Information for Medical AI Reporting): developing reporting standards for artificial intelligence in health care. J Am Med Inform Assoc. 2020;27(12):2011–5. https://doi.org/10.1093/jamia/ocaa088.
80. Barry N, Kendrick J, Molin K, et al. Evaluating the impact of the Radiomics Quality Score: a systematic review and meta-analysis. Eur Radiol. 2025;35(3):1701–13. https://doi.org/10.1007/s00330-024-11341-y.
81. Liu X, Cruz Rivera S, Moher D, et al. Reporting guidelines for clinical trial reports for interventions involving artificial intelligence: the CONSORT-AI extension. Nat Med. 2020;26:1364–74. https://doi.org/10.1038/s41591-020-1034-x.
82. Lekadir K, Osuala R, Gallin C, Lazrak N, Kushibar K, Tsakou G, Aussó S et al. FUTURE-AI: guiding principles and consensus recommendations for trustworthy artificial intelligence in medical imaging. 2021. arXiv preprint https://arxiv.org/abs/2109.09658.
83. Chen H, Gomez C, Huang CM, et al. Explainable medical imaging AI needs human-centered design: guidelines and evidence from a systematic review. npj Digit Med. 2022;5:156. https://doi.org/10.1038/s41746-022-00699-2.

84. Pinto-Coelho L. How artificial intelligence is shaping medical imaging technology: a survey of innovations and applications. Bioengineering (Basel). 2023;10(12):1435. Published 2023 Dec 18. https://doi.org/10.3390/bioengineering10121435.
85. Sahlsten J, Jaskari J, Wahid KA, et al. Application of simultaneous uncertainty quantification and segmentation for oropharyngeal cancer use-case with Bayesian deep learning. Commun Med. 2024;4(1) https://doi.org/10.1038/s43856-024-00528-5.
86. Roschewitz M, Khara G, Yearsley J, et al. Automatic correction of performance drift under acquisition shift in medical image classification. Nature Commun. 2023;14(1):6608. https://doi.org/10.1038/s41467-023-42396-y.
87. Kirillov A, Mintun E, Ravi N, Mao H, Rolland C, Gustafson L, Xiao, T, et al. Segment anything. In: Proceedings of the IEEE/CVF international conference on computer vision. 2023. pp. 4015–26.
88. Microsoft. BiomedCLIP-PubMedBERT_256-vit_base_patch16_224 [machine learning model]. Hugging Face. Published 2024. https://huggingface.co/microsoft/BiomedCLIP--PubMedBERT_256-vit_base_patch16_224. Accessed 25 Sept 2025.
89. PyCaret PyCaret: an open-source, low-code machine learning library in python [software]. PyCaret; April 2020–. https://pycaret.org/. Accessed 25 Sept 2025.
90. He Y, Yang D, Roth H, Zhao C, Xu D. Dints: differentiable neural network topology search for 3d medical image segmentation. In: Proceedings of the IEEE/CVF conference on computer vision and pattern recognition. 2021. pp. 5841–50.
91. Diaz-Pinto A, Alle S, Nath V, et al. MONAI label: a framework for AI-assisted interactive labeling of 3D medical images. Med Image Anal. 2024;95:103207. https://doi.org/10.1016/j.media.2024.103207.
92. Wasserthal J, Breit HC, Meyer MT, et al. TotalSegmentator: robust segmentation of 104 anatomic structures in CT images. Radiol Artif Intell. 2023;5(5):e230024. https://doi.org/10.1148/ryai.230024.
93. van Griethuysen JJM, Fedorov A, Parmar C, Hosny A, Aucoin N, Narayan V, Beets-Tan RGH, Fillon-Robin JC, Pieper S, Aerts HJWL. Computational Radiomics system to decode the radiographic phenotype. Cancer Res. 2017;77(21):e104–7. https://doi.org/10.1158/0008-5472.CAN-17-0339.
94. Fedorov A, Beichel R, Kalpathy-Cramer J, et al. 3D slicer as an image computing platform for the Quantitative Imaging Network. Magn Reson Imaging. 2012;30(9):1323–41. https://doi.org/10.1016/j.mri.2012.05.001.
95. LaBella D, Khanna O, McBurney-Lin S, et al. A multi-institutional meningioma MRI dataset for automated multi-sequence image segmentation. Sci Data. 2024;11:496. https://doi.org/10.1038/s41597-024-03350-9.
96. Chadha S, Weiss D, Janas A, Ramakrishnan D, Hager T, Osenberg K, Willms K, Zhu J, Chiang V, Bakas S, Maleki N, Sritharan DV, Schoenherr S, Westerhoff M, Zawalich M, Davis M, Malhotra A, Bousabarah K, Deusch C, Lin M, Aneja S, Aboian MS. Yale longitudinal dataset of brain metastases on MRI with associated clinical data (Yale-Brain-Mets-Longitudinal) (Version 1) [Data set]. The Cancer Imaging Archive. 2025. https://doi.org/10.7937/3YAT-E768.
97. Liew SL, Lo BP, Donnelly MR, et al. A large, curated, open-source stroke neuroimaging dataset to improve lesion segmentation algorithms. Sci Data. 2022;9(1):320. Published 2022 Jun 16. https://doi.org/10.1038/s41597-022-01401-7.
98. Andrearczyk V, Oreiller V, Abobakr M, et al. Overview of the HECKTOR challenge at MICCAI 2022: automatic head and neck tumor segmentation and outcome prediction in PET/CT. Head Neck Tumor Chall (2022). 2023;13626:1–30. https://doi.org/10.1007/978-3-031-27420-6_1.
99. IXI dataset. Brain Development. Funded by EPSRC GR/S21533/02.
100. Qure.ai. *qER*—AI Stroke & TBI Care (Head CT). Qure.ai website. https://www.qure.ai/product/qer. Accessed 26 Sept 2025.

101. U.S. Food and Drug Administration. *510(k) Premarket Notification—Qure.ai qER*. K200921. Published June 17, 2020. Accessed 26 Sept 2025.
102. Aidoc. Clinical AI solutions for healthcare providers (neurovascular). Aidoc website. https://www.aidoc.com/home/. Accessed 26 Sept 2025.
103. U.S. Food and Drug Administration. 510(k) Premarket Notification—Aidoc BriefCase (ICH). K180647. Published August 1, 2018. Accessed 26 Sept 2025.
104. Labelbox. How to automate medical imaging with AI. Labelbox Guides. Published March 6, 2024. https://labelbox.com/guides/how-to-automate-medical-imaging-with-ai. Accessed 26 Sept 2025.
105. V7 Labs. Auto-Annotate. V7 Docs. https://docs.v7labs.com/docs/auto-annotate. Accessed 26 Sept 2025.
106. Calabrese E, Villanueva-Meyer JE, Rudie JD, Rauschecker AM, Baid U, Bakas S, Cha S, Mongan JT, Hess CP. The UCSF preoperative diffuse glioma MRI (UCSF-PDGM) dataset. Radioly Artif Intell. 2022; https://doi.org/10.1148/ryai.220058.
107. Fedorov A, Beichel R, Kalpathy-Cramer J, Finet J, Fillion-Robin J-C, Pujol S, Bauer C, Jennings D, Fennessy FM, Sonka M, Buatti J, Aylward SR, Miller JV, Pieper S, Kikinis R. 3D slicer as an image computing platform for the quantitative imaging network. Magn Reson Imaging. 2012;30(9):1323–41. PMCID: PMC3466397.

Chapter 2
Implementing AI in Neuroradiology

Ramkumar Rajabathar Babu Jai Shanker, Amogh Shetty, and Daniel Thomas Ginat

Introduction

AI algorithms hold great promise to revolutionize neuroradiology in multiple ways, but translating them into clinical reality is not straightforward. More often than not, several underappreciated challenges can either make or break the model's success in practice. In particular, medical imaging, and neuroradiology in particular, is riddled with pitfalls, including multi-center variability, label and domain shift, segmentation variability, and small-sample uncertainties that are rarely visible in high-level summaries. The goal of this chapter is to provide an end-to-end walk-through of three representative pipelines that highlight practical considerations, methodological choices, and hidden traps, and to cover the research design from conception through internal validation and testing. Learning how to navigate these challenges is essential not only for developing robust AI tools but also for critically evaluating published studies and preparing models for clinical deployment.

R. R. Babu Jai Shanker (✉)
Biological Sciences Division, University of Chicago, Chicago, IL, USA

A. Shetty
Department of Biology, Rensselaer Polytechnic Institute, Troy, NY, USA

D. T. Ginat
Co-founder, Rad-Lab.ai, Chicago, IL, USA

D. T. Ginat (ed.), *Artificial Intelligence in Neuroradiology*,
https://doi.org/10.1007/978-3-032-24568-7_2

End-to-End Framework: Data, Development, and Deployment

While there are several ways in which research pipelines for machine learning algorithms can be defined, the basic underlying principles can be summarized using a standard framework (Fig. 2.1). Study design is the most important stage for any research project, but it is even more so for a machine learning project because it is at this stage that many key elements of the project are decided. Only when the machine learning task is clearly defined can the primary and secondary evaluation metrics be chosen appropriately. For example, if the research goal is to utilize CT radiomics of lymph nodes to predict if lymph nodes are metastatic, the machine learning task is a classification task and the evaluation metrics would be focused on measuring the model's discriminatory power such as AUROC, type-1 and type-2 errors, and calibration. On the other hand, if the research goal is to develop an auto-segmentation model that can segment gliomas from MRI images, then the task is a segmentation task and the evaluation metrics would be focused on evaluating the volumetric overlap and boundary agreement. If the research goal is to utilize LLMs to read radiology reports and come up with report labels or differential diagnosis, the machine learning task can either be a classification task or generative task. If we design it to be a generative task, the evaluation metrics would be focused on assessing how many of the essential findings are captured in the generated text. This can be evaluated quantitatively using metrics such as BLEU, ROUGE, and qualitatively using ordinal acceptability scores from a clinician, and error taxonomies.

Current research trends have shown that machine learning models tend to perform really well in single-center studies with hold-out test sets but often encounter a loss in performance when expanding to external test sets and centers. It is

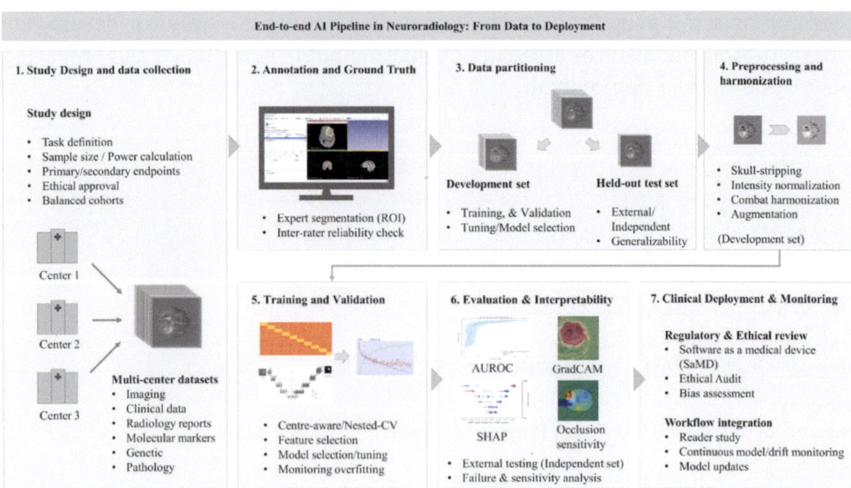

Fig. 2.1 End-to-end AI pipeline in neuroradiology, from data to deployment. (Example MRI images from BraTS-TCGA-GBM, licensed under CC-BY-3.0)

recommended that any research project involving machine learning models either have data collected from multiple institutions/hospitals (centers) or have the developed models validated (in this case, the term validation is used to refer to the testing step in the machine learning pipeline) using cases from an external center.

The second stage is to define the ground truths or reference standard. In the case of classification or lymph nodes classification, the gold standard of ground truth would be the nodal status from the histopathology exams (biopsy). In the case of segmentation and generative tasks, ground truths are often defined using inputs from the experts (neuroradiologists) in the form of manually labelled ROIs or report categories/differential diagnoses, respectively. If there are multi-parametric sequences or multimodal data, co-registration is done before annotation to bring the sequences into a common space. Multiple human annotators are preferred to not only improve the learning process but also to set a ceiling on expected performance from the machine learning model.

Data partitioning is carried out to split the dataset into a training set, which is used for training and internal validation, feature selection, hyperparameter tuning, classification probability threshold selection and other decisions, and a held-out test set, which is used solely for performance measurement to assess generalizability of the developed model. At this stage, it is essential to perform center-aware data partitioning, ensuring that data from any given center appear exclusively in either the development set or the held-out test set, but not in both.

Using the development set only, the preprocessing and harmonization steps are carried out. Preprocessing steps help the model learn only from relevant information. For example, z-score normalization or ComBat harmonization helps remove center-specific (site-of-acquisition) effects from the data. Without preprocessing and harmonization, models in multi-center settings tend to learn site-specific characteristics rather than biologically relevant features. Data augmentation is critical not only for increasing the training data size, but also to make the model more robust to noise and shifts.

Prior to model training, the cross-validation setup is defined, and this depends on the data at hand. K-fold cross-validation is a recommended step since neuroradiology datasets typically have a limited sample size. With a single train-test split of small datasets, the performance estimates may be quite unstable. In the case of segmentation, the folds can be split by stratifying on gross tumor volume so that each fold learns from a mix of various tumor sizes. Decisions around early stopping, hyperparameter tuning (grid search), and overfitting are also made with cross-validation.

One such use of cross-validation is for radiomics models, where the number of features is typically very high (where the number of features is higher than the number of samples) since they include shape, intensity, and texture features. In this setting, it is critical to select a limited set of parsimonious features that are stable. A nested cross-validation setup can help with feature selection, where only stable features (features selected across multiple inner folds) are selected. Specifically, feature selection is performed independently within each inner training fold, and features that are consistently selected across a majority of these folds are retained for model training, as their repeated selection indicates robustness to data resampling and reduced susceptibility to overfitting.

Another use-case of cross-validation is in choosing loss functions. Usually, loss functions are chosen according to the task so that the model learns the right patterns required to perform the task. For example, for large tumors, volumetric loss functions such as a combination of dice and cross-entropy loss work better. However, such volumetric loss functions can miss smaller tumors since the penalty for missing small volumes is generally low. Boundary loss functions are more sensitive to smaller tumors and perform better in segmenting the contours, thereby making the segmentations align better with clinical workflows. The cross-validation scores provide unbiased, stable estimates of performance within the development set. In this step, it is critical to avoid data leakage where some information from the internal validation set is inadvertently used for the training set. For example, methods to address missing values, outliers, and normalization, class imbalance should be applied only within the training portion of the outer/inner fold.

The next step involves putting the developed models to test using either a held-out test set or an external test set, preferably from a different center. These estimates are used to show how well the models would generalize to unseen data. During inference, the preprocessing steps that were identified during the training steps are applied using the same settings (for example, normalization ranges, missing values imputation values, etc.) and the predictions are derived for the test set. In certain cases, when the class imbalance is high, it is important to supplement performance estimates such as AUROC with the AUPRC and other metrics to show and estimate true performance. To assess clinical relevance, classifications should also be accompanied by their calibration scores to identify if the model is overconfident in certain circumstances.

One of the main challenges with AI models is that their inner workings are not very well understood by practitioners. For example, when a model predicts a lymph node to be metastatic, is it important to also understand why? In the case of generative algorithms, while using closed-weight networks such as GPT-4o and Gemini 1.5 Pro in the clinical setting, it is desirable to return outputs with supporting evidence (e.g., retrieved passages), uncertainty signals, and traceability. Therefore, a major part of user-adoption and acceptance is the presentation of explainable outputs (SHAP force plots, GradCAM transformations, Occlusion sensitivity, LLM reasoning) along with the output predictions. These outputs also help build trust with clinicians since they provide transparency into not only the model's strengths but also its weaknesses. Failures are investigated as to why they occur and whether there is a systemic reason behind them.

Finally, prior to clinical deployment, models must be evaluated for how they integrate into and interact with existing clinical workflows. This can be done through shadow ("silent") implementations, in which model outputs are presented to physicians without influencing clinical decision-making and are used solely for feedback collection, or through prospective pilot studies conducted in real-world settings. If the classification model is used for workload prioritization, the clinical metrics include concordance, time savings, interobserver consistency, and treatment plan outcomes. Prior to deployment, appropriate regulatory and ethical clearance must be obtained. Post-deployment, the performance of the model is monitored continuously for any drift so that the performance does not drop below acceptable limits.

Use-Case 1: Glioma Classification Using Radiomic Features

Radiomics-based Glioma classification is a common example of a noninvasive decision-support task. In this use-case, the study goal is to utilize radiomic features from glioblastoma (GBM) and low-grade glioma (LGG) segmentations on MRI. One of the key practical goals of this use-case, is to build a model that performs well beyond a single-center dataset and does not break or fail when deployed at a new hospital/institution. Through this use-case, we explore common pitfalls such as multi-center heterogeneity, class imbalance, and feature sensitivity to segmentation and preprocessing.

Multi-center Heterogeneity

The machine learning task is a binary classification task, and the evaluation metrics are AUROC, AUPRC, minimum acceptable sensitivity/specificity, and calibration (Brier) score. A key aspect of this dataset is the site confounding, where some of the centers only include either LGG or GBM data (Fig. 2.2).

One of the key practical goals of this study is to avoid the common pitfall with AI algorithms, where they perform really well in a single-center study, but their performance degrades when deployed at a new institution. So, in this study the multi-center heterogeneity is not a challenge but a feature. As illustrated in Fig. 2.2,

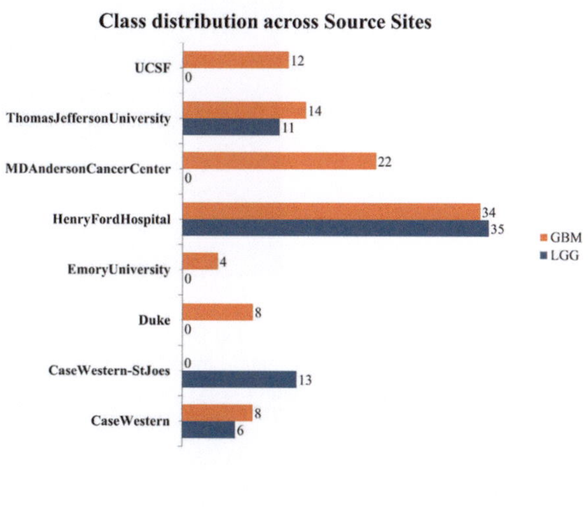

Fig. 2.2 Class distribution of glioma subtypes (GBM vs. LGG) across contributing source sites in the TCIA multi-institutional cohort. (Source: The Cancer Imaging Archive (TCIA))

the number of cases with Glioblastoma (GBM) is higher than those with low-grade glioma (LGG). Therefore, class imbalance is an important factor in this cohort.

Inter-observer Variability

The dataset is derived from the TCIA BraTS-TCGA-GBM collection that contains the segmentation labels and subsequently derived radiomic features for pre-operative multimodal MRI scans that were identified in the TCGA-GBM collection using radiological assessment (Fig. 2.3). Since radiomic features are highly sensitive to ROI definitions, the segmentations were first produced by an automated state-of-the-art model and later revised (misclassifications were manually corrected) by an expert board-certified neuroradiologist. It is worth noting that in many cases, ROI labeling is often performed without the help of baseline models directly on image editing solutions such as 3D Slicer. Recently, active learning, where the underlying models are trained while the ROIs are being annotated, has helped make the annotation process more time-efficient. Instead of manually contouring each region, the manual labeling process is reduced to a few clicks that either correct or specify new regions for the underlying model to further learn from. For example, MONAI Label uses DeepGrow, DeepEdit and Segment-Anything Model (SAM) to support the annotation process using active learning.

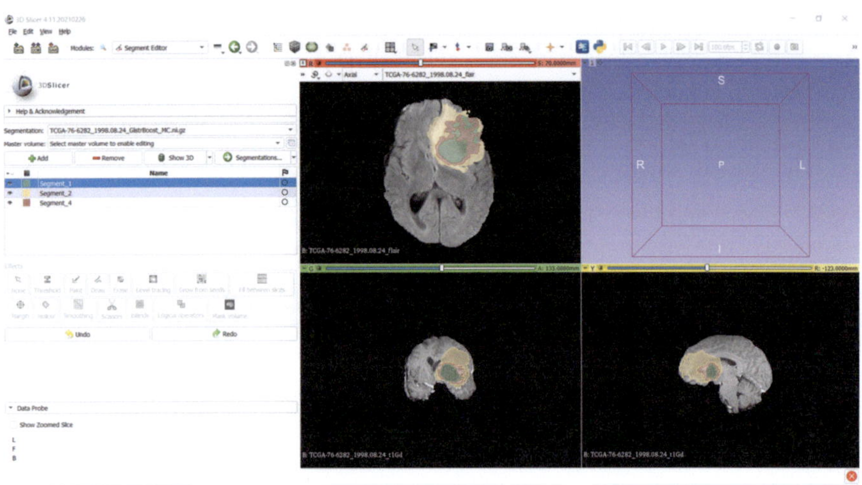

Fig. 2.3 Screenshot of the segmentation labeling tool 3D slicer illustrating the output labels for gliomas on MRI from the segmentation model used prior to manual correction. (Example from BraTS-TCGA-GBM, licensed under CC-BY-3.0)

Table 2.1 Sample splits using a center-aware nested cross-validation split with three outer folds and two inner folds

		Training set			Internal validation set		
Outer fold	Inner fold	Centers	GBM (n)	LGG (n)	Centers	GBM (n)	LGG (n)
A	A1	Case Western, Duke, Emory University	20	6	Thomas Jefferson University, UCSF	26	11
A	A2	Thomas Jefferson University, UCSF	26	11	Case Western, Duke, Emory University	20	6
B	B1	Thomas Jefferson University, UCSF	26	11	Case Western—St Joes, Emory University, MD Anderson Cancer Center	26	13
B	B2	Case Western—St Joes, Emory University, MD Anderson Cancer Center	26	13	Thomas Jefferson University, UCSF	26	11
C	C1	Case Western, Duke	16	6	Case Western—St Joes, MD Anderson Cancer Center	22	13
C	C2	Case Western—St Joes, MD Anderson Cancer Center	22	13	Case Western, Duke	16	6

Source: TCIA

Center-Aware Data Partitioning

In this multi-center dataset, performing a simple random patient-level split would leak site-specific information into both training and validation (internal) sets. This pitfall may produce inflated performance estimates that are not realistic. Therefore, one of the sites (for example, Henry Ford Hospital) is held out as an independent test set. The center-aware splitting needs to be performed even on the development set while partitioning the cross-validation folds (Table 2.1). This is to avoid unintentionally "peeking" at the validation (internal) data while tuning the hyperparameter and selecting features.

Missing Not at Random (MNAR)

In this example, for some patients, when the volume of enhancing tumor (ET) or edema (ED) is zero, the ET and ED-related radiomic features are all missing since they are not defined. In this case, it is important to treat these missing values as Missing Not at Random (MNAR). Commonly used missing value treatment techniques such as mean imputation or deletion may introduce significant bias and these values need to be treated using MNAR specific methods such as creating a new dummy variable (paired with the corresponding biological feature VOLUME_ET set to 0) to let the model know that such cases include imputed ET-related values that should not be treated the same way as the other cases. Additionally, these treatment methods. should be carried out only using the training portion of the inner-fold or outer fold to avoid data leakage.

Preprocessing and Harmonization

Some preprocessing steps such as skull-stripping and co-registration were carried out prior to passing the images through the segmentation model. For co-registration, rigid transformations with 6 degrees of freedom (DOF) are typically sufficient when the images are from the same session, but affine transformations with 12 DOF work better when there are motion changes. Symmetric Normalization (SyN) in Advanced Normalization Tools (ANTs), provides a powerful non-linear image registration method by finding the shortest, smoothest path between images without favoring a fixed/moving image.

Image transformations such as z-scoring or scaling are applied to place features on a comparable scale, given the diverse units and value ranges (e.g., volume in mm^3 vs. texture energies in arbitrary units). Combat harmonization is a method that adjusts the mean and standard deviation of feature distributions from different "batches" (in this case centers or scanners) to align them to a single reference.

In this specific dataset, the authors have used Brain Extraction Tool (BET), Multi-Atlas Skull-Stripping (MASS) and MUlti-atlas region Segmentation utilizing Ensembles (MUSE) for skull-stripping, FLIRT for co-registration and the radiomic features have been derived using CaPTk. However, other tools such as PyRadiomics are also commonly used for extraction of radiomic features. It is important to use software implementations that follow the technical guidelines of the Image Biomarker Standardization Initiative (IBSI) so that the radiomic features are consistently in a reproducible, benchmarked, harmonized and well-documented manner so that these models build the required trust among clinicians and regulatory bodies. This is necessary for integrating radiomics into routine clinical practice for diagnosis, prognostication, and treatment planning.

Model Complexity and Overfitting

Model training is the step where all the prior steps are put together for implementation. While typical machine learning pipelines that involve binary classification tasks carry out feature processing (removal of multicollinearity, dimensionality reduction, oversampling/undersampling, etc.) as part of the preprocessing step, in a radiomics ML pipeline, it is important to consider it within the model training step. This is because radiomics pipelines are natively high-dimensional (number of features typically much larger than number of samples) and feature selection is a step that is considered part of the tuning process, which determines the best performing classifier not only from discriminative performance but also from a model

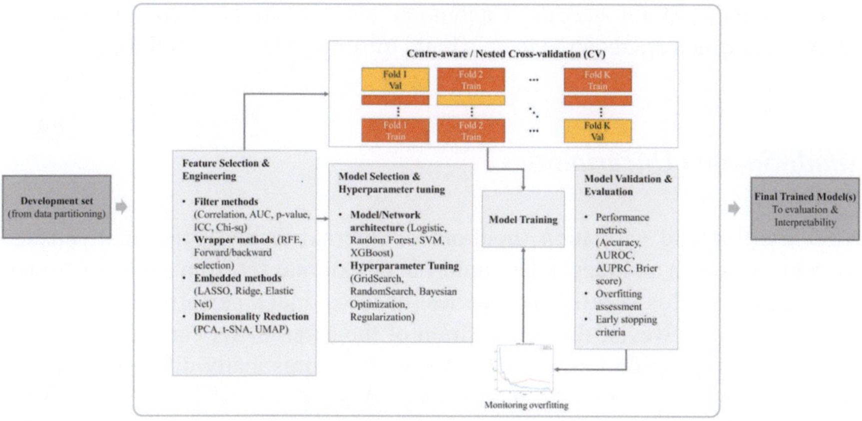

Fig. 2.4 Illustration of a training framework for a classification task using radiomic features

parsimony and stability standpoint. The radiomic features (typically along with features from other modalities such as clinical features, genomic features, etc.) are selected using filter-based methods, which assign independent scores to each feature, wrapper-based methods, which select optimal feature subsets from all possible subsets, and embedded methods, which use the feature selection as part of the model building directly.

Popular choices for binary classification tasks include traditional methods such as Logistic Regression, Random Forest, Support Vector Machines, Gradient boosting, and deep learning algorithms that include multi-layer neural networks (Fig. 2.4). Radiomics use-cases typically include case cohorts in the few hundreds of patients, which makes traditional methods a better fit. Deep learning architectures, which are of higher complexity, require larger cohorts and tend to overfit easily. Ensemble models, as used in random forests, have an advantage since they not only handle feature interactions better but also are more robust to overfitting. SVM is known for its ability to handle datasets with high dimensionality, as the algorithm optimizes the selection of a hyperplane in a high-dimensional space.

Preventing overfitting is a top priority for radiomics models since it is especially easy to select a group of features and a complex model architecture that works really well for the training set but fails to generalize well. Cross-validation ensures that the model performs well across folds and makes it easier to check that the performance does not drastically drop from the training set to the validation (internal) set. Data augmentations are relatively rare for radiomics studies since such features are highly sensitive to slight perturbations.

Class imbalance is addressed by using oversampling or undersampling methods. Models are also typically evaluated along multiple performance metrics (AUPRC in addition to AUROC) if class imbalance is a concern.

Calibration scores, which measure how well the model's prediction probabilities match its actual likelihood of outcomes, ensure the model is not consistently overestimating certain classes. Calibration curves can help spot over/under-confidence, which are required to help build trust in a clinical workflow.

Small-Sample Uncertainties

After training and validation (held-out or internal testing), the final selected model is tested on an independent hold-out or external set from a different institution/scanner. This is often the true test of the model's performance in a real-world setting. However, the composition of the external set can either be quite similar in composition to the development set or drastically different and caution is needed in interpreting such results. When point estimates are reported along with their 95% confidence intervals, it helps to address the small-sample uncertainties that come with a limited number of cases in the test sets. When confidence intervals are narrower, it signals a more reliable interpretation of performance.

Failure Analysis

In the clinical setting, it is important for practitioners to be aware of the limitations and failure modes of the machine learning model. Failure analysis examines the cases where the model predictions went wrong and explores the patterns behind why a model falsely classified an LGG as GBM (FP) or the other way around. SHAP plots (waterfall plots) provide explanations from the quantitative side, but it is important to correlate that with qualitative explanations from the MRI images.

Summary

To summarize, we discussed several challenges and pitfalls from a practical perspective and current best practices to address them.

Multi-center Data & Domain Shift Models trained on datasets from one center often underperform (fail to generalize) on datasets from another center, so it is recommended to use diverse training datasets that are large and heterogeneous.

Segmentation Variability Slight variations in the segmentation outlines can cause significant changes in subsequently extracted radiomic features. It is therefore recommended to use consistent, standardized segmentation guidelines, such as consensus methodology from multiple experts or manual editing of masks created by active learning algorithms (to reduce manual error). Intra/inter reader tests are required, and the feature stability should be reported using Intra-class correlation coefficients (ICC).

Feature Preprocessing Reproducibility of radiomic features (extraction, filtering, and discretization) is a challenge. It is recommended to use software implementations that follow IBSI standards to ensure standardization of features that facilitate clinical trust and adoption. Missing data for certain features that may not be missing at random (MNAR) should be addressed using appropriate imputation strategies. Always apply preprocessing steps (missing value imputation, feature scaling/normalization, feature selection ReliefF/LASSO) only on the training portion of the outer/inner splits to avoid "data leakage" and artificially inflating performance. Highly correlated features must be removed using correlation-filtering or LASSO methods.

Small Sample Challenges It is a major challenge to obtain high-quality labeled data for radiomics models. Small samples need extra attention to ensure the models are not too complex for the task (avoiding overfitting in high variance low bias situations) and small sample uncertainties are adequately reported using 95% CIs along with point estimates.

Interpretability AI algorithms are often considered "black-box" methods, but advancements in explainability methods are changing this belief. Explainability methods such as SHAP and LIME are demystifying the decision-making process within the model and also provide valuable insights into which radiomic features drove the model's predictions. It is recommended to use these methods to carry out failure analysis and explore the decision-making for common type-1 (false positive) or type-2 (false negative) errors. Further, correlating these findings with the underlying imaging and segmentations provides additional insights to the clinician who would eventually use such tools.

By carefully addressing these challenges, radiomics models can provide insightful results and be integrated well into the clinical workflow in line with emerging standards for trustworthy AI in medicine. A well-designed study is more likely to stand the test of external/independent multi-center test evaluation. Additionally, such models can also offer insight into novel features or biomarkers that can help improve knowledge of certain diagnostic features.

Use-Case 2: Automated Tumor Segmentation

Image segmentation is one of the most widely applied use-cases in radiology. In neuroradiology, most segmentation tasks involve isolating normal brain structures, delineating blood vessels and aneurysms, tumor segmentation, and lesion segmentation. Automated tumor segmentation using artificial intelligence can provide a time-efficient and consistent way to measure and characterize tumors (and tumor core, enhancing tumor, and edema) that is crucial for diagnosis, monitoring, and treatment planning. Tumor segmentation is a major focus of international challenges such as the Multimodal Brain Tumor Segmentation (BraTS) for the past decade. Unlike classification algorithms that produce a binary or multi-class prediction, segmentation algorithms produce a pixel-voxel output mask that indicates tumor vs. normal tissues. In this section, we will discuss an end-to-end deep learning segmentation pipeline for glioma segmentation and highlight some of the practical challenges and pitfalls that are unique to this task.

How Many Cases Are Needed for the Training Set?

During the study design phase, the machine learning task is defined along with the evaluation metrics. In this use-case, the machine learning task is to build a segmentation model that can segment brain tumors (gliomas) on input MRI sequences.

Data collection: While there is not one universal "required N," the general rule is to capture as much information as possible within the training set to help the deep learning architectures learn effectively. While power analysis can help calculate the required evaluation set size (testing/reader study) in hypothesis-testing, i.e., does the trained U-Net perform better than the baseline segmentation method, it is a poor fit for calculating the required sample size for the training set. Deep learning algorithms typically perform better with a higher number of cases, but it is also important to ensure the training set covers as much variance as possible, such as scanners, centers, tumor characteristics (grades, locations, size), and patient demographics. For example, the RSNA-ASNR-MICCAI-BraTS-2021 dataset contains brain MRI scans (T1, T1c, T2, T2-FLAIR) for 1480 glioma patients from multiple institutions (scanners/protocols) that reflect real-world heterogeneity. While some well-defined anatomies such as those requiring a lesser number of cases ~10–30 cases, some of the harder tasks such as tumor segmentation often require hundreds of cases.

Rigorous data collection is often the most valuable tool in addressing bias. Sampling bias, where the data collected is not representative of the target population, can be addressed by collecting data from multiple centers and by carrying out exploratory data analysis to ensure that the distribution of patients is representative of the overall target population.

Segmentation Variability

Manual segmentation is tedious and the annotations can vary between experts due to subjective judgment and imaging artifacts. Annotation guidelines that specify how commonly expected ambiguities can be resolved can help generate consistent segmentations. Additionally, some studies report using a third reviewer, who is often a more senior neuroradiologist, to help drive consensus between the annotations. Slight inter-observer variability may still remain even after consensus, since differentiating tumor margins or edema can be tricky, but robust algorithms should ideally be able to tolerate such slight variations. Some studies report the inter-rater Dice score and treat that as an upper benchmark for expected model performance. For example, if radiologists agree 90% on average, that is a realistic ceiling for segmentation performance.

Data Augmentations

Unlike radiomics classification models, data augmentations are imperative for segmentation algorithms since they not only help address low sample sizes and also make the model robust to slight variations or noise. In practice, data augmentations typically include a combination of spatial transforms (small rotations, translations, scaling or elastic deformations), intensity transforms (noise, blur, contrast/gamma changes), and simulated artifacts (low-resolution, k-spike noise, Rician noise, coarse dropout) (Fig. 2.5). Such augmentations are typically applied on-the-fly during training using a random setting (that is typically constrained using pre-defined ranges or guardrails). Spatial transforms are applied to the images, typically using a third-order spline interpolation, and to the masks using a nearest neighbor interpolation. It is very important during this stage to keep the augmentations realistic and avoid overly transforming the images, which can then create implausible anatomy and harm performance (Table 2.2).

Choosing an Appropriate Loss Function

Overlap-based metrics such as Dice loss are a better fit for segmentation tasks since they are not too sensitive to the class imbalance, thereby helping the network learn accurate boundaries (Table 2.3). For example, Dice loss (often

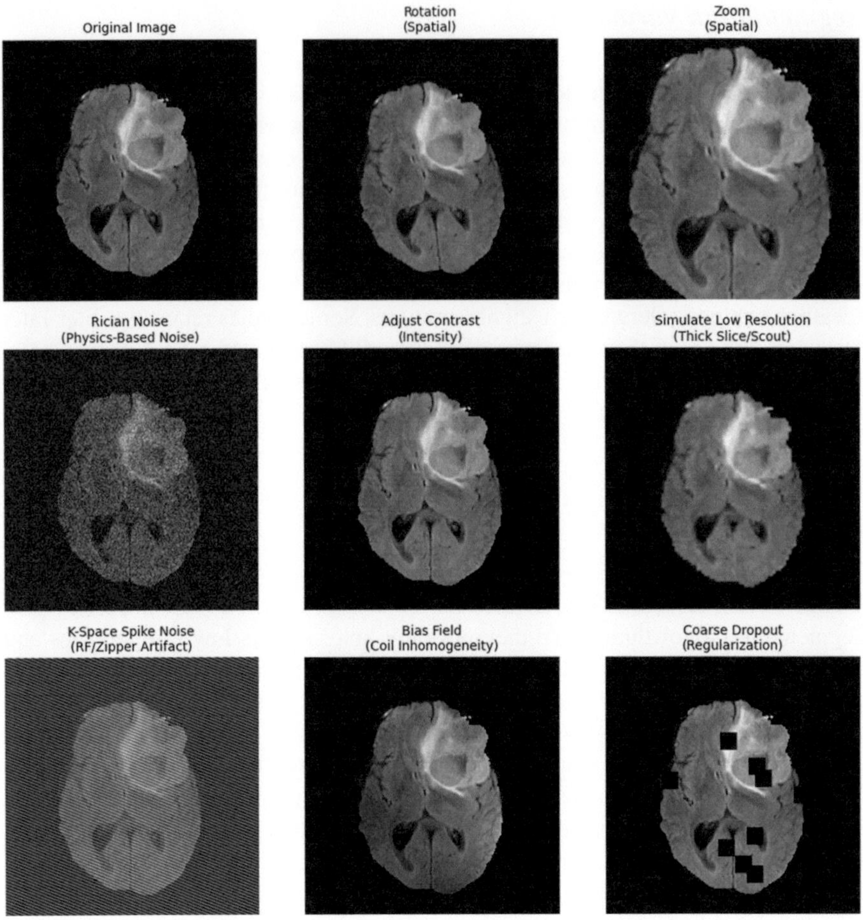

Fig. 2.5 Representative data augmentation techniques for neuroradiology implemented in MONAI. (Source: TCGA-GBM (Code: conv_04_brats_segmentation_unet.ipynb)) (Example Image from BraTS-TCGA-GBM, licensed under CC-BY-3.0)

combined with cross-entropy) is commonly used for segmentation models. In cases where there are multiple classes (tumor core, whole tumor, enhancing tumor), some pipelines use class-weighting or region-specific losses to avoid ignoring the small regions (e.g. enhancing tumor). Boundary-based losses work better when the tumors are smaller since volumetric losses work better for larger tumors. Losses such as the Cross-entropy loss tend to work for a wide variety of classes (since their gradients are much more well-defined and smoother), but their learning generally plateaus before the model can learn the task effectively. However, the best choice for a loss function is one that helps the model learn effectively and perform better on metrics that matter clinically.

Table 2.2 Data augmentations from MONAI transforms and nnU-Net data augmentation variant trainer

Augmentation	Function	Pros	Cons
Random geometric transformations	Randomly rotate, flip, scale, translate, or affine-transform images.	Improves invariance to patient positioning, scanner orientation, and field-of-view differences.	Can create anatomically implausible orientations if overused; may misalign labels if not applied consistently.
Random elastic and non-rigid deformations	Apply smooth, spatially varying warps to simulate tissue deformation.	Models realistic anatomical variability; improves generalization for soft tissues.	Risk of unrealistic distortions; computationally expensive; harder to tune.
Random intensity scaling and shifting	Adjust brightness and contrast by scaling or shifting intensity values.	Accounts for scanner gain differences and acquisition variability; simple and fast.	Can distort quantitative intensity relationships; may reduce physical or biological interpretability.
Random cropping and patch sampling	Randomly select spatial subregions or patches from images.	Increases sample diversity; mitigates class imbalance; reduces memory usage.	May remove global context; poor crop strategy can miss relevant anatomy.
Random intensity distribution changes	Modify histogram shape or remap intensity distributions.	Similar to intensity scaling, it improves robustness to contrast variability across scanners or protocols.	Can break modality-specific intensity meaning; may confuse models relying on absolute intensities.
Random blurring and smoothing	Apply smoothing or blur to reduce spatial detail.	Simulates resolution differences and partial-volume effects.	Loss of fine structural detail; may degrade performance on small objects.
Random noise injection	Add synthetic noise to simulate acquisition noise, independent of adjacent pixel intensities.	Improves robustness to low SNR and noisy clinical data.	Excessive noise harms learning; excessive noise may not match real data.
Random artifact simulation	Inject modality-specific artifacts (e.g., MRI k-space spikes, Gibbs ringing).	Enhances robustness to real-world imaging imperfections.	Highly modality-dependent; may introduce unrealistic artifacts if misused.
Probabilistic composition and selection	Randomly apply or select augmentations based on probabilities.	Prevents overfitting to a fixed augmentation pattern; increases data diversity.	Adds complexity; poorly chosen probabilities can reduce training stability.

Table 2.3 Loss functions from MONAI losses

Loss function type	What it optimizes	Common examples	Pros for brain tumor segmentation	Cons/common pitfalls
Cross-entropy	Per-voxel classification likelihood.	Binary Cross-Entropy (BCE), Categorical Cross-Entropy, Weighted Cross-Entropy	Stable gradients; easy to optimize; works well for large tumor regions and background separation.	Highly sensitive to class imbalance; background dominates loss; may ignore small tumor subregions; does not directly optimize spatial overlap.
Volumetric overlap (region)	Overlap between predicted and ground-truth regions.	Dice loss, Soft Dice, Jaccard (IoU) loss	Directly optimizes segmentation quality; robust to class imbalance; effective for small tumor cores and enhancing tumor regions.	Can be unstable early in training; insensitive to boundary accuracy; poor gradient when prediction is empty.
Tversky/ focal-Tversky	Asymmetric overlap with tunable false positives vs. false negatives.	Tversky loss, Focal Tversky loss	Allows explicit control over missing tumor vs. over-segmentation; excellent for highly imbalanced tumor subregions (e.g., enhancing tumor).	Hyperparameter tuning required; can over-penalize one error type; harder to interpret loss values.
Distance/ boundary-based	Distance between predicted and true boundaries.	Hausdorff loss, Boundary loss, Surface Dice loss	Improves boundary accuracy; captures tumor shape and extent; useful when margins are clinically relevant.	Sensitive to noisy labels; computationally expensive; weak supervision for interior regions.
Compound/ hybrid	Combination of complementary objectives.	Dice + Cross-Entropy, Dice + Focal, Dice + Boundary	Balances voxel-level accuracy and region overlap; stabilizes training; widely used in BraTS-style tasks.	Increased complexity; harder to debug; improper weighting can cause one term to dominate.

Stability of Model Performance

Cross-Validation Traditional ML algorithms utilize a data partition strategy where the overall dataset is split, typically using 80:20 ratio, into a train vs. test partition. However, the stability of such single train-test split depends heavily on the splitting strategy, which tends to provide unstable performance estimates when sample sizes are small. The current best practice is to further split the training set (development) using a cross-validation setup so that the performance does not change drastically between splits. For example, a ten-fold cross-validation setup ensures that the model performs reasonably well across all folds prior to evaluation on the held-out test set.

Point Estimates + Confidence Intervals While point estimates are incredibly useful to summarize overall accuracy, they often fail to convey the variability across patients. In segmentation tasks, when the dice score is reported along with the confidence intervals, they provide a more informative and reliable summary of model performance since they also convey the case-level heterogeneity, such as from tumor size, location, image quality, or scanner difference. This is especially important for use-cases when the sample size is relatively smaller as point estimates can be unstable or misleading.

Representativeness of Test Set

In order to present an unbiased evaluation, the test set (hold-out set) needs to be representative of the training set. However, this is not always realistically possible, especially in low N settings when only small sets of cases are carved out into a held-out test set. In these cases, it is important for the test set to have easy examples but also some of the tough ones. Data drift, also referred to in literature as domain shift, distributional shift, dataset bias, out-of-distribution generalization, and so on, is a potential source of generalization performance loss when there is a mismatch, either in the data features, target distribution or even the underlying relationships, between the conditions during the model training versus those during clinical use. When there are changes in the underlying relationship between the input variables and target variables, it is referred to as "concept drift" or "concept shift." For example, in the case of tumor segmentation, deep learning segmentation models work better for larger tumors and sometimes miss smaller tumors. If the test set has majorly larger tumors, for which the model works well, this may present an artificially inflated performance estimate. This is even more important when the model is evaluated on an independent test set, such as cases from a new hospital/center or from a different type of scanner. In this case, reporting the test set performance across tumor sizes can help provide a more realistic performance estimate. Most studies compare the test set distributions with the development set to provide a summary of how representative the test set is of the development set.

Self-Configuring Pipelines as Baseline

Deep 3-dimensional CNNs or Transformers are standard for most segmentation tasks. Frameworks such as nnU-Net, Auto3Dseg help provide a baseline that custom-defined architectures can try to beat. Segment Anything Model (MedSAM) for medical images, and Total Segmentator are other options to establish a baseline if the anatomy is already part of currently existing segmentation pipelines. Training a custom model from scratch can be unstable and requires multiple iterations to identify the right range of hyperparameters that enable the network to learn effectively.

Black Box vs. Explainable Models

Until recently, deep learning models were considered black-box models without any means to examine their inner-workings and reasoning. Explainability methods have significantly improved for traditional machine learning models and computer vision algorithms such as CNNs and Transformers. For CNNs, methods such as GradCAM, Attention Maps, LIME and Occlusion Sensitivity can provide valuable insights into the decision-making process behind the algorithm's final predictions. While it is still true that CNNs/Transformers often contain billions of parameters, we are now able to synthesize these parameters to come up with a reasoning that can accompany the model's predictions. For example in Fig. 2.6, the key reasons why enhancing tumor class typically achieves lower dice scores may be explained using the Grad-CAM visualizations which show that the U-Net model (without attention) failed to localize ET regions precisely when the masks were smaller size (sparse and fragmented) with thinner margins, or when tumor voxels for ET were potentially under-represented as compared to larger structures like edema. The activations for ET are diffuse and off target with less concentrated response over the scattered enhancing regions, and in contrast, the activations are contiguous and better defined for the tumor core and whole tumor masks.

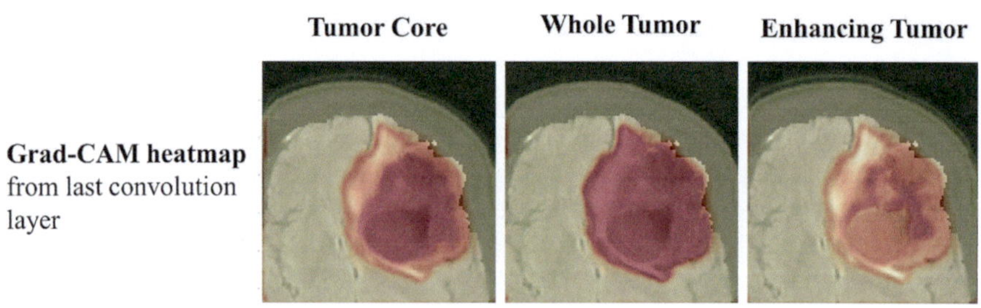

Fig. 2.6 Grad-CAM heatmaps from the final convolutional layer of an attention U-Net model are overlaid on a post-contrast axial brain MRI slice (Source: TCIA) for three segmentation targets: tumor core (left), whole tumor (middle), and enhancing tumor (right). Warmer colors (red) indicate regions of stronger activation guiding the model's predictions. Source: TCIA (Code: conv_04_brats_segmentation_unet.ipynb) (Example image from BraTS-TCGA-GBM, licensed under CC-BY-3.0)

Failure Analysis

Qualitative analysis of the model predictions can provide valuable insight into the performance of the segmentation algorithm by examining incorrectly segmented areas (CLAIM checklist Item 39) to identify any systematic model weaknesses. For example, we identified from the quantitative analysis that the dice scores were comparatively lower for enhancing the tumor than for the tumor core or whole. We could also infer from the GradCAM images that the model was struggling to precisely segment enhancing tumor areas where it was fragmented or scattered and the activations were diffuse and off target. From qualitative analysis, it can be observed that the predicted mask for enhancing tumor suffers from major under segmentation, which is the reason for poor dice scores. In contrast, the whole tumor and tumor regions have minor areas of over-segmentation and under-segmentation. The question of why such errors exist, if systematic, can be answered by looking under the hood at training setup configurations, such as the use of volumetric loss functions or lack of attention in U-Net, etc. These are important insights that the clinician or practitioner, who uses the output segmentations in their workflow, should be aware of to trust the underlying model. Aided with this information, the practitioner can appropriately plan the subsequent processes in their workflow (Fig. 2.7)

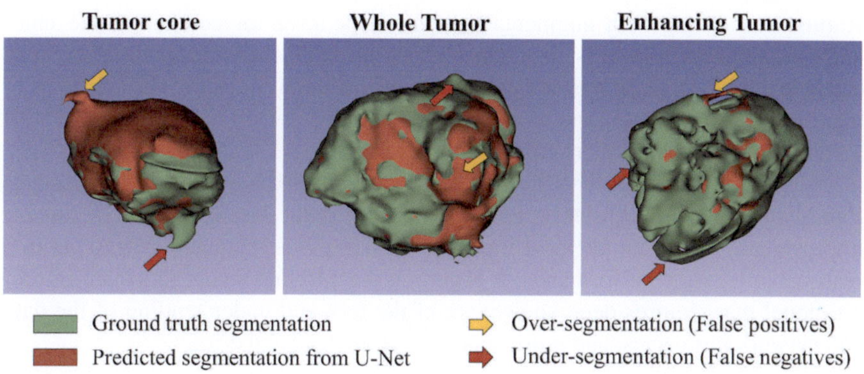

Fig. 2.7 Representative figures show examples of incorrectly segmented areas to aid reader understanding. (Code: conv_04_brats_segmentation_unet.ipynb) (Example ground truth segmentation from The Cancer Genome Atlas (TCGA) Glioblastoma Multiforme (GBM) collection (BraTS-TCGA-GBM), licensed under CC-BY-3.0) Visualized on 3D Slicer using 3D rendering with surface smoothing factor set to 0.5. Each subpanel uses an independently selected camera pose and magnification to emphasize error patterns; therefore, spatial orientation, scale, and apparent relative position are not directly comparable between panels

Summary

In summary, developing segmentation algorithms that are designed to perform well in clinical settings should carefully address common implementation challenges or pitfalls that may affect the model's effectiveness. A model with high performance on a development set does not necessarily mean that the model will perform well in practice.

Start with an Unbiased Heterogeneous Dataset Prioritize heterogeneity over size. While data collected from more cases definitely helps, it does not automatically help a model learn heterogeneity if they are all from an unrepresentative sample. The test set needs to be representative of the target population to present an unbiased evaluation of performance.

Inter-rater Variability While there are no universal rules to come up with the reference standard, there are some methods to get the ground truths as close as possible to the truth. The most common options are to have multiple annotators outline ROIs independently and use a third, more senior neuroradiologist to resolve consensus. Consensus can also be achieved programmatically using majority voting or statistically using methods such as STAPLE. Soft labels based on the fraction of raters can be used when more than two experts are available for manual labeling.

Data Augmentations Can Address Both Sample Size Limitations and Model Robustness While data augmentations are imperative for countering the challenges of small sample sizes, data transformations that include size scaling/rotations can help the model learn size and positional invariance. Introducing various types of intensity transforms and random noise helps the model learn to perform even with potentially protocol/scanner settings or artifacts.

Establish a Baseline Quickly In most cases, it is the last 20% of performance improvement that takes the most time (80%). While it is relatively easy to get to a reasonable baseline performance, it is getting the baseline model to a state-of-the-art model that requires deep knowledge of the task and understanding of the data and network intricacies, and most important of all, trial and error.

Qualitative Analysis While quantitative metrics can help summarize overall performance, qualitative analysis, in the form of reader studies, needs to be performed to evaluate common acceptance/rejection criteria.

Model Explainability and Failure Analysis One of the most important practical challenges is understanding the situations where the model is not performing well. Thoroughly investigate failure points and evaluate if the model's issues are systematic or random. For failures, investigate the underlying causes and summarize failure points that may require additional human-in-the-loop guardrails during the time of deployment.

Use-Case 3: LLMs for Radiology Report Classification

Radiology reports contain key clinical information, but the data is typically stored as free text, which may not support downstream workflows well. In this use-case, the study goal is to convert radiology reports into reliable structured outputs (e.g., labels, key findings, or standardized summaries). Structured outputs can then feed downstream steps like triage/worklists, longitudinal tracking of findings, registry building for research, quality audits, and operational reporting. Using this use-case, we explore key concerns with LLM outputs such as model choice, hallucinations, reproducibility, reasoning and privacy/workflow constraints.

Zero-Shot vs. Fine-Tune

As it stands today, most of the open-source and closed-source LLMs are not trained using a representative radiology reports corpus. While natural language conversation/instruction level tasks can be trained using public datasets in natural language, radiology tasks need to account for unique language complexities such as synonyms, ellipses, and double negations. For example, BioMedCLIP is a vision language model that uses 15 million figure caption pairs from PubMed Central. Similarly, the MedGemma 27B model released by Google was pre-trained using various public and private multimodal datasets such as MIMIC-CXR, TCGA, etc. Other off-the-shelf LLMs with open-source weights need to be fine-tuned such as the Llama using methods such as Low-Rank-Adaptation (LoRA) to be expected to perform for specialized neuroradiology tasks. Fine-tuning availability depends on the vendor and model version. Some proprietary models support fine-tuning in specific products (e.g., via provider platforms), while others may only support prompting or RAG. However, prompt engineering techniques such as zero-shot or few-shot methods can explain the reasoning using chain of thoughts to get the LLMs to work for custom tasks.

Retrieval Augmented Generation (RAG)

LLMs can hallucinate, where they invent findings or references and may amplify errors in the data. Grounding the model is imperative and can be implemented using a retrieval layer (Fig. 2.8), which finds data from trusted sources and injects it into the prompt for the LLM to use, thereby reducing hallucinations and inaccuracies. Training or fine-tuning the LLM on domain-specific datasets and using Retrieval Augmented Generation pipelines can address this issue. While RAG can improve grounding and often reduce hallucinations, the output still needs verification. LLMs

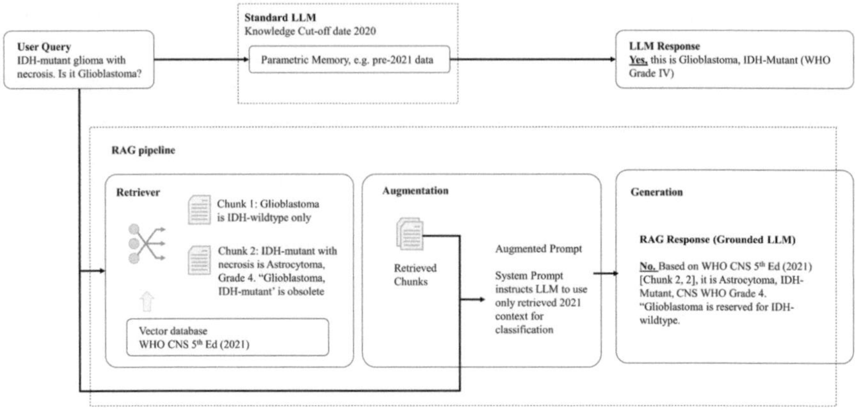

Fig. 2.8 Illustration of a sample RAG pipeline that shows the steps involved in grounding the LLM using a database from WHO CNS 5th Ed, to provide reliable and accurate responses

Table 2.4 Prompt-types for reasoning and improved accuracy

Prompt type	Concept	Strengths	Weaknesses
Input-output (IO)	Model maps input directly to output with no explicit reasoning steps.	Fast, simple, low token cost; works well for straightforward tasks.	Poor performance on multi-step reasoning; opaque reasoning.
Chain of thoughts (CoT)	Model is prompted to generate intermediate reasoning steps before the final answer.	Improves performance on reasoning, math, logic, and multi-step problems; more interpretable.	Longer responses; higher token cost; reasoning may still be incorrect.
Self-consistency with CoT (majority voting)	Model generates multiple CoT solutions and selects the most common final answer.	Reduces random errors; improves robustness and accuracy on reasoning tasks.	Computationally expensive; still fails if all paths share the same flaw.
Tree of thoughts (ToT)	Model explores multiple reasoning paths in a tree structure with evaluation and pruning.	Better global search; handles complex planning and decision-making tasks.	Very expensive; complex to implement; slower inference.

have also been shown to ground their responses better when the prompt explicitly asks the LLM to cite its sources (Table 2.4).

Qualitative Evaluation

Commonly used quantitative metrics for generative algorithms involve measuring the concordance between the ground truth and generated output using metrics such as BLEU or ROUGE. However, these scores are agnostic to meaning, and while these concordance scores can be high, some significant errors, such as missing a significant impression or diagnosis, may still slip between the cracks without appropriate qualitative evaluation. A reader study, where radiologists provide a qualitative score on an ordinal scale of 1–5, can provide valuable insights into the clinical meaning of the generated output.

Reasoning

Transformers, which are the underlying neural network architecture we discussed in Chap. 1, are known for their self-attention mechanism and excel at parallel processing and long-range word dependencies. However, in order for them to function in the desired manner, it is important to break down complex problems into intermediate steps, especially when dealing with multi-step tasks prevalent in neuroradiology. This can be done during the prompt engineering phase, as shown in Fig. 2.9, where the latent reasoning steps are verbalized so that the model's thought process follows a desired structured path. Therefore, when the model responds with its outputs along with the underlying reasoning process, it can reduce logical mistakes and help spot logical errors more easily, thereby making the output more reliable.

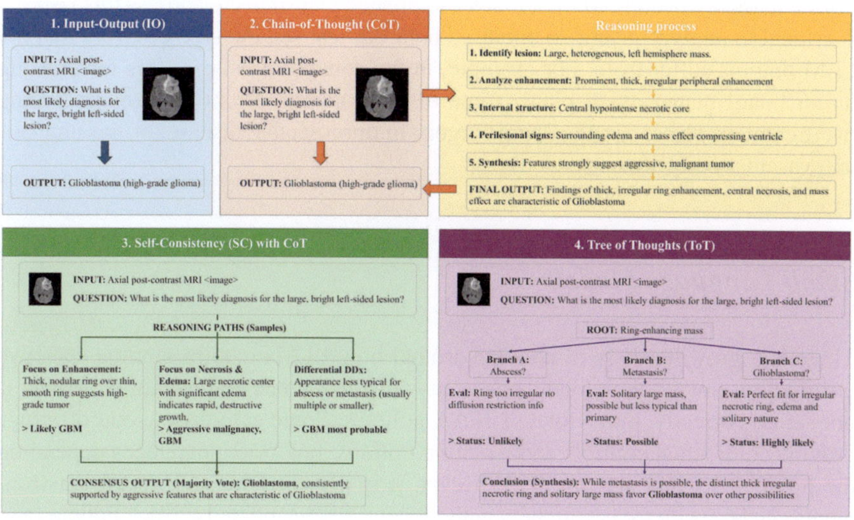

Fig. 2.9 Illustration of reasoning types for explainable VLMs (Sample image from The Cancer Genome Atlas (TCGA) Glioblastoma Multiforme (GBM) collection (BraTS-TCGA-GBM), licensed under CC-BY-3.0). (Sample image and text used in this figure are only intended as examples to show the inner working of the prompt types).

Reproducibility

Inconsistent outputs that vary every time the model runs inference can drastically alter clinical decisions. Reproducible results build trust, provide reliable diagnoses, and improve patient safety. One of the easiest ways to ensure the results are reproducible is to set the LLMs hyperparameters to an appropriate value. For example, setting the temperature hyperparameter, which controls the level of creativity or randomness, to zero would help favor deterministic, consistent responses. While lower temperatures usually reduce randomness and help reproducibility, determinism is not guaranteed, so it is important to keep track of the model version and system fingerprints wherever possible. Additionally, this is a significant challenge since many of the closed-source models are updated with new training data and knowledge cut off behind the scenes. Open-source models, whose weights are fixed and released with version control, may be a better fit for tracking the specific state of the model that was used for generating responses.

Error Analysis

LLMs, just like any other predictive algorithm, can provide incorrect predictions. However, the nuance here is that LLMs can confidently provide incorrect predictions and there are currently not many established guardrails to address this issue. It is critical to analyze, using an unbiased held-out test set, the type of errors that the LLM outputs suffer from. For example, in the context of using LLMs for drafting tumor board management plans, some of the common errors involved providing overtreatment plans, or suggesting surgery in unresectable disease, or missing certain vascular involvements.

Small Language Models

There is a growing body of concern around how LLMs require sending sensitive information over to the cloud, sometimes outside the hospital networks, which, if not set up correctly, may violate HIPAA policies. Some enterprise cloud offerings provide contractual controls and isolation options, but exact guarantees depend on the product tier and agreement. However, it is unclear how such secure environments can be set up for researchers without centrally negotiated privacy policies and whether such current privacy policies would stay that way in the future.

Small Language Models, which are also based on the transformer architecture but with significantly fewer parameters, can be trained using LoRA methods and with data specific to an institution and the inference of such models can be run on light-weight compute environments as found in a typical laptop used by a clinician. Smaller models, such as the Open pre-trained transformers (OPT-350M), can often run on modest hardware (sometimes CPUs, often with quantization), making local deployment more feasible. Most importantly, the user queries and computations are all processed within the hospital environment without sending data to external networks.

LLMs in the Workflow

Some use-cases such as support for differential diagnoses can help junior radiology residents more than senior neuroradiologists. Additionally, in certain cases, when a probabilistic output is shown in front of an experienced neuroradiologist before their impressions or decisions are recorded, it is possible that there might be some anchoring biases in play. Moreover, the clinical application of the LLM would dictate the level of tolerance to different types of errors.

Summary

In summary, reliable, state-of-the-art solutions involving LLMs for neuroradiology use-cases require careful study design, extensive training datasets, comprehensive evaluation, and engineered guardrails prior to implementation.

Fine-Tuning vs. Off-the-Shelf While off-the-shelf LLMs from closed-source providers (GPT-4o, Gemini) can be used for tasks that involve natural language text, applying them to radiology use-cases often involves using LLMs trained using neuroradiology datasets (BioMedCLIP, MedGemma). As an alternative, open-source models such as Llama or DeepSeek can be fine-tuned using LoRA methods to improve their reliability and performance for neuroradiology tasks.

Ground LLMs Using RAG This is crucial because LLM/VLM responses need to be factual and anchored in current, authoritative medical knowledge. RAG can help reduce hallucinations (LLM makes up incorrect facts). Additionally, RAG techniques can provide LLMs with access to the latest research, guidelines and protocols that can help overcome the static nature of their training data.

Identify Failure Points LLMs can produce incorrect results with high confidence. It is important to identify if there is a systemic cause for such errors using error analysis. While quantitative scores such as BLEU, ROUGE can help assess overall accuracy, rigorous evaluations need to be carried out by including qualitative evaluation in the form of user studies.

Establish Appropriate Guardrails While LLMs have shown promising results in some use-cases, they have also been shown to produce unsupported evidence. Clinical settings should utilize an appropriate Human-in-the-loop deployment pipeline to counter LLMs' limitations.

Consider Small-Language-Models Individual researchers or labs without extensive resources may find it challenging to interact with LLMs in a privacy-safe manner. Consider training and deploying SLMs, which may provide the required performance but without the computational overhead and privacy risks.

Conclusion

Artificial intelligence has the potential to meaningfully augment neuroradiology across classification, segmentation, and generative tasks, but successful clinical translation depends far more on rigorous study design and implementation choices than on model novelty alone. The use-cases presented in this chapter demonstrate that common pitfalls such as multi-center heterogeneity, segmentation variability, small-sample uncertainty, data leakage, and limited interpretability are often the primary reasons for failure when models are deployed beyond controlled research settings. Addressing these challenges requires an end-to-end perspective that spans data curation, annotation strategy, preprocessing and harmonization, model selection, validation methodology, and post-deployment monitoring. Equally important is the integration of explainability and failure analysis to ensure transparency, build clinician trust, and define appropriate guardrails for real-world use. While the specific technical details may vary by application, the overarching framework and best practices outlined here are broadly applicable to neuroradiology AI workflows and serve as a practical guide for developing robust, generalizable, and clinically meaningful AI systems that can withstand external validation and ultimately improve patient care.

Suggested Reading

1. Winder AJ, Stanley EA, Fiehler J, Forkert ND. Challenges and potential of artificial intelligence in neuroradiology. Clin Neuroradiol. 2024;34(2):293–305. https://doi.org/10.1007/s00062-024-01382-7.
2. Choi Y, Yu W, Nagarajan MB, et al. Translating AI to clinical practice: overcoming data shift with explainability. Radiographics. 2023;43(5):e220105. https://doi.org/10.1148/rg.220105.
3. Bento M, Fantini I, Park J, Rittner L, Frayne R. Deep learning in large and multi-site structural brain MR imaging datasets. Front Neuroinform. 2022;15:805669. Published 2022 Jan 20. https://doi.org/10.3389/fninf.2021.805669.
4. Karimi D, Dou H, Warfield SK, Gholipour A. Deep learning with noisy labels: exploring techniques and remedies in medical image analysis. Med Image Anal. 2020;65:101759. https://doi.org/10.1016/j.media.2020.101759.

5. Mongan J, Moy L, Kahn CE Jr. Checklist for Artificial Intelligence in Medical Imaging (CLAIM): a guide for authors and reviewers. Radiol Artif Intell. 2020;2(2):e200029. Published 2020 Mar 25. https://doi.org/10.1148/ryai.2020200029.
6. Yu AC, Mohajer B, Eng J. External validation of deep learning algorithms for radiologic diagnosis: a systematic review. Radiol Artif Intell. 2022;4(3):e210064. Published 2022 May 4. https://doi.org/10.1148/ryai.210064.
7. Fortin JP, Cullen N, Sheline YI, et al. Harmonization of cortical thickness measurements across scanners and sites. NeuroImage. 2018;167:104–20. https://doi.org/10.1016/j.neuroimage.2017.11.024.
8. Abgrall G, Holder AL, Chelly Dagdia Z, Zeitouni K, Monnet X. Should AI models be explainable to clinicians? Crit Care. 2024;28(1):301. Published 2024 Sep 12. https://doi.org/10.1186/s13054-024-05005-y.
9. Reyes M, Meier R, Pereira S, et al. On the interpretability of artificial intelligence in radiology: challenges and opportunities. Radiol Artif Intell. 2020;2(3):e190043. Published 2020 May 27. https://doi.org/10.1148/ryai.2020190043.
10. OpenAI. Hello GPT-4o. OpenAI. Published May 13, 2024. https://openai.com/index/hello-gpt-4o/. Accessed 23 Dec 2025.
11. Hassabis D, Gemini Team. Introducing Gemini 1.5, Google's next-generation AI model. Google Blog. Published February 15, 2024. https://blog.google/technology/ai/google-gemini-next-generation-model-february-2024/. Accessed 23 Dec 2025.
12. Lundberg SM, Lee S. A unified approach to interpreting model predictions. In: Neural information processing systems. 2017.
13. Selvaraju RR, Das A, Vedantam R, Cogswell M, Parikh D, Batra D. Grad-CAM: visual explanations from deep networks via gradient-based localization. Int J Comput Vis. 2016;128:336–59.
14. Zeiler MD, Fergus R. Visualizing and understanding convolutional networks. In: Fleet D, Pajdla T, Schiele B, Tuytelaars T, editors. Computer vision—ECCV 2014. ECCV 2014, Lecture notes in computer science, vol. 8689. Cham: Springer; 2014. https://doi.org/10.1007/978-3-319-10590-1_53.
15. Wei J, Wang X, Schuurmans D, Bosma M, Chi EH, Xia F, Le Q, Zhou D. Chain of thought prompting elicits reasoning in large language models. 2022. ArXiv, abs/2201.11903.
16. Rosenbacke R, Melhus Å, McKee M, Stuckler D. How explainable artificial intelligence can increase or decrease clinicians' trust in AI applications in health care: systematic review. JMIR AI. 2024;3:e53207. https://ai.jmir.org/2024/1/e53207. https://doi.org/10.2196/53207.
17. van der Vegt AH, Scott IA, Dermawan K, Schnetler RJ, Kalke VR, Lane PJ. Implementation frameworks for end-to-end clinical AI: derivation of the SALIENT framework. J Am Med Inform Assoc. 2023;30(9):1503–15. https://doi.org/10.1093/jamia/ocad088.
18. Kwong JCC, Erdman L, Khondker A, et al. The silent trial—the bridge between bench-to-bedside clinical AI applications. Front Digit Health. 2022;4:929508. Published 2022 Aug 16. https://doi.org/10.3389/fdgth.2022.929508.
19. Vasey B, Nagendran M, Campbell B, et al. Reporting guideline for the early-stage clinical evaluation of decision support systems driven by artificial intelligence: DECIDE-AI. Nat Med. 2022;28(5):924–33. https://doi.org/10.1038/s41591-022-01772-9.
20. Do HM, Spear LG, Nikpanah M, et al. Augmented radiologist workflow improves report value and saves time: a potential model for implementation of artificial intelligence. Acad Radiol. 2020;27(1):96–105. https://doi.org/10.1016/j.acra.2019.09.014.
21. World Health Organization. Ethics and governance of artificial intelligence for health. Published June 28, 2021. https://www.who.int/publications/i/item/9789240029200. Accessed 23 Dec 2025.
22. US Food and Drug Administration. Methods and tools for effective postmarket monitoring of artificial intelligence (AI)-enabled medical devices. content current as of June 10, 2024. https://www.fda.gov/medical-devices/medical-device-regulatory-science-research-programs-conducted-osel/methods-and-tools-effective-postmarket-monitoring-artificial-intelligence-ai-enabled-medical-devices. Accessed 23 Dec 2025.

23. Bakas S, Akbari H, Sotiras A, Bilello M, Rozycki M, Kirby J, Freymann J, Farahani K, Davatzikos C. (2017) Segmentation labels and Radiomic features for the pre-operative scans of the TCGA-LGG collection [Data set]. The Cancer Imaging Archive. https://doi.org/10.7937/K9/TCIA.2017.GJQ7R0EF.
24. Bakas S, Akbari H, Sotiras A, Bilello M, Rozycki M, Kirby J, Freymann J, Farahani K, Davatzikos C. Segmentation labels for the pre-operative scans of the TCGA-GBM collection [data set]. The Cancer Imaging Archive. 2017. https://doi.org/10.7937/K9/TCIA.2017.KLXWJJ1Q.
25. Fedorov A, Beichel R, Kalpathy-Cramer J, et al. 3D Slicer as an image computing platform for the Quantitative Imaging Network. Magn Reson Imaging. 2012;30(9):1323–41. https://doi.org/10.1016/j.mri.2012.05.001.
26. Diaz-Pinto A, Alle S, Nath V, et al. MONAI label: a framework for AI-assisted interactive labeling of 3D medical images. Med Image Anal. 2024;95:103207. https://doi.org/10.1016/j.media.2024.103207.
27. Sakinis T, Milletari F, Roth H, Korfiatis P, Kostandy P, Philbrick K, Akkus Z, Xu Z, Xu D, Erickson BJ. Interactive segmentation of medical images through fully convolutional neural networks. 2019. arXiv preprint arXiv:1903.08205.
28. Diaz-Pinto A, et al. Deepedit: deep editable learning for interactive segmentation of 3d medical images. In: Nguyen HV, et al., editors. Data augmentation, labelling, and imperfections. Cham: Springer Nature Switzerland; 2022. p. 11–21.
29. Ma J, He Y, Li F, Han L, You C, Wang B. Segment anything in medical images. Nat Commun. 2024;15(1):654. Published 2024 Jan 22. https://doi.org/10.1038/s41467-024-44824-z.
30. Groenwold RH, White IR, Donders AR, Carpenter JR, Altman DG, Moons KG. Missing covariate data in clinical research: when and when not to use the missing-indicator method for analysis. CMAJ. 2012;184(11):1265–9. https://doi.org/10.1503/cmaj.110977.
31. Tustison NJ, Cook PA, Holbrook AJ, et al. The ANTsX ecosystem for quantitative biological and medical imaging. Sci Rep. 2021;11(1):9068. Published 2021 Apr 27. https://doi.org/10.1038/s41598-021-87564-6.
32. Smith SM. Fast robust automated brain extraction. Hum Brain Mapp. 2002;17(3):143–55. https://doi.org/10.1002/hbm.10062.
33. Doshi J, Erus G, Ou Y, Gaonkar B, Davatzikos C. Multi-atlas skull-stripping. Acad Radiol. 2013;20(12):1566–76. https://doi.org/10.1016/j.acra.2013.09.010.
34. Doshi J, Erus G, Ou Y, et al. MUSE: MUlti-atlas region Segmentation utilizing Ensembles of registration algorithms and parameters, and locally optimal atlas selection. NeuroImage. 2016;127:186–95. https://doi.org/10.1016/j.neuroimage.2015.11.073.
35. Smith SM, Jenkinson M, Woolrich MW, Beckmann CF, Behrens TEJ, Johansen-Berg H, Bannister PR, De Luca M, Drobnjak I, Flitney DE, Niazy R, Saunders J, Vickers J, Zhang Y, De Stefano N, Brady JM, Matthews PM. Advances in functional and structural MR image analysis and implementation as FSL. NeuroImage. 2004;23(S1):208–19.
36. Davatzikos C, Rathore S, Bakas S, et al. Cancer imaging phenomics toolkit: quantitative imaging analytics for precision diagnostics and predictive modeling of clinical outcome. J Med Imaging (Bellingham). 2018;5(1):011018. https://doi.org/10.1117/1.JMI.5.1.011018.
37. van Griethuysen JJM, Fedorov A, Parmar C, et al. Computational radiomics system to decode the radiographic phenotype. Cancer Res. 2017;77(21):e104–7. https://doi.org/10.1158/0008-5472.CAN-17-0339.
38. Zwanenburg A, Vallières M, Abdalah MA, et al. The image biomarker standardization initiative: standardized quantitative Radiomics for high-throughput image-based phenotyping. Radiology. 2020;295(2):328–38. https://doi.org/10.1148/radiol.2020191145.
39. Moons KG, Altman DG, Reitsma JB, et al. Transparent reporting of a multivariable prediction model for Individual Prognosis or Diagnosis (TRIPOD): explanation and elaboration. Ann Intern Med. 2015;162(1):W1–W73. https://doi.org/10.7326/M14-0698.

40. Hesamian MH, Jia W, He X, Kennedy P. Deep learning techniques for medical image segmentation: achievements and challenges. J Digit Imaging. 2019;32(4):582–96. https://doi.org/10.1007/s10278-019-00227-x.
41. Hsu WC, Meuschke M, Frangi AF, Preim B, Lawonn K. A survey of intracranial aneurysm detection and segmentation. Med Image Anal. 2025;101:103493. https://doi.org/10.1016/j.media.2025.103493.
42. Dorfner FJ, Patel JB, Kalpathy-Cramer J, Gerstner ER, Bridge CP. A review of deep learning for brain tumor analysis in MRI. NPJ Precis Oncol. 2025;9(1):2. Published 2025 Jan 3. https://doi.org/10.1038/s41698-024-00789-2.
43. Zeng C, Gu L, Liu Z, Zhao S. Review of deep learning approaches for the segmentation of multiple sclerosis lesions on brain MRI. Front Neuroinform. 2020;14:610967. Published 2020 Nov 20. https://doi.org/10.3389/fninf.2020.610967.
44. Menze BH, Jakab A, Bauer S, et al. The multimodal Brain Tumor Image Segmentation Benchmark (BRATS). IEEE Trans Med Imaging. 2015;34(10):1993–2024. https://doi.org/10.1109/TMI.2014.2377694.
45. Balki I, Amirabadi A, Levman J, et al. Sample-size determination methodologies for machine learning in medical imaging research: a systematic review. Can Assoc Radiol J. 2019;70(4):344–53. https://doi.org/10.1016/j.carj.2019.06.002.
46. Baid U, Ghodasara S, Mohan S, et al. The RSNA-ASNR-MICCAI BraTS 2021 benchmark on brain tumor segmentation and radiogenomic classification. 2021; arXiv preprint https://arxiv.org/abs/2107.02314.
47. Narayana PA, Coronado I, Sujit SJ, Wolinsky JS, Lublin FD, Gabr RE. Deep-learning-based neural tissue segmentation of MRI in multiple sclerosis: effect of training set size. J Magn Reson Imaging. 2020;51(5):1487–96. https://doi.org/10.1002/jmri.26959.
48. Fang Y, Wang J, Ou X, et al. The impact of training sample size on deep learning-based organ auto-segmentation for head-and-neck patients. Phys Med Biol. 2021;66(18). Published 2021 Sep 14. https://doi.org/10.1088/1361-6560/ac2206.
49. Vokinger KN, Feuerriegel S, Kesselheim AS. Mitigating bias in machine learning for medicine. Commun Med (Lond). 2021;1:25. https://doi.org/10.1038/s43856-021-00028-w.
50. Rouzrokh P, Khosravi B, Faghani S, et al. Mitigating bias in radiology machine learning: 1. Data handling. Radiol Artif Intell. 2022;4(5):e210290. Published 2022 Aug 24. https://doi.org/10.1148/ryai.210290.
51. Visser M, Müller DMJ, van Duijn RJM, et al. Inter-rater agreement in glioma segmentations on longitudinal MRI. Neuroimage Clin. 2019;22:101727. https://doi.org/10.1016/j.nicl.2019.101727.
52. Pati S, Verma R, Akbari H, et al. Reproducibility analysis of multi-institutional paired expert annotations and radiomic features of the Ivy Glioblastoma Atlas Project (Ivy GAP) dataset. Med Phys. 2020;47(12):6039–52. https://doi.org/10.1002/mp.14556.
53. Moawad AW, Janas A, Baid U, et al. The Brain Tumor Segmentation-Metastases (BraTS-METS) Challenge 2023: Brain Metastasis Segmentation on Pre-treatment MRI. Preprint ArXiv 2024;arXiv:230600838v3 Published 2024 Dec 9.
54. De Sutter S, Dirks I, Raes L, et al. Interobserver ground-truth variability limits performance of automated glioblastoma segmentation on [18F]FET PET. EJNMMI Phys. 2025;12(1):54. Published 2025 Jun 6. https://doi.org/10.1186/s40658-025-00767-y.
55. Cardoso MJ, Li W, Brown R, Ma N, Kerfoot E, Wang Y, Murrey B, Myronenko A, Zhao C, Yang D, Nath V. Monai: an open-source framework for deep learning in healthcare. 2022. arXiv preprint https://arxiv.org/abs/2211.02701.
56. Isensee F, Jaeger PF, Kohl SAA, Petersen J, Maier-Hein KH. nnU-Net: a self-configuring method for deep learning-based biomedical image segmentation. Nat Methods. 2021;18(2):203–11. https://doi.org/10.1038/s41592-020-01008-z.
57. Varma S, Simon R. Bias in error estimation when using cross-validation for model selection. BMC Bioinformatics. 2006;7:91. Published 2006 Feb 23. https://doi.org/10.1186/1471-2105-7-91.

58. Vabalas A, Gowen E, Poliakoff E, Casson AJ. Machine learning algorithm validation with a limited sample size. PLoS One. 2019;14(11):e0224365. Published 2019 Nov 7. https://doi.org/10.1371/journal.pone.0224365.
59. El Jurdi R, Varoquaux G, Colliot O. Confidence intervals for performance estimates in brain MRI segmentation. Med Image Anal. 2025;103:103565. https://doi.org/10.1016/j.media.2025.103565.
60. Tejani AS, Klontzas ME, Gatti AA, et al. Checklist for artificial intelligence in medical imaging (CLAIM): 2024 update. Radiol Artif Intell. 2024;6(4):e240300. https://doi.org/10.1148/ryai.240300.
61. Sahiner B, Chen W, Samala RK, Petrick N. Data drift in medical machine learning: implications and potential remedies. Br J Radiol. 2023;96(1150):20220878. https://doi.org/10.1259/bjr.20220878.
62. Wasserthal J, Breit HC, Meyer MT, et al. TotalSegmentator: robust segmentation of 104 anatomic structures in CT images. Radiol Artif Intell. 2023;5(5):e230024. Published 2023 Jul 5. https://doi.org/10.1148/ryai.230024.
63. Akinci D'Antonoli T, Stanzione A, Bluethgen C, et al. Large language models in radiology: fundamentals, applications, ethical considerations, risks, and future directions. Diagn Interv Radiol. 2024;30(2):80–90. https://doi.org/10.4274/dir.2023.232417.
64. Reichenpfader D, Müller H, Denecke K. A scoping review of large language model based approaches for information extraction from radiology reports. NPJ Digit Med. 2024;7(1):222. Published 2024 Aug 24. https://doi.org/10.1038/s41746-024-01219-0.
65. Cai T, Giannopoulos AA, Yu S, et al. Natural language processing technologies in radiology research and clinical applications. Radiographics. 2016;36(1):176–91. https://doi.org/10.1148/rg.2016150080.
66. Peng Y, Wang X, Lu L, Bagheri M, Summers R, Lu Z. NegBio: a high-performance tool for negation and uncertainty detection in radiology reports. AMIA Jt Summits Transl Sci Proc. 2018;2017:188–96. Published 2018 May 18.
67. Callen AL, Dupont SM, Price A, et al. Between always and never: evaluating uncertainty in radiology reports using natural language processing. J Digit Imaging. 2020;33(5):1194–201. https://doi.org/10.1007/s10278-020-00379-1.
68. Zhang S, Xu Y, Usuyama N, et al. BiomedCLIP: a multimodal biomedical foundation model pretrained from fifteen million scientific image-text pairs. arXiv 2023. https://doi.org/10.48550/arXiv.2303.00915.
69. Sellergren et al. MedGemma technical report. 2025. arXiv preprint arXiv:2507.05201.
70. Johnson AEW, Pollard TJ, Berkowitz SJ, et al. MIMIC-CXR, a de-identified publicly available database of chest radiographs with free-text reports. Sci Data. 2019;6(1):317. Published 2019 Dec 12. https://doi.org/10.1038/s41597-019-0322-0.
71. Cancer Genome Atlas Research Network, Weinstein JN, Collisson EA, et al. The cancer genome atlas pan-cancer analysis project. Nat Genet. 2013;45(10):1113–20. https://doi.org/10.1038/ng.2764.
72. Hu EJ, Shen Y, Wallis P, et al. LoRA: low-rank adaptation of large language models. 2021. arXiv https://doi.org/10.48550/arXiv.2106.09685
73. Touvron H, Lavril T, Izacard G, et al., LLaMA: open and efficient foundation language models. 2023. arxiv https://doi.org/10.48550/arXiv.2302.13971.
74. Voinea ŞV, Mămuleanu M, Teică RV, Florescu LM, Selişteanu D, Gheonea IA. GPT-driven radiology report generation with fine-tuned llama 3. Bioengineering (Basel). 2024;11(10):1043. Published 2024 Oct 18. https://doi.org/10.3390/bioengineering11101043.
75. Dietrich N, Bradbury NC, Loh C. Prompt engineering for large language models in interventional radiology. AJR Am J Roentgenol. 2025;225(2):e2532956. https://doi.org/10.2214/AJR.25.32956.
76. Weinert DA, Rauschecker AM. Enhancing large language models with retrieval-augmented generation: a radiology-specific approach. Radiol Artif Intell. 2025;7(3):e240313. https://doi.org/10.1148/ryai.240313.

77. Wada A, Tanaka Y, Nishizawa M, et al. Retrieval-augmented generation elevates local LLM quality in radiology contrast media consultation. NPJ Digit Med. 2025;8(1):395. Published 2025 Jul 2. https://doi.org/10.1038/s41746-025-01802-z.
78. Pingua B, Sahoo A, Kandpal M, et al. Medical LLMs: fine-tuning vs. retrieval-augmented generation. Bioengineering (Basel). 2025;12(7):687. Published 2025 Jun 24. https://doi.org/10.3390/bioengineering12070687.
79. Louis DN, Perry A, Wesseling P, et al. The 2021 WHO classification of tumors of the central nervous system: a summary. Neuro-Oncology. 2021;23(8):1231–51. https://doi.org/10.1093/neuonc/noab106.
80. Li CY, Chang KJ, Yang CF, et al. Towards a holistic framework for multimodal LLM in 3D brain CT radiology report generation. Nat Commun. 2025;16(1):2258. Published 2025 Mar 6. https://doi.org/10.1038/s41467-025-57426-0.
81. Jarrett PC, Hill J, Howell M, et al. Piloting temperature-driven variability in emergency diagnostic accuracy using a leading large language model. Cureus. 2025;17(10):e94476. Published 2025 Oct 13. https://doi.org/10.7759/cureus.94476.
82. Kim SH, Wihl J, Schramm S, et al. Human-AI collaboration in large language model-assisted brain MRI differential diagnosis: a usability study. Eur Radiol. 2025;35(9):5252–63. https://doi.org/10.1007/s00330-025-11484-6.
83. Jajodia A, Gupta K, Latinovich MF, Patlas MN, Elbanna KY. Optimizing clinical decision-making in pancreatic cancer: the role of GPT-4o and DeepSeek V3 large language models. Presented at the Radiological Society of North America (RSNA) annual meeting, November 30–December 4, 2025, Chicago.
84. Dennstädt F, Hastings J, Putora PM, Schmerder M, Cihoric N. Implementing large language models in healthcare while balancing control, collaboration, costs and security. NPJ Digit Med. 2025;8(1):143. Published 2025 Mar 6. https://doi.org/10.1038/s41746-025-01476-7.
85. Zheng G, Kamel P, Jacobs MA, Braverman V, Parekh V. One SLM is all you need: adaptive, privacy-preserving small language models for multi-task clinical assistance. Presented at the Radiological Society of North America (RSNA) annual meeting, November 30–December 4, 2025, Chicago.
86. Zhang S, Roller S, Goyal N, et al., OPT: open pre-trained transformer language models. 2022. Arxiv https://doi.org/10.48550/arXiv.2205.01068.
87. Schramm S, Le Guellec B, Ziegelmayer S, et al. The expertise paradox: who benefits from LLM-assisted brain mRI differential diagnosis? Presented at the Radiological Society of North America (RSNA) annual meeting, November 30–December 4, 2025, Chicago.
88. Liu A, Feng B, Xue B, Wang B, Wu B, Lu C, Zhao C, Deng C, Zhang C, Ruan C, Dai D Deepseek-v3 technical report. 2024. arXiv preprint https://arxiv.org/abs/2412.19437.

Chapter 3
Artificial Intelligence for Head and Neck Anatomy and Lesion Segmentation

Mathew Illimoottil, Andrew Kunz, Yauheniya Makarevich, Marius Staring, and Daniel Thomas Ginat

Against this backdrop, artificial intelligence (AI) has emerged as a transformative tool for medical image segmentation. Over the past decade, the field has rapidly evolved from atlas-based auto-contouring methods to machine learning and now deep learning-based segmentation. Modern deep learning algorithms, particularly convolutional neural networks (CNNs), have demonstrated the ability to produce highly accurate and consistent contours with significantly reduced human effort. Early studies showed that deep learning auto-segmentation can achieve contour accuracy on par with human experts and often exceeding older atlas methods. Specifically in the head and neck region, where many critical structures are packed in close proximity, AI-based segmentation has shown great promise in handling the complexity and reducing the workload on clinicians. Multiple studies have highlighted that auto-segmentation can harmonize contours between observers and institutions, thereby improving consistency of care. Furthermore, substantial time savings have been reported: contemporary deep learning models have reduced contouring time by over 75% in head and neck cases compared to manual delineation. In one multi-institutional report, an AI system achieved up to a 90% reduction in clinicians' workload for head and neck organ segmentation, with the vast majority of its auto-generated contours requiring only minor edits for clinical acceptance. These gains translate to hours of physician time saved per patient, which can be redirected toward direct patient care or other critical tasks.

M. Illimoottil
University of Missouri Kansas City, Kansas City, MO, USA

A. Kunz
University of Chicago, Chicago, IL, USA

Y. Makarevich · M. Staring
Leiden University, Leiden, The Netherlands

D. T. Ginat (✉)
Co-founder, Rad-Lab.ai, Chicago, IL, USA

D. T. Ginat (ed.), *Artificial Intelligence in Neuroradiology*,
https://doi.org/10.1007/978-3-032-24568-7_3

This chapter explores the principles and applications of AI-driven segmentation for head and neck anatomy and lesions. We begin with foundational concepts—the imaging modalities used, the anatomical challenges unique to the head and neck region, and the evolution from manual and atlas-based methods to current AI techniques. We then delve into state-of-the-art segmentation models, discussing the **U-Net** architecture and its variants that underpin many solutions. Performance metrics such as the **Dice similarity coefficient (DSC)** and **95th-percentile Hausdorff distance (HD95)** are explained as key measures of segmentation quality. With this foundation, we survey the current landscape of AI applications: automatic delineation of normal tissues (OARs) for radiotherapy, tumor segmentation in imaging for diagnostics and planning, and the integration of these tools into clinical workflows. Both commercial software packages and open-source tools are presented (with summary tables) to give readers a clear view of available solutions. We also discuss real-world implementation considerations—from regulatory approval and validation requirements to the practical aspects of deploying AI in a hospital setting, including user training and quality assurance. To enrich the narrative, boxed elements are included: a **Case Study** illustrating a real-world use of AI segmentation, a **Math Moment** unpacking the mathematics of evaluation metrics, and a **Key Challenges** summary highlighting ongoing hurdles in the field. The chapter concludes with a summary of take-home points and a set of review questions and research prompts to encourage further exploration of this topic.

Learning Objectives

By the end of this chapter, readers (radiologists, researchers, and physician-scientists) should be able to:

- **Understand the role of imaging modalities** (CT, MRI, PET) in head and neck anatomy segmentation and why each modality presents unique challenges.
- **Recognize the anatomical and technical challenges** of head and neck segmentation, including complex anatomy, variability between patients, and imaging artifacts.
- **Describe the evolution of segmentation methods**, from manual contouring and atlas-based techniques to modern AI-driven approaches.
- **Explain the fundamental architecture of U-Net** and similar deep learning models used for medical image segmentation, and why they are well-suited to head and neck tasks.
- **Identify key performance metrics** for segmentation quality (Dice coefficient, Hausdorff distance, etc.) and interpret what these metrics imply about model performance.
- **Survey current applications** of AI in segmenting head and neck structures, including auto-segmentation of organs-at-risk for radiotherapy planning and lesion (tumor) segmentation for diagnosis and treatment monitoring.

- **Compare commercial and open-source segmentation tools**, knowing examples of each, their capabilities, and how they integrate into clinical workflows.
- **Discuss real-world implementation considerations** such as integrating AI into existing clinical software (PACS/TPS), regulatory approvals (e.g., FDA clearance), the necessity of human review of AI-generated contours, and strategies for local validation of models.
- **Appreciate the potential impact and limitations** of AI segmentation in clinical practice, including how it can improve efficiency and consistency, and what challenges (data, acceptance, out-of-distribution cases) remain to be addressed.
- **Critically evaluate an AI segmentation study or tool**, understanding the study design elements (training data, validation, multi-institutional testing) and how to assess whether an AI model is ready for clinical use.

Key Terms and Definitions

- **Organ-at-Risk (OAR)**—A normal organ or tissue (e.g., parotid gland, optic nerve) that is sensitive to radiation. In radiotherapy planning, OARs must be contoured so that radiation dose to them can be limited to avoid complications.
- **Gross Tumor Volume (GTV)**—The visible or imaged tumor volume. In head and neck oncology, GTV often refers to the primary tumor or involved lymph nodes that should be targeted by treatment. Segmentation of GTV on imaging is crucial for radiotherapy targeting and surgical planning.
- **Auto-Segmentation**—Automatic delineation of structures or lesions by a computer algorithm. In the context of AI, this typically refers to using trained models to generate contours without manual drawing, subject to later human review.
- **Convolutional Neural Network (CNN)**—A class of deep learning models particularly adept at image analysis. CNNs apply learned filters (convolutions) across images to detect features. They form the backbone of most medical image segmentation networks.
- **U-Net**—A widely used CNN architecture for biomedical image segmentation, characterized by an encoder-decoder structure with skip connections. The U-Net can capture both coarse context and fine details, making it effective for delineating anatomical structures in images. Variants of U-Net (2D, 3D, multi-scale, etc.) are the basis of many head and neck segmentation models.
- **Dice Similarity Coefficient (DSC)**—A statistic used to gauge the similarity between two segmentations. It ranges from 0 to 1 (or 0% to 100%), where 1 indicates perfect overlap. Mathematically, $DSC = 2|X \cap Y| / (|X| + |Y|)$, where X and Y are the sets of voxels (or pixels) in the predicted and ground-truth segmentation, respectively. It is also known simply as the **Dice coefficient** or Dice score.
- **Hausdorff Distance (HD)**—A measure of distance between two contours or surfaces, defined as the maximum distance of a point on one contour to the closest point on the other contour. In segmentation evaluation, a **95th-percentile Hausdorff Distance (HD95)** is often used to reduce sensitivity to outlier points. HD95 represents a robust measure of the worst-case contour discrepancy, ignor-

ing the most extreme 5% of outlier distances. It is reported in physical units (e.g., millimeters) and provides a sense of how far apart boundaries can be.

- **Atlas-Based Segmentation**—An earlier auto-segmentation approach where a predefined atlas (an image with expert-drawn contours) is deformably registered to a new patient's scan to propagate the contours. Multiple atlases can be used (multi-atlas segmentation) to improve robustness. While historically important and still used, atlas-based methods are generally slower and less accurate than current deep learning methods.
- **Inter-Observer Variability**—Differences in the way multiple experts delineate the same structure on an image. High inter-observer variability in head and neck contouring (each physician contouring slightly differently) has been well-documented. Auto-segmentation seeks to reduce this variability by providing a consistent starting contour.
- **Segmentation Pipeline**—The end-to-end process of turning an input image (or set of images) into output contours. A typical AI segmentation pipeline may include preprocessing (normalizing intensities, cropping), running the deep learning model to get a raw segmentation, post-processing (e.g., removing small artifacts), and exporting the result into a format (DICOM-RT structure) compatible with clinical systems.
- **Clinical Workflow Integration**—The incorporation of AI tools into routine clinical practice. For segmentation AI, this means the ability to retrieve images from PACS or scanners, run the model (often via a software interface or within the treatment planning system), and allow clinicians to easily review/edit the AI-generated contours. Effective integration requires the AI tool to fit seamlessly into how radiologists or radiation oncologists already work, without causing major delays or complexity.
- **Regulatory Clearance**—Approval by regulatory bodies (such as the U.S. Food and Drug Administration—FDA, or CE marking in Europe) for clinical use of a medical device or software. AI-based segmentation software intended for patient care usually must undergo this process, demonstrating safety and effectiveness. For example, several AI contouring tools for head and neck OARs have received FDA 510(k) clearance in recent years (e.g., an MRI-based OAR segmentation tool by GE Healthcare cleared in 2025, capable of delineating 37 head, neck, and pelvic structures). Regulatory clearance is a key step before AI tools can be widely adopted in hospitals.

Foundational Principles of Head and Neck Imaging and Segmentation

Imaging Modalities in Head and Neck Anatomy

Multiple imaging modalities are employed in the head and neck region, each with strengths and limitations for anatomical and lesion segmentation. **Computed Tomography (CT)** is commonly used, especially in radiotherapy planning, because it provides electron density information needed for dose calculations and a reasonably good depiction of bony anatomy and some soft tissues. CT is fast and widely available, but differentiating soft-tissue structures in the head and neck (e.g., salivary glands, lymph nodes, muscle groups) can be challenging due to relatively low soft-tissue contrast. **Magnetic Resonance Imaging (MRI)** offers superior soft tissue contrast and is often the imaging modality of choice for delineating tumors and certain organs (like the optic nerves or brainstem) in the head and neck. For example, MRI is better at defining the extent of a nasopharyngeal carcinoma or an oropharyngeal tumor in relation to muscle and fat planes. However, MRI segmentation must contend with varying sequences (T1, T2, contrast-enhanced, etc.), and the images may have lower spatial resolution or more deformation (patient swallow or motion artifacts) compared to CT. **Positron Emission Tomography (PET)**, usually combined with CT (PET/CT), is another modality particularly useful in identifying metabolic activity of tumors or lymph nodes. PET highlights cancerous lesions (e.g., with FDG uptake) and can assist segmentation by providing functional boundaries, but PET resolution is low and it is rarely used alone for detailed anatomical segmentation. In practice, PET is often used in conjunction with CT; for instance, PET/CT auto-segmentation methods have achieved higher tumor segmentation accuracy (dice scores above 0.7) than MRI-alone methods for certain head and neck cancers. Lastly, **Ultrasound** is occasionally used for certain neck structures (like thyroid or lymph nodes), but it is not a primary modality for comprehensive head and neck segmentation due to its limited field of view and operator dependence. In summary, **multimodality imaging** is common—a head and neck cancer patient may have a planning CT, diagnostic MRI, and PET. Each modality's data can be leveraged by AI models, but also poses integration challenges (different resolutions, needing image registration if used together, etc.). Most current AI segmentation efforts in this domain focus on CT (for OARs) and MRI or PET/CT (for tumor segmentation), reflecting their prevalent use in therapy planning and diagnostics, respectively.

Anatomical Complexity and Segmentation Challenges

The head and neck region encompasses a dense array of organs, tissues, and tumors in a relatively small volume, presenting unique challenges for segmentation. Key normal structures include vital organs-at-risk such as the **optic nerves and chiasm, eyes, inner ears, salivary glands (parotid, submandibular), thyroid, spinal cord, brainstem, mandible, larynx, pharyngeal muscles**, and many lymph node levels—among others. These structures vary greatly in size, shape, and contrast on imaging. For example, the parotid glands are large and fairly discernible on CT/MRI, whereas the optic nerves are thin tubular structures that can be difficult to distinguish. Many OARs are in close proximity; the border between, say, a tumor and adjacent muscle, or between the parotid gland and surrounding soft tissue, can be subtle. This proximity demands high precision in segmentation to avoid "leaking" one structure's contour into another. Another challenge is **patient-specific variability**: normal anatomical variations (one patient's lymph node anatomy or vascular anatomy may differ from another's), as well as differences due to pathology (tumors can deform or obscure normal anatomy, or prior surgeries may remove or alter structures). Imaging artifacts are also problematic—dental fillings, for instance, cause streak artifacts on CT that can obscure anatomy in the oral cavity and oropharynx, confounding both humans and algorithms. Similarly, patient motion or swallowing during scanning can blur boundaries. The **class imbalance problem** is evident in lesion segmentation: tumors (target volumes) often occupy a much smaller volume than normal tissues in the head and neck; an AI model must learn to detect a relatively tiny abnormal region in an image dominated by normal anatomy. Additionally, some structures may only be present on one side or not at all (e.g., unilateral neck dissections or congenital absence), requiring algorithms to handle optional anatomy robustly. These factors make manual contouring labor-intensive—the clinician must navigate slice by slice, carefully differentiating each organ. It is reported that the complexity and sheer number of OARs to delineate in head and neck cases contribute to significant workload for planners. Moreover, **inconsistent delineation criteria** add to variability; despite published contouring guidelines (such as those by expert groups), studies have shown considerable inter-observer differences in how experts draw boundaries. For example, one physician might include certain small muscles or lymph node levels that another might contour differently, even when following the same instructions. This variability not only affects the quality of care but also complicates the training of AI models (since the "ground truth" itself may be inconsistent across institutions). In summary, the head and neck region epitomizes the challenges of medical image segmentation: it demands fine-grained precision, must handle a multitude of structures, and requires consistency amid variability.

Traditional Segmentation Approaches (Manual and Atlas-Based)

Prior to the deep learning era, two primary methods were used for head and neck segmentation in clinical practice: **manual contouring** and **atlas-based auto-segmentation**. Manual contouring, as noted, is painstaking and depends on the skill and experience of the clinician. In the 2000s and early 2010s, to alleviate some of this burden, researchers and vendors developed atlas-based solutions. **Atlas-based segmentation** involves using previously contoured patient scans (atlases) and deformably registering them to the new patient's scan to automatically propagate the contours. In head and neck radiotherapy, companies offered atlas libraries of "template" patients where all major OARs were pre-contoured; the software would morph those contours onto the new CT. While this approach could provide a reasonable starting point, it had limitations. Accuracy would drop if the new patient's anatomy diverged too much from the atlas anatomy, or if there were significant pathology-induced distortions. Atlas methods also tended to struggle with **registration errors**, sometimes yielding misplaced or oddly shaped contours that required substantial manual correction. Studies comparing atlas-based auto-segmentation to manual have shown mixed results—while atlas contours can save time, clinicians often still spend non-trivial time editing them for correctness. Notably, an early randomized trial in head and neck cancer found that an atlas-assisted approach did speed up contouring and could be non-inferior to manual in terms of plan quality, but it did not eliminate the need for careful review. **Machine learning methods** prior to deep learning (like statistical shape models or shallow classifiers) saw limited use in this region due to the complexity of shapes involved. Thus, through the 2010s, manual and atlas-based methods were the mainstay. However, as computing power and algorithms improved, **the stage was set for deep learning**—by around 2015, convolutional neural networks had revolutionized image recognition tasks, and pioneers began applying CNNs to medical segmentation, including head and neck OARs. One early CNN application in this field by Ibragimov and Xing demonstrated that a trained neural network could segment several head and neck organs (like mandible, spinal cord, parotids) with accuracy approaching that of experts. The success of these initial studies galvanized interest in AI solutions, leading to the current generation of deep learning-based auto-segmentation tools. By 2018–2020, multiple teams had reported CNN models outperforming atlas-based methods in accuracy for head and neck OARs, firmly establishing deep learning as the new gold standard approach for this task.

AI-Driven Segmentation Techniques

Deep Learning and the U-Net Architecture

At the core of modern AI segmentation is **deep learning**, specifically convolutional neural networks trained on large collections of annotated images. The workhorse architecture for biomedical segmentation is the **U-Net**, introduced by Ronneberger and colleagues in 2015. U-Net has an **encoder-decoder** structure shaped roughly like a "U": the encoder path progressively downsamples the image while learning abstract feature representations (e.g., detecting edges, textures, shapes), and the decoder path upsamples back to the original resolution, using the learned features to output a segmentation map. Crucially, U-Net introduced skip connections that pass high-resolution details from the encoder to corresponding decoder layers, preserving fine spatial information that would otherwise be lost. This design allows U-Net models to achieve both localization precision and contextual understanding—ideal for tasks like delineating a small nerve (fine detail) in the context of an entire CT neck scan (global context). Since 2015, numerous **variants and extensions** of U-Net have been proposed and applied to head and neck segmentation. For instance, **3D U-Net** architectures process whole image volumes (or thick slices) instead of 2D slices, capturing 3D spatial context of structures; this is beneficial for organs like the spinal cord or brainstem, which span multiple slices. Studies have shown that 3D convolutional networks can improve segmentation consistency across slices, albeit at the cost of higher memory usage. Another variation is the **multi-view CNN**, which trains separate 2D U-Nets on different anatomical planes (axial, sagittal, coronal) and combines their outputs. This approach can approximate a 3D understanding while using simpler 2D models, and has been used, for example, to better segment tumors on MRI, where leveraging multiple orientations helps capture complex shapes. **Attention mechanisms** have also been added to U-Nets (e.g., Attention U-Net) to help the network focus on relevant regions and ignore irrelevant background. More recently, researchers have explored **transformer-based architectures** (inspired by the success of Transformers in natural language processing and vision) for segmentation. These models, often called things like "TransUNet" or using **Vision Transformers (ViTs)**, can model long-range dependencies in the image. While promising, they typically require very large training datasets and have only begun to be applied in niche segmentation tasks—as of this writing, CNN-based U-Nets still dominate head and neck segmentation literature due to their efficiency and strong performance on moderate-sized datasets.

One important contribution to the field was the development of **nnU-Net** (no-new-Net) by Isensee et al. in 2021, a self-configuring framework that automatically tunes U-Net models for a given dataset. The nnU-Net approach is noteworthy because it won numerous medical segmentation challenges by using a robust pipeline rather than novel network layers. For head and neck applications, nnU-Net can automatically select appropriate 2D vs. 3D U-Net configurations, data augmentations, and training hyperparameters, often achieving top-tier performance without manual tweaking. Moreover, nnU-Net automatically adapts to multi-modal inputs, such as combining CT with PET as stacked channels, allowing the network to jointly leverage complementary structural and metabolic information. The takeaway is that architectural optimizations and training strategies are as important as the base network. In practice, many current head/neck segmentation tools under the hood are U-Net variants or ensembles of U-Nets. Figure **(Placeholder: U-Net diagram)** illustrates a generic U-Net architecture that could be employed for segmenting a head and neck CT: the input image is downsampled through convolutional layers to extract features (like edges of organs), then upsampled with skip connections to produce a mask labeling each voxel as belonging to a certain organ or not. The final layer might have multiple output channels if segmenting multiple structures in one go (multi-class segmentation)—some AI models segment all OARs with one network, whereas others train separate networks for each organ and combine results. Both approaches exist in the literature. Multi-class segmentation is efficient, but single-class models can sometimes be optimized better for each organ. For example, one open-source project trained **11 separate U-Nets**, one per OAR, to contour common head and neck structures and found that performance exceeded a single multi-class network on some organs. Regardless of approach, it is clear that deep learning has enabled a step-change in segmentation capability: what once required engineered features and deformable templates is now achieved with learned representations from data.

Training Data and Annotation Considerations

A supervised deep learning model is only as good as the data it is trained on, and this maxim holds true for head and neck segmentation. Creating a high-quality training dataset is a major undertaking: one needs numerous patient scans with accurate annotations (contours) for each structure of interest. In radiotherapy contexts, many institutions have archives of CTs with manual OAR contours, which can serve as ground truth. However, these may come from different physicians with different styles; consistency in training labels is crucial. Some studies address this by having one expert or a consensus re-delineate all cases to use as training truth, though this is time-consuming. Data augmentation techniques (randomly shifting, rotating, and adding noise to images during training) are employed to make models more robust to variations and limited sample sizes. For head and neck, augmentation may also simulate different contrast levels or add synthetic artifacts to teach the model to handle real-world imaging issues. **Public datasets and challenges** have contributed significantly to data availability. For instance, the MICCAI 2019 HECKTOR challenge provided PET/CT images for head and neck tumor segmentation, and the Open Segmentation Challenge had a Head-Neck task for OARs on CT and MRI. These allow researchers to train models on multi-institution data and benchmark performance against others. Another consideration is **label scope**: as mentioned, some models aim to segment dozens of OARs, including very small structures (like the inner ear cochlea or tiny lymph node stations), while others focus on a subset (e.g., only the major salivary glands, spinal cord, brainstem, etc.). Including more classes can make the task harder for the model (more chances for confusion), especially if some classes have very little training volume (class imbalance). Techniques like loss function weighting can help (e.g., giving more importance to small structures in the training objective). A notable example, **SOARS** (Stratified Organ At Risk Segmentation) system by Ye et al. tackled 42 head and neck OARs by stratifying them into groups and training specialized models for different subsets, achieving high accuracy across the board. They carefully managed the training process with 176 patients and validated it on 1327 patients from multiple institutions. The result was a model robust enough that in their tests, 98% of its contours required only minor or no adjustments to be clinically acceptable—an impressive feat underlining what ample data and thoughtful model design can accomplish. Finally, beyond images and labels, training an AI segmentation model also requires choosing hyperparameters (learning rate, number of epochs), and often using a **validation set** to prevent overfitting. Cross-validation or testing on independent cohorts from other hospitals is highly recommended, given that CT scanners, MRI sequences, and patient demographics can differ. A model trained only on one hospital's scans might perform worse on another's due to subtle differences (this is known as the domain shift problem). For this reason, recent work emphasizes **multi-institutional training and testing** to ensure generalizability. In summary, assembling a diverse, well-annotated dataset and following best practices in training is foundational to any successful AI segmentation project.

Performance Metrics for Segmentation

How do we know if an AI segmentation is good? This is where **evaluation metrics** come in. The **Dice similarity coefficient (DSC)** is the most commonly reported metric in segmentation studies. As defined in Key Terms, it measures overlap between the AI-generated segmentation and the ground-truth segmentation. A Dice of 1 (or 100%) indicates perfect overlap, whereas 0 indicates no overlap. In head and neck OAR segmentation, Dice scores typically range from about 0.7 to 0.9 for major structures when the AI is performing well; values in the 0.8–0.9 range usually indicate the AI contour is very close to expert-drawn. For instance, auto-segmentation of a large organ like the brainstem or mandible might achieve Dice ~0.90 because these structures have clear boundaries and contrast on CT. In contrast, a small or hard-to-see structure like an optic chiasm might yield Dice ~0.70–0.80 even for a good model, because a one-voxel difference in boundary could significantly affect the overlap proportion (and inter-expert Dice might not be much higher either, due to inherent ambiguity in where the boundary lies). It's worth noting that Dice is **insensitive to where errors occur**—missing a chunk of contour in the middle versus slightly misaligning the entire contour can result in similar Dice values, even though the latter might be clinically more acceptable than the former. To address spatial accuracy, **surface distance metrics** are used. The **Hausdorff Distance (HD)** is one such measure: it looks at the maximum error between the surfaces of AI and ground truth. A variant, **HD95**, calculates the 95th percentile of distances, which effectively ignores a few outlier points and gives a more robust measure of the "worst case" error. For example, an HD95 of 5 mm for a parotid gland segmentation means that except for possibly a few isolated points, the AI contour is within 5 mm of the true contour everywhere—a decent result since 5 mm is within typical inter-observer variability. If an AI overshoots into an adjacent structure badly, the HD95 would increase accordingly. Another metric seen in literature is the **mean surface distance (MSD)**, which averages the distance errors over the surface; this gives a sense of overall boundary agreement in physical units (mm). In the context of head and neck, one might see a result like: "DSC = 0.85, HD95 = 3 mm, MSD = 1 mm" for an organ, indicating substantial overlap and very tight boundary alignment on average, with at most a 3 mm deviation at the worst parts. When tumor volume itself is an important clinical decision point, the **Relative Volume Error** becomes relevant, although it is less reported in the literature. It is defined as the difference between the ground truth and the AI-generated volume of the segmentations, divided by the ground truth volume. For tumor segmentation (lesions), often besides Dice and HD, **precision and recall** (or sensitivity) may be reported to evaluate how well the model identifies the tumor voxels versus including false positives. Overestimation (false positives) is a common problem in tumor auto-segmentation on MRI—the model might "spill" beyond the actual tumor. In such cases, a moderate Dice might hide the fact that the model captured the tumor but also some extra areas; looking at precision (percent of AI segmentation that is correct) and recall (percent of true tumor captured) can be informative. A high recall but low precision means the model found the tumor but also added much extra that needs deletion. Another approach in evaluation is **qualitative expert scoring**—e.g., having physicians rate AI contours as acceptable, minor edit needed, major edit needed, or unusable. Such scales directly measure clinical acceptability. Some studies combine these: for example, an AI might achieve high Dice on average, but if an important structure is missed entirely for one patient, the Dice metric (averaged over a test set) might not reflect that catastrophic failure. Therefore, researchers also count **failure cases** or compute the percentage of structures where the AI contour was within some acceptable threshold. In clinical deployment, consistency is key—it's often better to have slightly lower average Dice if that means avoiding large errors that require re-contouring from scratch. One example: in a cross-center study, the auto-segmentation of most OARs had no statistically significant differences from manual contours in terms of Dice and other metrics, implying the AI was essentially as good as human-drawn for those metrics; but the true test was that when these AI contours were used as a starting point, after physician edits the resulting contours had reduced inter-observer variability compared to fully manual ones. This hints that beyond pure numbers, **AI can serve to standardize** the outcome by providing a consistent baseline, which humans then fine-tune. In summary, evaluating segmentation involves a **basket of metrics**: overlap (Dice), boundary accuracy (HD95, MSD), possibly region-based stats (volume difference, etc.), and increasingly important—human evaluation of whether the contour is clinically acceptable or how much time savings it provides. The next section provides a "Math Moment" to clarify how one of these metrics, the Dice coefficient, is calculated and interpreted.

Math Moment: Dice Similarity Coefficient (DSC) The Dice coefficient quantifies how well two regions overlap. If we denote A as the set of voxels in the ground truth contour and B as the set of voxels in the AI-generated contour, the Dice is defined as:

$$DSC = \frac{2|A \cap B|}{|A| + |B|}$$

In other words, it's twice the number of overlapping voxels divided by the total number of voxels in both contours. The factor of 2 ensures that if one contour is a perfect subset of the other, the Dice will be <1 unless they're identical—it penalizes both misses and false positives symmetrically. As an example, suppose an expert delineated a lymph node tumor of volume 10 cm^3, and an AI model segmented a volume of 9 cm^3, of which 8 cm^3 correctly overlaps with the expert's area. The Dice would be $2 \times 8/(10 + 9) = 16/19 \approx 0.84$ (84%). A Dice of 0.84 is quite good, though it indicates the AI missed part of the tumor and also included a non-tumor area. If the Dice were 1.0 (100%), it would mean the AI's segmentation exactly matches the expert's. If Dice is 0, the AI and expert segmentations do not overlap at all (a complete failure or perhaps segmenting entirely different regions). In practice, a "good" Dice score depends on the context—for large well-defined structures (like the brain in neuroimaging) one might expect >0.9, but for small, ambiguous structures in head and neck (like certain lymph node levels or small glands), a Dice of 0.75 might be an acceptable result given that even two experts might only agree to that extent. It's important to remember Dice is a **global overlap measure** and does not directly tell you where the discrepancies are—hence it is often paired with surface distance metrics like HD95, which might say (for instance) that the worst-case boundary error is 5 mm. Together, these numbers help assess if the segmentation is accurate enough for clinical use.

Model Architectures and Advancements

U-Net and CNN Variants As detailed, U-Net is ubiquitous in biomedical segmentation. Many head and neck segmentation models in research are essentially U-Nets with tweaks. For example, **DeepMedic** (a 3D CNN originally developed for brain lesions) has been adapted for head and neck by using multi-scale inputs. Some architectures incorporate **residual blocks** (like in ResNet) into the U-Net backbone for potentially improved feature learning. Others incorporate **dense connections** (like in DenseNet) for better gradient flow. However, one consistent finding in the community is that no single exotic architecture has completely supplanted U-Net; rather, careful training and data handling often matter more. A 2019 study by van Rooij et al. compared a deep learning model to atlas-based results and provided geometric/dosimetric evaluation; it used a straightforward U-Net and still showed clear advantages over the atlas method in accuracy. **Two-Stage Models**: Another approach is cascaded models—for instance, one network first roughly identifies a region of interest (like where the parotid gland is), and a second network then does a fine segmentation within that cropped region. This can improve results for small structures, as the second stage can focus on a smaller area at higher resolution. Such two-stage or "coarse-to-fine" pipelines have been used especially in research on tumors, where first a network finds the tumor region and then another delineates its precise boundary. **Ensemble models** are also seen: combining outputs of multiple networks (say, one 2D U-Net and one 3D U-Net, or several models initialized differently) can often boost performance by averaging out individual model quirks (Fig. 3.1).

Transformers and Emerging Methods Transformer-based segmentation models (often called **Segmentation Transformers** or incorporating modules like a self-attention layer into U-Net, e.g., TransUNet, Swin-Unet) are an active area of

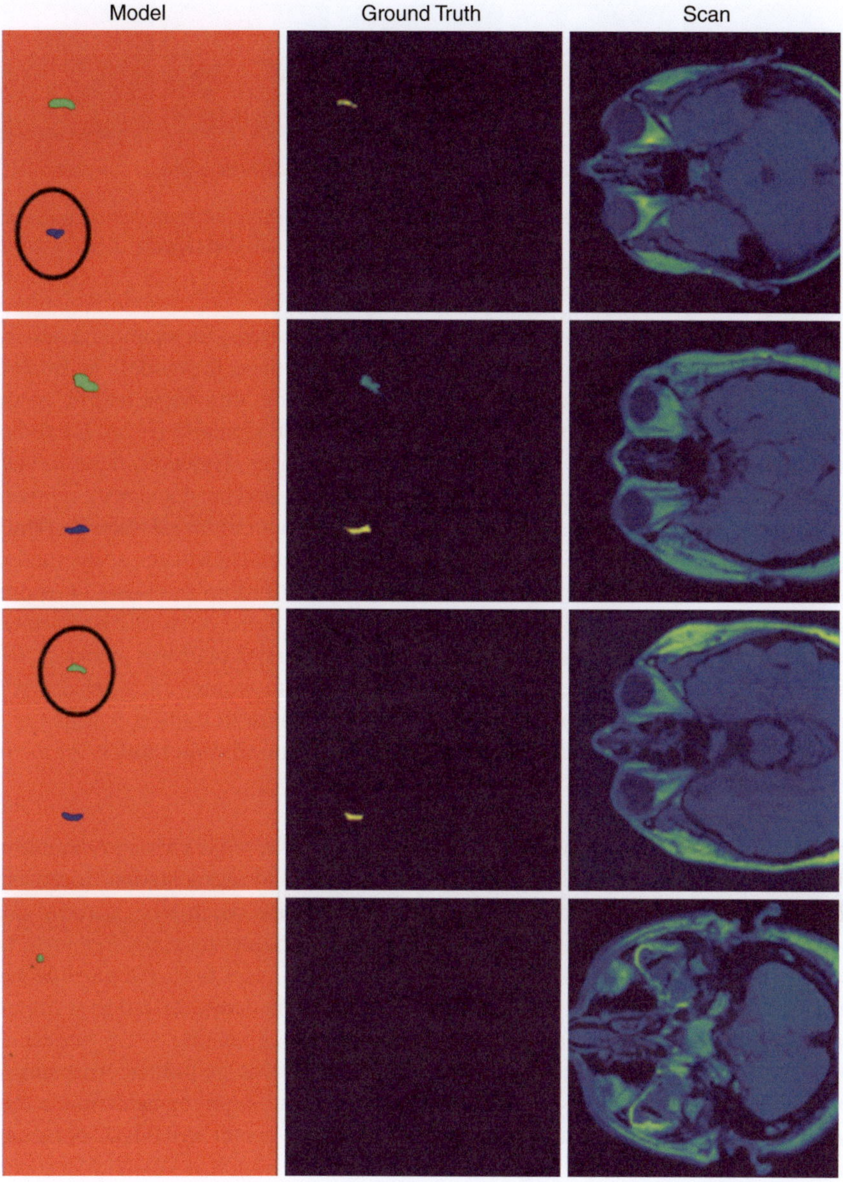

Fig. 3.1 Unet was used for automated segmentation of the lacrimal glands on MRI in this example

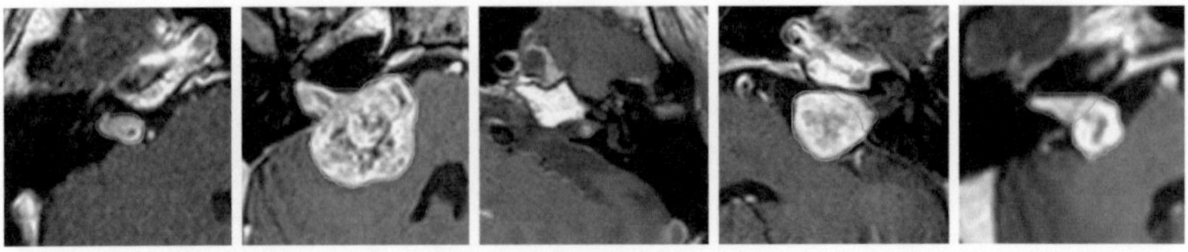

Fig. 3.2 Representative examples of fully automated three-dimensional vestibular schwannoma segmentation on contrast-enhanced T1-weighted MRI, using the nnU-Net pipeline. Red: intrameatal component; green: extrameatal component

research. They potentially handle long-range context better—for example, knowing that if a certain structure is identified in one part of the image, the model can "attend" to distant but related features. In head and neck imaging, this might help in ensuring, say, that left and right parotid glands are segmented similarly or that if a tumor is found in one slice, it pays attention to connected slices. However, these models require large training datasets to realize their potential, and head and neck segmentation data, while growing, is not as plentiful as, say, natural image datasets. Thus, as of 2025, transformers are not yet standard in commercial head/neck segmentation tools, but we might expect to see more of them as institutions pool data or as pre-training on big datasets (like using models initially trained on whole-body organ segmentation) becomes feasible. Indeed, one commercial platform approach has been to pre-train a model on millions of contours from various sites (head, neck, body) and then fine-tune to a specific clinic's data—akin to transfer learning at a large scale. This can be thought of as moving towards **foundation models** for medical imaging segmentation.

AutoML and Self-Configuring Pipelines The nnU-Net we discussed is an example of automated machine learning (AutoML) applied to segmentation. It reduces the need for an engineer to manually decide things like patch size, learning rate schedule, etc., thereby making it easier to deploy AI in new contexts. In a hospital setting, this means one could feed their own annotated cases to such a pipeline and get a decent model without extensive AI expertise. This democratization is important for widespread adoption and for niche tasks (like segmenting a very rare structure) where a bespoke model might be needed but resources are limited. An example of such is the work by Neve et al. on vestibular schwannoma segmentation, a rare intracranial tumor, who trained the nnU-Net on multi-center MRI data, obtaining accurate delineation results (Fig. 3.2).

Continuous Learning A final note on model development: some systems now support **continuous learning** or **adaptive learning**, where corrections made by clinicians on AI-generated contours can be fed back to retrain or fine-tune the model. For instance, a tool might notice that a clinician consistently enlarges the AI's contour for the larynx; this feedback could be used to adjust the model. There are challenges here—one must avoid drift or learning from erroneous edits—but conceptually this closes the loop to improve performance over time and adapt to individual physician preferences or demographic differences in patient population. A related concept is **incremental learning for new structures**: e.g., adding an ability to segment a new organ without forgetting how to segment the original ones (known as avoiding catastrophic forgetting). Techniques from machine learning are being brought in to handle these.

In summary, the architectural and algorithmic toolkit for AI segmentation is rich and evolving, but the common thread is that nearly all successful approaches leverage CNN-based segmentation networks (especially U-Net style) as a backbone. The differences lie in how they are optimized, how data is augmented and fed, and how they might incorporate new ideas like attention or multi-stage refinement. The result of these innovations is reflected in the performance metrics we see in literature—steadily improving Dice scores and decreasing editing times—which we will explore in the context of specific studies and applications next.

Applications of AI Segmentation in Head and Neck

Auto-Segmentation of Organs-at-Risk (OARs) for Radiotherapy

One of the most mature and impactful applications of AI in head and neck imaging is the auto-segmentation of organs-at-risk for radiotherapy treatment planning. In a standard head-and-neck radiotherapy case, a clinician must contour numerous critical structures on the planning CT (and sometimes MRI)—these contours inform how the radiation beams are shaped and optimized. AI-driven auto-segmentation serves as an AI assistant, providing an initial set of contours that the clinician can then review and edit rather than drawing everything from scratch. This application has rapidly gained traction in clinics worldwide because of its clear efficiency benefits and the relatively straightforward integration into the treatment planning workflow. Many commercial treatment planning systems or add-on software now offer auto-contouring plug-ins. Nowadays, beyond auto-contouring, plan prediction (to calculate the radiation dose) has also become the domain of AI and is starting to find its way to commercial Treatment Planning Systems.

Efficiency and Time Savings Clinical studies consistently report significant time savings using AI auto-segmentation. For example, a study by Doolan et al. evaluated five commercial AI contouring systems and found that for head and neck cases, using any of the AI solutions reduced contouring time by on the order of **70–90 min per case** on average. Considering that manual head/neck contouring might take 2–3 h, this is a roughly 40–50% reduction in time. Another multi-institutional trial reported overall time savings of **42% and 49%** in two separate phases of their study when using AI vs. manual. The magnitude of saved time can vary by structure: larger, easier structures (like brain or bone) might be almost entirely AI-drawn with minimal edits, whereas very small or tricky structures (certain lymph node levels, for instance) might still require manual refinement, thus yielding less time saved. Interestingly, Pang et al. noted that lymph node levels I and some Level IV subdivisions showed no significant time savings in their study—at some centers, editing the AI's nodal contours took as long as manual drawing would have. This highlights that not every structure benefits equally from current AI; the simpler and more well-defined OARs currently reap the most benefit. Since the clinical acceptance and use of auto-contouring tools has sharply risen, Mody et al. recently created an "AI-pencil" that can efficiently correct (rather than create from scratch) contours with the help of AI. They conducted a comparison study on head and neck imaging data and found that experts were 16–97% faster with the AI-pencil than without it.

Accuracy and Consistency In terms of contour accuracy, deep learning models have largely surpassed atlas-based methods. Gibbons et al. demonstrated that a deep learning auto-segmentation system achieved higher geometric accuracy (compared to reference manual contours) than an atlas approach across head and neck OARs. Typical Dice scores for AI vs. expert in head/neck OAR are in the high 0.8s for many organs, which is often on par with the inter-observer agreement between two human experts. For instance, in Doolan et al.'s multivendor study, the median Dice scores for head and neck OARs were reported around 0.82–0.88 for the various AI systems. All systems thus produced "good" contours, and indeed the variability between different AI vendors was small compared to the variability between human observers. This suggests a certain level of **maturation** in the technology—multiple independent groups have managed to reach a similarly high performance level, likely because they all leverage similar network architectures (U-Net variants) and have access to training on large datasets. One concern, however, is **error modes** of AI: while average performance is high, occasionally an AI might completely miss a structure or confuse it (especially if the anatomy is unusual). For example, if a patient has had surgery and lacks a left parotid gland, an AI trained mostly on patients with two parotids might hallucinate a contour where tissue once was. Awareness of such failure modes is important. Clinically, it is emphasized that **auto-segmentation outputs must be reviewed by clinicians**. If an AI contour needs only minor tweaking, great—but if a contour is substantially off and requires as much time to fix as drawing anew, then the AI hasn't helped for that structure. This is why some evaluations (including Doolan et al.) specifically measure correction time. Ideally, the sum of AI contour generation time plus user correction time is much less than manual time; if it approaches manual time, the AI might not be worth using for that particular structure or scenario.

Clinical Acceptance An important measure beyond pure geometry is whether the AI-drawn contours are clinically acceptable after editing. In many studies, physicians rate the final contours or simply note if they would use them for planning. Lucido et al. conducted a validation of a deep-learning autosegmentation for head/neck OARs and found that after minimal edits, the contours were within acceptable clinical tolerances in the vast majority of cases. Ye et al. reported that 98% of their model's OAR contours needed only minor or no edits to be accepted, which is an exceptionally high rate. These results are very promising—they imply that for routine cases, an AI could essentially pre-contour everything and the doctor just does a quick check and minor adjustment, rather than laboring through each structure. Also notable is the effect on **inter-observer variability**. When multiple clinicians each manually contour a case, their results can differ (sometimes markedly). But if they all start from the same AI contour and just edit, their final results tend to be more similar to each other than purely manual results. This was shown in Pang's multicenter study: when physicians edited AI contours, the variation between centers in how structures were contoured decreased, compared to when each did it manually in their usual way. Such harmonization is a subtle but important benefit: it can lead to more uniform treatment planning and potentially make outcomes more comparable across institutions. It is even useful for clinical trials, where consistent contouring is needed for a fair comparison of treatments. An important clinical marker for contour quality is also dependent on the downstream task, i.e., how the contours are used. In the case of radiotherapy as a treatment modality, many studies therefore adopt metrics derived from the dose distribution that was derived from the segmentations. To that end the so-called Dose Volume Histogram is computed and measures such as D_{max}, the maximum dose within a region, and $V_{95\%}$, the percentage of a region receiving at least 95% of the prescription dose, are derived and compared with clinical guidelines.

Lymph Node Levels and Special Cases Head and neck radiotherapy often requires contouring not just organs but also target volumes like lymph node regions (elective nodal levels). Auto-segmentation of nodal levels is tricky since those are anatomical regions rather than distinct organs. Some AI solutions have tackled it by training on physician-drawn nodal station contours. Early work on atlas-based segmentation of nodal levels showed a reduction in inter-observer variation, and recent AI methods continue that trend with better accuracy. However, as mentioned, some nodal levels benefit less from automation because they can be ambiguous and vary by clinical judgment. In practice, many clinics still draw nodal target volumes manually to ensure they cover exactly the tissue at risk as per clinical criteria. The AI might assist in suggesting a volume, but radiation oncologists often modify it heavily due to oncologic reasoning (like patterns of spread that an AI, which only sees images, might not fully infer). Therefore, current AI segmentation is predominantly used for **OARs** rather than gross tumor volumes (GTVs) or clinical target volumes (CTV nodal levels). OAR segmentation is a natural fit because it's well-defined anatomically and doesn't require oncologic decision-making beyond identification. Still, as AI models get more sophisticated and incorporate, say, PET information, they might take on more of the target delineation in the future (see next section for tumor segmentation).

In summary, auto-segmentation of normal structures in the head and neck is a real-world success of AI in medical imaging. It addresses a clear clinical pain point (time and variability in contouring), and extensive validation shows that contemporary models can produce high-quality, clinically usable contours. Table 3.1 below

Table 3.1 Selected commercial AI segmentation tools for head & neck

Product (company)	Description & features	Regulatory status	Notes
Contour ProtégéAI (Mirada Medical)	Deep learning auto-contouring software that covers a wide range of OARs (including head, neck, etc.) and some target volumes. Often integrated via treatment planning systems as a plug-in.	FDA 510(k) cleared (Nov 2023) as "Contour ProtégéAI" for clinical use. CE-marked in EU.	Provides ~100+ contours including lymph node levels. Known for user-friendly editing interface.
MVision AI Contouring (MVision)	A cloud-based auto-segmentation service: the CT is uploaded to MVision's platform, which returns contours for head & neck and other sites. Emphasizes multi-institution training data and continuous learning.	CE-marked; FDA clearance for certain sites (e.g., prostate)—head & neck model in use in Europe.	Used globally in clinics; requires internet connection to use. Offers a subscription model.
AutoContour (Radformation)	An AI segmentation tool integrated with planning systems (works with Eclipse via scripting). Focuses on common structures in head & neck, breast, etc.	FDA-cleared (as of 2023) for multiple anatomies including head/neck OARs.	Strength in tight integration with existing TPS workflow (Radformation also provides automation tools).
RayStation DLC (RaySearch Laboratories)	RayStation treatment planning system's Deep Learning Contouring (DLC) models. Built into the TPS—user selects which organs to auto-segmentation and the model (trained on large datasets) generates them within RayStation.	CE-marked; pending FDA (RayStation as a whole is cleared, DLC models clearance varies by release).	Convenient for RayStation users; covers many structures but only for those with models provided (67+ contours in head & neck as per 2023).
TheraPanacea (ART-Plan)	A suite including AI autosegmentation (known as **Harmony** Segmentation). Uses deep learning to contour OARs and some targets, with emphasis on adaptive radiotherapy integration.	CE-marked; in clinical use in EU/Asia. Not yet widely FDA cleared.	Multi-organ model (reports ~80+ head/neck structures). Strong academic collaborations, e.g., used in multi-institution studies.
Siemens AI-Rad Companion Organs RT (Siemens Healthineers)	Automated segmentation for radiotherapy planning, including head & neck CT and MR. Can segment numerous organs and export them to DICOM RT structure sets.	FDA 510(k) cleared (2022) for multiple anatomies; CE-marked.	Available as part of Siemens software ecosystem; uses both CT and MR models.

(continued)

Table 3.1 (continued)

Product (company)	Description & features	Regulatory status	Notes
GE Healthcare MR Contour ~ DL (GE)	MRI-based auto-segmentation tool focusing on leveraging MR imaging for improved soft-tissue delineation (37 organs in head, neck, and pelvis).	FDA 510(k) cleared (2025).	Useful for MR-only planning or MRI-guided radiotherapy. Showcased at ESTRO 2025, indicating a new trend to incorporate MRI in planning.

Notes: All the above systems offer **significant time savings** in practice, on the order of tens of minutes per case. They generally allow editing of results and do not require AI expertise to operate. Pricing and licensing vary; many are licensed per machine or per institution, and cloud ones may be usage-based. Also, most vendors continually update their models, so performance improves over time (e.g., adding new organs, refining accuracy with more training data)

lists some **commercial AI OAR segmentation solutions** and their characteristics, as well as **open-source or academic tools** available for this task.

Tumor and Lesion Segmentation

Beyond normal anatomy, AI is also applied to segment **pathologic lesions** in the head and neck, such as primary tumors, metastatic lymph nodes, or other abnormalities (e.g., cysts, vascular lesions on imaging). This application can support radiologists in measuring tumor volumes, assist radiation oncologists in defining gross tumor volume for planning, or help surgeons and oncologists in treatment assessment (like tracking tumor shrinkage on therapy). However, tumor segmentation is inherently more challenging than OAR segmentation for several reasons: tumors vary widely in shape, size, location, and imaging appearance, and there is no fixed "template" like there is for an organ. Additionally, tumors can blend with surrounding tissues, especially on modalities like MRI. As a result, the performance of AI for lesion segmentation in head and neck has been more mixed and generally not as advanced as for OARs.

Segmentation on CT vs. MRI vs. PET The modality used drastically affects outcomes. On **contrast-enhanced CT**, many head and neck tumors are visible, but others (especially when the tumor's density is similar to muscle) can be hard to delineate even for experts. AI models trained on CT alone can miss the extent that a radiologist would catch by also considering MRI or clinical exam. On **MRI**, the tumor is often well delineated due to contrast differences (e.g., a T2-weighted MRI shows a nasopharyngeal carcinoma clearly against surrounding tissue). However, AI on MRI has struggled historically because MRI datasets were smaller and varied (different sequence parameters). A study by Schouten et al. attempted automatic segmentation of primary head and neck tumors on MRI using a multi-view

CNN. They reported an average Dice of only **0.49** (49%) for the tumor segmentation, which indicates moderate overlap at best. Small tumors (<3 cm^3 volume) had especially low Dice (~0.26), whereas larger tumors (>15 cm^3) reached about 0.63. The model tended to **overestimate** tumor volume and had false positives in healthy structures. This points to a common problem: ensuring that the AI is precise in distinguishing tumors from normal tissues. **PET/CT** approaches have generally shown better results for certain tumors (like FDG-PET, highlighting metabolically active tumors can reach Dice >0.70, as noted in Schouten's background). There have been MICCAI challenges (HECKTOR) focusing on segmenting head and neck cancers using PET/CT, and top algorithms often combine CNNs that use both the metabolic PET signal and the anatomical CT to get the best of both worlds. Some commercial tools also incorporate PET for tumor auto-contouring, especially for nasopharyngeal or oropharyngeal cancers, where PET can help delineate nodes and primary better than CT alone.

Clinical Integration for Tumors In clinical practice, most physicians still manually delineate GTVs (tumors) because this task is nuanced—it requires integrating knowledge of how the cancer spreads. For example, knowing that a certain lymph node is involved or not might depend on size criteria or other context that a generic image segmentation AI might not handle. That said, AI can assist as a second pair of eyes: e.g., highlighting lymph nodes on a CT that are abnormally enlarged or suggestive, which the physician can then review. Some AI research tools perform **lymph node detection and segmentation** in head/neck CTs, which could be useful for diagnostic radiology as well (finding abnormal nodes on scans). For primary tumors, an AI might provide a preliminary contour that the physician adjusts. A scenario where this could be especially helpful is in adaptive radiotherapy—if a tumor shrinks significantly mid-treatment, one may re-scan and re-contour; having AI generate the new tumor contour for the shrunken tumor could save time.

Outcomes and Radiomics Segmented tumor volumes can be used to derive quantitative features (a field known as **radiomics**). Although not the main focus of this chapter, it's worth noting that having consistent tumor segmentations via AI can enable better radiomic analysis for predicting outcomes or feeding into AI models that predict prognosis. In research, some have used AI to segment tumors and then used those volumes to model patient outcomes like response to chemoradiotherapy. High-quality segmentation is a prerequisite for reliable radiomic features (like shape, texture of the tumor). Thus, improving AI for tumor segmentation could have downstream benefits in personalized medicine for head and neck cancer.

Current Performance and Challenges In summary, for **OARs** we have near-clinical-grade AI solutions widely used; for **tumors**, AI tools exist but are usually adjuncts rather than replacements for human delineation. The challenges include obtaining enough training data (especially for rare tumor sites or variations), dealing with imaging modality differences, and achieving the level of precision a clinician would trust. Some promising approaches involve **multi-modal AI**—e.g., combining CT, MRI, and PET inputs in a unified model to leverage all information. Another line of work is **using prior knowledge or shape constraints**, since tumors don't have consistent shapes, one could incorporate knowledge like "tumors are contiguous regions" to avoid scattered false positives. The goal in the coming years is to push tumor auto-segmentation closer to the reliability of OAR auto-segmentation. Even if not fully automatic, a robust tumor AI could highlight areas of probable tumor for the physician, which might expedite the process or catch regions that might be overlooked (especially in large, complex cases).

Integration into Clinical Workflow

For AI segmentation to provide value, it must integrate smoothly into the clinical workflow of radiologists and radiation oncologists. Workflow integration includes both technical integration (software) and human factors (how users incorporate it in their routine).

Technical Integration Many hospitals use Picture Archiving and Communication Systems (PACS) for radiology images and dedicated Treatment Planning Systems (TPS) for radiotherapy. AI solutions can integrate in a few ways: **Built-in TPS Modules:** Some treatment planning software (e.g., Varian Eclipse, Elekta Monaco, RayStation) now have AI segmentation features either built-in or as plug-ins. For instance, RayStation's AI segmentation uses a built-in model (RaySearch has developed machine learning models) and can automatically contour structures once the planning CT is loaded, requiring just a button click. This tight integration is convenient for users as they don't have to switch software. **Third-Party Software and PACS Integration:** Other solutions act as separate applications. For example, a clinician can send a CT scan from PACS to a dedicated AI software (say, Mirada Medical's software or MVision's cloud platform). The AI processes the image (some cloud solutions can do this in a couple of minutes) and returns the contours, which are then imported into the planning system or viewed on PACS. GE Healthcare's recently FDA-cleared **MR Contour ~ DL** for MRI-based segmentation is an example: it would take MRI images and output contours of head & neck organs, which can be sent to planning systems. Similarly, some cloud-based offerings allow uploading DICOM images to a web portal and then downloading the resulting DICOM RT structure set. **Open-Source Platforms:** Tools like 3D Slicer (a free medical image analysis application) with the **MONAI Label** plug-in enable integration of AI models into the imaging software radiologists use for segmentation. A radiologist could load an MRI into Slicer, click "run model" for head & neck tumor segmentation, and get an initial contour which they can refine with Slicer's editing tools, then save or push to PACS. This approach is in pilot in some research settings.

User Interaction and Acceptance Introducing AI into workflow requires careful user training and setting expectations. Many departments have developed protocols where the AI segmentation is used as a first draft. The clinician then reviews each structure. If a contour is good, great—if not, they correct it. Some clinics initially double-check every contour meticulously (essentially treating it as if they were contouring, just faster). As confidence in the tool grows, some editing tasks may be delegated to junior staff or the review might become faster. It's generally emphasized that **AI does not eliminate the need for an expert**, but rather re-focuses the expert's effort from drawing to verifying and fine-tuning. There can be a learning curve: radiotherapy staff must become familiar with the typical quirks of their AI system (e.g., "it usually undercontours the larynx cartilage – keep an eye on that" or "it sometimes confuses the sternocleidomastoid muscle as a lymph node"). When users know these tendencies, they can quickly correct them.

Interactivity Some emerging tools allow interactive refinement—for instance, the user can click on a region to indicate "this is tumor" or "this is not tumor" and the AI will update the segmentation on the fly. Such human-in-the-loop systems can combine the speed of AI with the intuition of a human, leading to a segmentation process that's faster than manual but more accurate than a one-shot AI. This is particularly useful for complex tumor cases where an initial auto-segmentation might be rough; a few corrections can steer it right. An example of such a tool is the "AI-pencil" by Mody et al.

Quality Assurance (QA) Many institutions treat AI-generated contours the same as those from another human source—they undergo QA like any other contour. For example, if a clinic has peer review meetings of contours, they will look at AI-assisted cases just like manual ones to ensure nothing is missed. Over time, if AI proves very reliable for certain structures, the QA might be streamlined (but not removed). Additionally, if a major discrepancy is found (e.g., AI missed half of a structure), it's valuable to feed that back to vendors or developers to improve future versions.

IT and Infrastructure Implementing AI in practice requires appropriate hardware if on-premises (GPUs for local model inference if not using cloud) and dealing with patient data transfer (ensuring de-identification if using cloud services, or that the cloud service is compliant with health data regulations). Some hospitals choose on-premises solutions to keep data internal, while others use secure cloud offerings for ease of updates and maintenance. The decision often involves the IT department, legal/privacy teams, and cost considerations. Cloud solutions often operate on a software-as-a-service model, potentially charging per use or per patient set, whereas on-premises might be a one-time purchase or license.

Regulatory and Liability Aspects With FDA- or CE-cleared tools, using them clinically is generally allowed as per the clearance. However, clinicians remain responsible for the final contours. It's analogous to any other tool—for instance, a spell-checker in word processing: it catches many errors but the writer is responsible for the final text. If an AI segmentation error leads to a significant issue (like a critical organ not being spared enough dose), it would still be the treatment team's responsibility if they failed to catch it. This is why human review is essential and also why AI output is often locked for editing (not just accepted blindly). Some regulatory bodies or professional societies have issued guidelines: for example, the American Association of Physicists in Medicine (AAPM) suggests thorough local validation of auto-segmentation models and periodic checks to ensure they remain accurate after any software updates. In addition to FDA- and CE-marking, which is typically the domain of industry, within the European Union, for example, it is allowed to use locally created AI tools as well, but only when a process defined in the Medical Device Regulations (MDR) is followed.

Institution-Specific Customization One insight from studies like Pang 2025 is that **institution-specific commissioning** of auto-segmentation is needed to maximize benefit. This means each clinic should test the tool on a sample of their own cases, measure how much time it really saves, ensure the contours meet their physicians' standards, and possibly adjust parameters (some tools allow tweaking the aggressiveness of contouring or which structures to contour). If the tool performs sub-optimally on certain organs in their setting, they might decide to only use it for the organs it's good at, and contour the others manually or using a different method. Also, institutions often maintain their own contouring standards (some may contour certain lymph node levels that others do not); they must configure the AI or supplement it to adhere to those standards.

In conclusion, integrating AI segmentation into clinical practice is as much a process issue as it is a technical one. The technology is there to produce the contours, but getting it to smoothly work within clinical operations—and having the human clinicians trust and efficiently use it—determines the actual impact on patient care. Done well, integration can lead to a faster, more consistent planning workflow, as evidenced by numerous centers now routinely using AI for head and neck cases without slowing down throughput (in fact often speeding it up). In the next section, we will enumerate some of the prominent **tools and platforms** available, which exemplify how these integrations are implemented.

Tools and Platforms: Commercial and Open-Source

The growing demand for AI segmentation in head and neck oncology has spurred a variety of tools. **Commercial solutions** are typically user-friendly, validated products that come with support and regulatory clearance, whereas **open-source solutions** offer flexibility and transparency for research or institutions with the necessary expertise to implement them. Tables 3.1 and 3.2 provide overviews of selected examples in each category:

Table 3.2 Selected open-source/academic segmentation tools

Tool/framework	Description	Accessibility	Notes
nnU-Net (Isensee et al.) [Framework]	An open-source self-configuring segmentation method. While not specific to head & neck, it has been applied to it. Users can train on their data and get a ready model. Code available in Python (MIT license).	Free, open-source (GitHub). Requires coding skills to train on own data. Pretrained models from challenges sometimes available.	nnU-Net won the MICCAI 2021 Head & Neck segmentation challenge, demonstrating top performance. Often the starting point for researchers.
HeadNeck AutoSeg	A ready-to-use deep learning tool for 11 common head & neck OARs, provided by researchers as a packaged solution (with pre-trained models and a web interface).	Free, via GitHub. Comes with Docker and instructions; requires modest hardware.	Focused on CT OAR segmentation. The authors showed it performed better than an atlas tool and released it for others to adopt.
TotalSegmentator (Wasserthal et al.)	A robust tool that segments a comprehensive set of organs in CT (total body) using deep learning. Though not tailored to head & neck, it includes head/neck organs in its outputs (e.g., lenses, eyes, optic nerves, etc.).	Free for research (Apache 2.0 license). Pre-trained model available that runs on any CT image.	Useful for quickly labeling many structures. Might not be as fine-tuned for small H&N structures as dedicated models, but very convenient.
3D Slicer + MONAI Label	3D Slicer is an open-source imaging workstation. MONAI Label is a plug-in that allows deploying AI models for interactive segmentation. Several community-contributed H&N models (e.g., for salivary glands, tumors) exist.	Free. Slicer is cross-platform; MONAI Label server (Python) is free.	Allows a clinician to click and get AI suggestions inside Slicer. Good for research or centers building their own AI. Requires some setup to host the model.
Plastimatch Automated Segmentation (MABS)	An open-source multi-atlas segmentation tool (non-AI) as part of Plastimatch toolkit, sometimes used as a baseline in research or when deep learning is not available.	Free (Apache 2.0). Included in Plastimatch, which can be used via command line or through 3D Slicer.	While not a learning-based AI, it's a legacy open method that is still used in open-source planning systems (e.g., CERR or SlicerRT) for comparison. Much slower than CNNs and accuracy varies by atlas quality.

(continued)

Table 3.2 (continued)

Tool/framework	Description	Accessibility	Notes
Carina IntContour (research use)	Carina is a platform focusing on bringing AI autosegmentation to low-resource settings. IntContour is their tool that was used in a study for Africa (not fully open-source, but academic collaboration).	Collaborative access (not publicly downloadable as of 2024).	Demonstrates the use of AI via the web for contouring in remote setups. Emphasizes training on diverse data.

Notes: Open-source solutions are valuable for innovation and customizability. However, they require technical know-how to implement, and they do not come with formal regulatory approval (they are typically "research use only"). Some clinics with strong medical physics or informatics teams incorporate these into internal research pipelines or for non-critical tasks. For example, an academic center might use an open model to generate contours for retrospective studies or as a second-check tool, even if the primary clinical workflow uses a commercial FDA-cleared tool.

It should be mentioned that **not all tools are equal**—accuracy can vary, and one should refer to publications or benchmarks. For instance, the performance of the five commercial systems was found to be broadly similar in one study, but a different study might find nuances (e.g., one might be slightly better on optic nerves, another on parotids, etc.). Open-source models similarly range in quality; the advantage is that one can potentially fine-tune them on local data to improve them.

Choosing a tool often depends on the clinical context: A busy radiotherapy center might opt for a commercial solution with support and integration for reliability. A research group could lean on open-source frameworks to experiment with new methods or to segment imaging for analyses. Some centers may use a hybrid: e.g., use a commercial model for OARs, but a custom research model for a novel task (like segmenting perineural tumor spread on MRI) that no commercial tool covers.

Finally, when deploying any tool, ongoing **validation and monitoring** are key. If patient demographics or scanner protocols change, the model's performance should be reassessed. Many clinics maintain a log of AI segmentation outcomes (time saved, any notable errors) to ensure quality remains high. With time, we expect these tools to further improve and perhaps even converge—one can envision a future where an all-in-one AI model, perhaps provided by the treatment planning system vendor or an open consortium, handles all routine segmentation with minimal intervention.

Case Study: Accelerating Radiotherapy Planning with AI

Dr. Elena Rossi is a radiation oncologist at a comprehensive cancer center. Before AI, she would spend nearly 2 h contouring each head and neck cancer patient's CT scan—outlining critical organs like the brainstem, optic nerves, salivary glands, esophagus, etc., as well as the tumor. With a busy clinic, this often meant coming in early or staying late to complete contours before the physics team could plan treatment.

In 2023, her department implemented an FDA-cleared deep learning auto-segmentation tool integrated into their planning system. In a typical case (oropharyngeal carcinoma), the auto-segmentation now produces contours for 25 OARs in about 2 min. Dr. Rossi then spends about 20 min reviewing and fine-tuning them: she might adjust the spinal cord contour if it was a slice or two off at the top, or erase a small portion of a parotid gland contour that included a bit of tumor. The gross tumor volume she still contours manually, but now with all OARs done, she focuses her attention fully on the tumor and nodal volumes.

The impact was immediately felt. "It's like having a junior colleague pre-contour everything consistently," she says. In the first month, they audited cases and found that no critical structure was missed by the AI. Dice similarity between the AI and her final edited contours was above 0.85 for most organsm, which gave her confidence. More importantly, she noticed that even when multiple doctors treated patients, the contours looked more uniform than before. This harmonization came from everyone starting from the same AI suggestion. Now, 6 months later, Dr. Rossi cannot imagine going back. "For straightforward cases, AI saves me at least an hour. For complex cases, it saves my mental energy so I can concentrate on the tricky decisions rather than the mundane anatomy."

One particular patient, an elderly man with extensive disease, had a very distorted anatomy post-surgery. The AI struggled with a few structures (for instance, it contoured a missing left parotid by mistake), but Dr. Rossi easily deleted that and continued. She finds that the AI is not perfect, but its imperfections are predictable and manageable. The department estimated a 40% overall reduction in contouring time per case, in line with published studies. They also observed that plan quality and consistency improved, as reported by their dosimetrists.

This case study illustrates how AI auto-segmentation, when properly integrated and validated, can substantially enhance efficiency in a real-world clinical workflow, benefitting both providers and patients (through faster turnaround times and potentially more consistent treatment planning).

Key Challenges and Future Directions

Despite the significant progress and real-world successes of AI in head and neck segmentation, several challenges remain. Some are technical, others logistical or ethical:

- **Limited Generalizability:** A model trained on one dataset may not perform equally well on another—differences in scanner calibration, patient population (e.g., average body habitus or prevalence of certain surgeries), or imaging protocols can lead to drops in accuracy. Ensuring models generalize or can be quickly adapted (via transfer learning) to new settings is crucial, especially for global deployment. Initiatives for more diverse training data and federated learning (training on data from multiple hospitals without sharing patient data) are underway to address this.

- **Small Structures and Extreme Cases:** Certain tiny structures (e.g., cochlea, optic nerves) or unusual anatomies (patient with surgical alterations, rare anomalies) are still challenging. Models sometimes miss or inaccurately segment these because they occupy few voxels or are underrepresented in training. Dedicated networks or incorporating high-resolution images (like a focused MRI for inner ear) might help in the future. Additionally, lesions that invade bone or sinus cavities, etc., can confuse models—multimodality input could help here (e.g., using both CT and MRI together to distinguish tumor from normal).
- **Ground Truth Quality:** For training and evaluation, the "ground truth" contours are usually those drawn by humans, which can be imperfect. If those contours are inconsistent or suboptimal, the AI will learn those imperfections. There is ongoing research into using the consensus of multiple experts or even using AI to flag potential errors in human contours during the curation of training data. Some studies explore uncertainty estimation: having the AI indicate regions where it's less confident, which often coincide with where even humans might disagree. International implementation of a consensus guideline on head and neck delineation, like the HNCIG group, is also instrumental towards a unified ground truth and deep learning models derived from that.
- **Clinical Acceptance and Trust:** Not all clinicians readily trust AI outputs. Some may be biased to either over-trust ("the AI gave it, it must be right") or under-trust ("I will redo it anyway"). Proper training, demonstration of the tool's performance, and involving end-users in tool selection can mitigate this. It helps to show that the tool has been validated on cases from their own institution or to start with a trial period where contours are double-checked more rigorously to build confidence.
- **Regulatory and Legal Issues:** Each new version of an AI model might be considered a new device requiring approval. This can slow down deployment of the latest algorithms, especially if regulations aren't agile. Moreover, liability in case of an AI-related error is a gray area—currently, since clinicians must approve contours, the liability remains with them/the clinic. In the future, if AI gets more autonomous, this will be an important area to clarify. Also, data privacy laws affect how training data is shared; thus, large-scale datasets that could improve models may be siloed. Frameworks for privacy-preserving training (like federated learning) are being explored so that models can learn from multi-institution data without directly sharing patient scans.
- **Maintenance and Monitoring:** After deployment, models might face "drift" in performance if imaging practices change (e.g., a new CT scanner or protocol). Ongoing QA is needed. A challenge is that, unlike a static device, AI software can update or "learn"—balancing model updates with the need for re-validation at each site is non-trivial. Some vendors push updates frequently; each update might necessitate a quick QA check by the clinic to ensure nothing regressed. Resource-strapped clinics might find this burdensome.

- **Expanding Scope:** There are opportunities to extend AI segmentation beyond the current scope. For instance, integrating AI segmentation into adaptive radiotherapy, where, during treatment, the patient might be re-scanned and the plan adapted, relies on very fast, reliable segmentation of new scans. Some research prototypes are looking at real-time or online segmentation (even on MRI machines during treatment). Another area is combining segmentation with **dose prediction**—once structures are contoured, AI might also assist in automatically generating a draft radiation plan. That extends beyond our chapter's scope, but segmentation is the first domino.
- **Educational and Workforce Impact:** As segmentation becomes easier, trainees (residents, dosimetrists in training) might get fewer repetitions of manual contouring. Some have raised concerns that over-reliance on AI could erode skills. On the other hand, if AI takes away the grunt work, trainees can spend more time on higher-level planning and decision-making. It will be important to still teach anatomy and contouring principles, maybe using AI as a teaching tool (e.g., having students critique AI contours to learn).

In the near future, we can expect **hybrid models** that integrate symbolic or prior knowledge with the data-driven approach. For example, if AI proposes a contour that violates an anatomical rule, such as a contour of the optic nerve that is discontinuous, a rule-based system could catch and correct that. We may also see more use of **3D generative models or diffusion models** that can model variability in shapes and produce more refined predictions. As computational power and datasets increase, a plausible goal is an AI that can segment an entire head & neck scan—all organs and any visible tumors—with expert-level accuracy consistently. The journey is ongoing, but the progress to date already signals a positive change in how head and neck imaging is handled in practice.

Summary

In this chapter, we examined how artificial intelligence, particularly deep learning, is revolutionizing the segmentation of head and neck anatomy and lesions. We started with the fundamentals: CT, MRI, and PET are key imaging modalities, each presenting unique information and challenges for delineation. The head and neck region's complexity—with numerous small, adjacent structures—historically made manual contouring a laborious and variable process. Traditional atlas-based auto-segmentation offered some relief but had limitations. The advent of deep learning and the U-Net architecture brought a step change in capability. By learning directly from annotated data, AI models can now contour organs-at-risk with speed and accuracy approaching that of human experts, while greatly reducing inter-observer variability.

We discussed the U-Net and its many adaptations (3D U-Net, attention U-Net, multi-view CNNs), highlighting why this architecture is well-suited to medical segmentation. Key performance metrics like Dice and HD95 were introduced to quantify segmentation quality, alongside the importance of physician review and clinical acceptability. Current applications in radiology and radiotherapy are broad: from auto-segmentation of normal organs for treatment planning (the area of most immediate clinical impact) to the more challenging task of tumor segmentation for diagnostic and planning purposes. Integration of AI into workflows has proven feasible and beneficial—numerous commercial tools are now FDA-cleared and in routine use, enabling clinicians to save time and focus on critical decisions. We listed several such products and noted open-source alternatives, giving readers a panorama of options and what they entail.

The chapter also presented a case study demonstrating real-world use of AI to accelerate radiotherapy planning, a math breakout to solidify understanding of the Dice coefficient, and a candid look at remaining challenges. These challenges, including generalizability, small structure accuracy, user trust, and regulatory considerations, define the frontier for research and development. Real-world implementation needs careful validation and human oversight, but the trajectory is clear—AI-assisted segmentation is becoming a standard component of head and neck imaging practice. It not only streamlines workflows but also holds promise for improving consistency and potentially outcomes (e.g., by enabling more consistent OAR sparing or more quantified tumor assessments).

In conclusion, AI for head and neck segmentation exemplifies the synergy of advanced technology with clinical expertise. Radiologists and radiation oncologists armed with AI tools can perform their tasks more efficiently, but their role remains pivotal in guiding the AI, checking its outputs, and making the ultimate judgments that affect patient care. As AI models continue to improve and accumulate real-world experience, one can envision a future where tedious manual contouring is largely a thing of the past, and where segmentation—once a bottleneck—becomes a rapid, reliable stepping stone towards personalized and precise head and neck cancer treatment. The key to this future is continued collaboration across clinicians, researchers, and engineers to ensure these tools are robust, validated, and aligned with clinical needs.

Review Questions and Research Prompts

1. **Fundamentals:** Why is manual segmentation of head and neck structures considered challenging? List at least three reasons related to anatomy or imaging that make this task difficult without AI.

   Hints: Consider the number of structures, their sizes, and variability between patients.
2. **Imaging Modalities:** How do different imaging modalities (CT, MRI, PET) contribute to head and neck segmentation? Provide one strength and one limitation for each modality in the context of segmentation (either by humans or AI).

3. **Architecture Insight:** Describe the U-Net architecture and its relevance to medical image segmentation. Why do the skip connections in U-Net matter, and how do they improve segmentation of fine structures like nerves or small tumors?
4. **Metrics Calculation:** Given two segmentations—one by an AI and one by an expert—that overlap substantially, how would you calculate the Dice coefficient between them? If the AI missed a small portion of the structure and also included a small false region elsewhere, explain qualitatively how that would affect the Dice score.
5. **Application & Tools:** Name two commercial auto-segmentation tools for head and neck anatomy and two open-source tools or frameworks. For each, provide a brief note on how it is used (e.g., integrated in a planning system, standalone software, or a coding framework).
6. **Performance Evaluation:** What is the Hausdorff Distance (HD) and specifically HD95, and why is it important in evaluating segmentation quality? Give an example scenario where two segmentations could have a high Dice similarity but a large HD95, and explain what that means in practice.
7. **Clinical Workflow:** Outline the steps of how an AI-generated contour would be used in a radiotherapy planning workflow. Who reviews it and what actions are taken from image acquisition to treatment plan regarding these contours?
8. **Real-world Impact:** Summarize findings from one key study that evaluated AI auto-segmentation in a clinical setting (e.g., multi-institution trial or a vendor comparison study). What were the time savings and any noted limitations or requirements highlighted by that study?
9. **Future Directions:** Identify one major challenge for AI segmentation in head and neck that is not fully solved yet. Propose a research idea or technical improvement that could address this challenge (for example, improving tumor segmentation on MRI, or better generalizing models across hospitals).
10. **Ethical/Regulatory Consideration:** If an AI segmentation model makes a significant mistake that a clinician fails to catch, what are the potential consequences and who is held accountable? Discuss how current practice mitigates this risk and what steps are taken before an AI tool is allowed to be used on patients (think validation and regulatory approval).

Suggested Reading

1. Ye X, Guo D, Ge J, et al. Comprehensive and clinically accurate head and neck cancer organs-at-risk delineation on a multi-institutional study. Nat Commun. 2022;13:6137. Introduces the SOARS deep learning system for 42 head & neck OARs, trained on multi-institution data. Demonstrated >3 hour manual contour time for 24 OARs and achieved up to 90% workload reduction with AI, with 98% of auto-contours needing only minor/no edits for clinical acceptance.
2. Cardenas CE, Yang J, Anderson BM, Court LE, Brock KB. Advances in auto-segmentation. Semin Radiat Oncol. 2019;29(3):185–97. A review of auto-segmentation techniques in radio-

therapy, covering atlas-based methods through deep learning. Discusses the evolution and the improvements deep learning brought to segmentation workflows.
3. Pang EPP, Tan HQ, Wang F, et al. Multicentre evaluation of deep learning CT autosegmentation of the head and neck region for radiotherapy. NPJ Digit Med. 2025;8:312. A seven-institution study assessing a commercial auto-segmentation tool (HARMONY) for head & neck. Found 42–49% contouring time reduction on average, with variations among structures (some LN levels saw no time saved). Also showed reduced inter-observer variability when using AI-generated contours. Emphasized need for institution-specific validation.
4. Rong Y, et al. NRG oncology assessment of artificial intelligence deep learning-based auto-segmentation for radiation therapy: current developments, clinical considerations, and future directions. Int J Radiat Oncol Biol Phys. 2024;119(2):261–80. Guidance from NRG Oncology on the status of AI auto-segmentation in RT. Reviews performance, integration considerations, and suggests best practices for evaluation and clinical implementation of auto-segmentation models.
5. Gibbons E, Kouznetsova T, Fripp J, et al. Clinical evaluation of deep learning and atlas-based auto-segmentation for critical organs-at-risk in radiation therapy. J Med Radiat Sci. 2023;70(S2):15–25. Comparative study showing that a deep learning auto-segmentation outperformed an established atlas-based system in accuracy for head & neck, thoracic, and pelvic OARs. Provided evidence that AI contours were closer to manual reference than atlas contours, supporting the shift to deep learning methods.
6. van Dijk LV, van den Bosch L, Aljabar P, et al. Improving automatic delineation for head and neck organs at risk by deep learning contouring. Radiother Oncol. 2020;142:115–23. An early deep learning study for head & neck OAR segmentation. Demonstrated that a CNN (U-Net) could significantly improve contour accuracy over previous methods. Noted that model performance for some organs approached the variability seen between human experts.
7. Doolan PJ, Ryan EM, Wynne C, et al. A clinical evaluation of the performance of five commercial artificial intelligence contouring systems for radiotherapy. Front Oncol. 2023;13:1213068. Benchmarked five commercial AI auto-segmentation solutions (Mirada, MVision, Radformation, RayStation, TheraPanacea) on 80 patients across breast, head & neck, lung, and prostate. Found all systems produced high-quality contours with median Dice ~0.8–0.88 and substantial time savings (~40 minutes on average per head & neck case). Concluded that all could improve workflow efficiency, highlighting also the importance of user review to correct any errors.
8. Lucido JJ, et al. Validation of clinical acceptability of deep-learning-based automated segmentation of organs-at-risk for head-and-neck radiotherapy treatment planning. Front Oncol. 2023;13:1137803. Validated a deep learning OAR segmentation model by assessing whether its output (after minimal editing) was clinically acceptable. Reported significant time savings (>75% reduction in contouring time) and that virtually all auto-segmented structures were deemed acceptable or needed only minor adjustments, aligning with the high acceptance rate noted in other studies.
9. Schouten JPE, Noteboom S, Martens RM, et al. Automatic segmentation of head and neck primary tumors on MRI using a multi-view CNN. Cancer Imaging. 2022;22:8. Research article focusing on delineating primary head & neck squamous cell carcinoma on MRI with a multi-view convolutional neural network. Found moderate accuracy (average Dice ~0.49) with better performance on larger tumors and a tendency of the model to over-segment. Highlights the difficulty of MRI-based tumor segmentation and the need for improved methods to reduce false positives.
10. Hall J. FDA clears MRI-based AI segmentation of organs at risk during radiation therapy. Diagn Imaging, May 2, 2025. News article on the FDA 510(k) clearance of GE Healthcare's MR Contour DL software. Notes that it can segment 37 organs/structures in head, neck, and pelvis using MRI, illustrating regulatory progress in AI tools. Quotes GE reps on the importance of advancing MR for RT planning. An example of a vendor integrating AI with MRI to complement CT-based planning.

11. Asbach JC, Le AH, Londyn SM, et al. Deep learning tools for the cancer clinic: an open-source framework with head and neck contour validation. Radiat Oncol. 2022;17:28. Describes the development and validation of an open-source deep learning auto-contouring framework for head & neck OARs. Trained on 229 patients (11 OARs) and compared against a commercial atlas-based tool, showing improved quantitative metrics and reduced correction time for the DL model. The authors released their code and model publicly, aiming to help other clinics adopt AI with transparency.
12. Ibragimov B, Xing L. Segmentation of organs-at-risks in head and neck CT images using convolutional neural networks. Med Phys. 2017;44(2):547–57. One of the pioneering studies applying CNNs to segment multiple head & neck OARs (parotids, larynx, etc.) on CT. Achieved promising results compared to atlas-based methods of that time. This paper demonstrated the feasibility of deep learning for multi-organ segmentation and paved the way for subsequent research in this area.
13. Walker GV, Awan MJ, Tao R, et al. Prospective randomized double-blind study of atlas-based organ-at-risk autosegmentation-assisted radiation planning in head and neck cancer. Radiother Oncol. 2014;112(3):321–5. Earlier clinical trial evaluating atlas-based auto-contouring in head & neck planning. Found that while atlas assistance could reduce contouring time and some variability, it did not fully replace careful manual editing. This provides historical context on what auto-segmentation could (and could not) achieve pre-deep-learning, highlighting the progress made since.
14. Ronneberger O, Fischer P, Brox T. U-Net: convolutional networks for biomedical image segmentation. Proceedings of MICCAI 2015, LNCS Volume 9351, 2015. The seminal paper introducing the U-Net architecture. Although focusing on cell microscopy in the original paper, U-Net became the foundation for countless medical imaging segmentation tasks including head & neck anatomy. The paper details the encoder-decoder with skip connections design that enables precise localization with context, and reports impressive results on biomedical segmentation challenges.
15. Neve OM, Chen Y, et al. Fully automated 3D vestibular schwannoma segmentation with and without gadolinium-based contrast material: a multicenter, multivendor study. Radiol Artif Intell. 2022;4(4):e210300. Presents a fully automated nnU-Net-based pipeline for VS segmentation trained and validated across multiple centers and MRI vendors, achieving clinician-level performance for both T1 contrast-enhanced and T2 high resolution sequences, with separate delineation of intrameatal and extrameatal tumor components.
16. Mody PP. Automated quality assurance of deep learning contours in head-and-neck radiotherapy. PhD thesis, Chapter 5, Leiden University Medical Center, January 2026. https://hdl.handle.net/1887/4287843
17. Mody PP, et al. Large-scale dose evaluation of deep learning organ contours in head-and-neck radiotherapy by leveraging existing plans. Phys Imaging Radiat Oncol. 2024;30:100572.
18. Ye X, Guo D, Ge J, et al. Comprehensive and clinically accurate head and neck cancer organs-at-risk delineation on a multi-institutional study. Nat Commun. 2022;13(1):6137.
19. Pang EPP, Tan HQ, Wang F, Niemelä J, Bolard G, Ramadan S, Kiljunen T, Capala M, Petit S, Seppälä J, Vuolukka K, Kiitam I, Zolotuhhin D, Gershkevitsh E, Lehtiö K, Nikkinen J, Keyriläinen J, Mokka M, Chua MLK. Multicentre evaluation of deep learning CT autosegmentation of the head and neck region for radiotherapy. NPJ Digit Med. 2025;8(1):312.
20. Asbach JC, Singh AK, Matott LS, Le AH. Deep learning tools for the cancer clinic: an open-source framework with head and neck contour validation. Radiat Oncol. 2022;17(1):28.
21. Neve OM, Chen Y, et al. Fully automated 3D vestibular schwannoma segmentation with and without gadolinium-based contrast material: a multicenter, multivendor study. Radiol Artif Intell. 2022;4(4):e210300.

Chapter 4
AI and Radiomics for Tumor Characterization and Prognosis in Neuroimaging

Golnaz Lotfian

Background

Radiomics has revolutionized neuroimaging by enabling the extraction of detailed quantitative information from routine medical images. These characteristics, such as tumor texture, shape, intensity, and heterogeneity, provide a wealth of information that is not immediately visible to the human eye. Radiomics provides a rare chance to improve prognostication, improve tumor characterization, and customize treatment plans for each patient by transforming pictures into high-dimensional data.

Advanced analysis techniques are required due to the complexity of radiomic data, and artificial intelligence has quickly emerged as a key component in this field. Because radiomics is a high-dimensional field, machine learning and deep learning algorithms are particularly well-suited to handle it. They can identify subtle patterns and create prediction models that can greatly enhance clinical decision-making. These AI-powered methods have already demonstrated promise in enhancing patient outcomes, forecasting therapy responses, and boosting diagnostic accuracy.

This chapter explores the intersection of radiomics and AI in neuroimaging, focusing on their applications in tumor characterization and prognosis. Key sections will define foundational radiomics concepts, detail methodologies for tumor characterization, and discuss the integration of AI in these workflows. Furthermore, we will explore how AI methodologies, including machine learning and deep learning, are driving innovation in this space, with a spotlight on commercially available tools currently making strides in clinical practice. This integration of radiomics and AI represents a paradigm shift, offering neuroradiologists the potential to deliver more precise and personalized care.

G. Lotfian (✉)
Department of Diagnostic Radiology and Nuclear Medicine, Rush University Medical Center, Chicago, IL, USA

D. T. Ginat (ed.), *Artificial Intelligence in Neuroradiology*,
https://doi.org/10.1007/978-3-032-24568-7_4

Discussion

Basics of Radiomics in Neuroimaging

In the expansive domain of neuroimaging, radiomics is redefining the possibilities of medical imaging by harnessing the power of high-throughput extraction techniques to gather vast quantities of quantitative data from images. This transformative approach explores the intricacies of medical scans, employing sophisticated algorithms to reveal a multitude of features that, although imperceptible to the human eye, provide crucial insights into the pathology, physiology, and genetics of tissues.

At the beginning of image acquisition, the precision of medical imaging technologies like MRI, CT, and PET scans plays a foundational role in the workflow of radiomics. Here, the fidelity of the data captured—ensured through standardized imaging protocols—sets the stage for the reliability of the entire radiomic analysis. As the process advances to segmentation, the focus sharpens on delineating regions of interest like tumors from the surrounding tissues. Whether through manual, semi-automated, or fully automated methods, the accuracy of this segmentation directly impacts the quality of the data extracted and is thus pivotal.

Emerging from segmentation, the journey of data characterization moves to feature extraction. In this crucial phase, the previously segmented images are processed to compute a diverse array of quantitative features, ranging from simple first-order statistics to complex textural and higher-order statistical features. These features are meticulously derived through a variety of mathematical algorithms, each designed to quantify different aspects of the image data.

The final leg of the radiomic workflow is the analysis phase, where the extracted features undergo thorough scrutiny to decode patterns and relationships tied to critical clinical outcomes like disease diagnosis, progression, and response to treatment. This stage often integrates sophisticated statistical analyses and leverages the prowess of machine learning models, highlighting features that predict clinical outcomes with notable precision.

Throughout each step, the meticulous execution of the radiomic workflow not only ensures the robustness and validity of the analysis but also paves the way for the integration of artificial intelligence. AI and machine learning are not merely adjuncts in this context but are central to amplifying the capabilities of radiomics. By automating the interpretation of complex data and learning from vast datasets, AI technologies hold the promise of significantly advancing the field of radiomics. They enrich the process by enhancing the precision of diagnostics and prognostics, leading to more personalized and effective treatment plans. This symbiosis of radiomics and AI is poised to further revolutionize the landscape of neuroimaging, setting new standards for the early detection, characterization, and management of neurological disorders and cancers.

Radiomic Features: The Foundation of Tumor Characterization

Radiomic features are crucial for extracting valuable clinical information from standard medical images, which traditional visual assessment might overlook. These features can be broadly classified into several categories, each providing unique insights into the tumor's characteristics.

Texture Features

Texture features aim to quantify the spatial distribution and patterns of pixel/voxel intensities in an image. These patterns reflect tissue heterogeneity and microstructural organization, which can often reveal critical insights into tumor behavior and biology. They can be classified into three broad categories as described:

1. Statistical Texture Features: Measuring intensity distribution and relationships using statistics.
   - First-order statistics: Analyzes individual voxel intensities without considering spatial relationships (e.g., kurtosis, skewness, mean, standard deviation, entropy).
   - Second-order statistics: Evaluates spatial relationships between neighboring voxels. These are often derived from matrices like:
     - Gray-Level Co-occurrence Matrix (GLCM): Quantifies how often pairs of intensity values occur at a specified spatial relationship.
     - Run-Length Matrix (RLM): Measures the length of consecutive runs of voxels with the same intensity in a specific direction.
     - Size Zone Matrix (SZM): Assesses the size of homogeneous zones of voxel intensities within an ROI.
     - Neighborhood Gray Tone Difference Matrix (NGTDM): Quantifies the difference between a voxel's intensity and the average intensity of its neighbors.
2. Transform-Based Texture Features: Applying mathematical transformations to the image to enhance certain spatial patterns or frequencies before texture analysis. Examples include:
   - Wavelet transform: decomposes the image into frequency sub-bands to analyze texture at different scales and orientations.
   - Fourier transform: evaluates the frequency domain of the image to identify repetitive patterns or structures.
3. Structural-Based Texture Features: Derived by modeling the image's spatial structure or morphology. Examples include:

- Fractal Features: Measure the complexity of a structure across different scales, often linked to tumor microarchitecture.
- Derived Textures: Features extracted from filtered images (e.g., Laplacian, Sobel filters) to emphasize edges or other structural characteristics.

Shape and Size Features

Quantitative measurements such as volume, surface area, and sphericity provide critical information on tumor growth kinetics and morphological changes. These parameters can help characterize tumor aggressiveness and progression, such as in gliomas, where irregular shapes might indicate more invasive types.

- Volume: Measures the three-dimensional size of the tumors, correlating with their growth and treatment response.
- Surface Area: Reflects the total area of the tumor's surface, which is important for assessing boundary irregularities.
- Sphericity: Evaluates how closely the shape of a tumor resembles a sphere, with deviations often indicating invasive growth.
- Elongation and Flatness: describes the degree to which the tumor shape deviates from being round, providing insights into growth patterns.
- Surface Regularity: Highlights the smoothness of the tumor's surface, calculated as the ratio of the actual surface area to the surface area of a sphere with the same volume. Tumors with highly irregular surface areas are often expected to exhibit more aggressive biological behavior.

Intensity Features

These involve the statistical distribution of pixels or voxel intensities within the tumor, including metrics like mean, median, skewness, and kurtosis. Intensity features are particularly useful in identifying and quantifying the physiological properties of tumors, such as necrotic versus active tumor regions.

Higher-Order Features

Derived from advanced mathematical models applied to the image, such as wavelet transforms or Laplacian of Gaussian filters, these features can capture additional details about the tumor's microenvironment and vascular characteristics. These details are often correlated with malignant potential and therapeutic response.

While enumerating these radiomic features provides critical insight into tumor characterization, it also lays the groundwork for integrating AI into radiomics. The complexity and volume of data derived from these features necessitate advanced analytical approaches that exceed conventional capabilities. AI plays a crucial role in this situation. AI's capability to process and interpret these high-dimensional datasets enables the development of more sophisticated, efficient, and accurate tools for tumor characterization and prognosis. By integrating AI, the potential of radiomics is not only expanded but also optimized, allowing for predictive models and analyses that can revolutionize personalized medicine.

Leveraging AI to Enhance Radiomic Analysis

In the domain of neuroimaging, AI plays a crucial role in refining the analysis and interpretation of radiomic features from brain scans. This integration not only enhances precision but also significantly speeds up the diagnostic process, with substantial improvements in predictive capabilities essential for effective management of neurological disorders.

AI-Driven Feature Selection and Optimization

Differentiating between different brain disorders, such as benign meningiomas and malignant gliomas, is crucial in neuroimaging. AI greatly improves diagnostic and prognostic capacities by painstakingly sorting through large amounts of radiomic data to find the most instructive elements. AI, for instance, has shown that it can reduce the dimensionality of radiomic data by as much as 30%, which significantly increases the focus and effectiveness of analysis.

This optimized selection process is particularly critical in neurology, where specific biomarkers play a pivotal role in clinical decision-making. Biomarkers such as apparent diffusion coefficient (ADC) values from diffusion-weighted imaging can help differentiate high-grade gliomas, which often show lower ADC values due to higher cellularity, from lower-grade or benign tumors. Additionally, relative cerebral blood volume (rCBV) derived from perfusion MRI offers insights into the vascular properties of tumors, where higher rCBV values may indicate more aggressive malignancies like glioblastomas.

Furthermore, AI can leverage textural features extracted from standard MRI scans to identify subtle patterns that correlate with tumor types or genetic profiles, such as the presence of MGMT methylation in glioblastomas, which is associated with a better response to certain chemotherapies. By integrating these biomarkers into AI models, clinicians can not only distinguish between different types of brain tumors more accurately but also predict therapeutic outcomes, enhancing the precision and effectiveness of treatment planning.

Thus, the integration of AI in feature selection and optimization allows for a more targeted analysis, focusing on biomarkers that provide critical insights into the tumor's behavior and potential response to therapy. This capability underscores the transformative potential of AI in neuroimaging, enabling a more personalized approach to neurooncology.

Pattern Recognition and Classification in Tumor Characterization

AI's capacity for advanced pattern recognition, particularly through deep learning techniques like convolutional neural networks (CNNs), has markedly advanced the characterization of tumors in neuroimaging. These models are not only proficient in detecting and classifying subtle radiomic signatures but are also pivotal in distinguishing between benign and malignant tumors, enhancing the diagnostic precision.

For example, CNNs have been employed with over 90% accuracy in classifying complex radiomic patterns that differentiate between various types of brain tumors, significantly outperforming traditional visual assessments. This capability extends to identifying tumor grades and predicting treatment response based on textural and morphological features derived from MRI scans.

A noteworthy application of this approach can be seen in the context of head and neck tumors. Recent studies have utilized CNNs for the segmentation and classification of head and neck squamous cell carcinoma using multiparametric MRI data. These models effectively analyze radiomic features such as T2* signal intensities and texture patterns to identify tumor boundaries with remarkable precision. For instance, CNN-based segmentation achieved a Dice Similarity Coefficient (DSC) of up to 65%—quantifying the overlap between the AI-predicted segmentation and ground truth—on seven MRI contrasts, highlighting the potential of AI to complement traditional diagnostic workflows.

By leveraging these AI-driven insights, clinicians can better understand tumor behavior and progression, which is crucial for optimizing therapeutic strategies. Automating the analysis of these intricate patterns not only accelerates the diagnostic process but also enhances the overall efficiency of clinical workflows in oncology, reducing the time required for image evaluation by about 50%.

Predictive Modeling

AI's capabilities in predictive modeling are particularly transformative in the field of neuroradiology when integrated with radiomic features. By combining these detailed radiomic profiles with historical clinical data, AI models can forecast disease progression and response to treatments with an accuracy rate exceeding 85%. For example, AI-driven models that analyze the complex interplay of radiomic features have been crucial in predicting the growth trajectories of malignant gliomas. These predictions enable clinicians to devise earlier and more tailored treatment strategies, significantly improving patient outcomes. Such predictive models leverage the detailed textural, shape, and intensity features unique to radiomics, ensuring that the forecasts are not only precise but also deeply reflective of the underlying pathology.

Other Quantifiable Benefits

The use of AI in neuroimaging has improved diagnostic accuracy and reliability while also speeding up the processing of complex imaging data by up to 70%. There have been reports of up to 40% reductions in diagnostic errors, indicating AI's capacity to have a substantial influence on clinical judgment. Better patient care results from these developments because they enable doctors to start treatment earlier and with more assurance.

AI's integration into radiomic analysis in neuroimaging marks a significant advancement in the neurological field, revolutionizing how conditions like gliomas, meningiomas, and multiple sclerosis are diagnosed and managed. As AI technologies continue to evolve, they promise to bring even more profound improvements in the precision, efficiency, and personalization of medical diagnostics and treatments.

Prognostic Value of Radiomics

By offering quantitative evaluations that precisely forecast patient outcomes like survival rates and illness recurrence, radiomics is transforming prognostic modeling in neuroimaging. In order to manage a variety of neurodegenerative and oncologic disorders, it is essential to identify risk stratifications and prognostic indications through the integration of complicated imaging data patterns that are frequently invisible to the human eye. Texture analysis of brain tumors, for example, has been demonstrated to be a potent non-invasive diagnostic technique with the ability to predict patient survival with an accuracy of up to 80% when made possible by sophisticated software such as the XD3 platform (Mirada Medical, Oxford, UK).

Survival Analysis and Recurrence Prediction

Radiomic features are critical to creating robust models that predict patient longevity with high precision. In glioblastoma cases, advanced imaging biomarkers derived from MRI and PET imaging have been identified as critical indicators of tumor aggressiveness and patient prognosis. Specific biomarkers, such as enhanced T1-weighted intensity heterogeneity, increased tumor necrosis ratio, and elevated choline-to-N-acetylaspartate ratios, are associated with shorter survival times and higher tumor grade.

These biomarkers, when analyzed by AI platforms like IntelliSpace Discovery (Philips Healthcare, Amsterdam, Netherlands), enable the development of quantitative models that tailor treatment plans to individual patients, having been shown to improve survival rates by as much as 25% in targeted patient groups. For example, hyperintense signal abnormalities on T2-weighted and FLAIR sequences that extend beyond the enhancing tumor margins have been linked to aggressive tumor infiltration, helping clinicians identify candidates for more intensive interventions.

Additionally, radiomic signatures are proving valuable in predicting tumor recurrence. Features such as texture irregularities (e.g., entropy and contrast measures) and vascular permeability patterns provide early warnings of likely recurrence, often before visible changes on standard imaging. Analyzed using software such as Watson Health Imaging (IBM, Armonk, New York), these biomarkers have demonstrated the ability to detect subtle changes that signal recurrence.

Integrating Clinical Data

Prognostic models are improved by the combination of radiomic characteristics with comprehensive clinical data, including patient demographics, medical history, and genetic profiles. This allows for a more comprehensive approach to patient management. The effectiveness of targeted treatments has been demonstrated to increase by up to 30% when this data is combined with platforms such as Edison (GE Healthcare, Chicago, Illinois), which enables the customization of medicines based on the genetic makeup of tumors. Additionally, this integration has increased disease progression models' predictive accuracy by about 20%, enabling more accurate risk assessments tailored to individual patients.

AI-Driven Approaches to Enhancing Prognostic Models

The advancements in AI, particularly through deep learning and machine learning, are profoundly enhancing prognostic models in neuroimaging. Tools such as Clara AI (NVIDIA, Santa Clara, California) and DeepMind Health (Google, Mountain View, California) utilize convolutional neural networks to process and learn from large-scale imaging data, extracting in-depth radiomic features that significantly improve outcome predictions. Machine learning algorithms, such as those implemented in AI-Rad Companion (Siemens Healthineers, Erlangen, Germany), analyze combined data from imaging and clinical records to forecast patient outcomes with an accuracy often exceeding 85%. These continually evolving models ensure that prognostic capabilities improve over time with the accumulation of new data.

The integration of AI into radiomic prognostic modeling, supported by commercially available software, marks a significant advancement for neuroimaging. These tools not only enhance the accuracy and adaptability of predictions but also streamline clinical workflows, fundamentally changing the landscape of neurological diagnostics and treatment. As AI technologies and radiomic applications continue to evolve, they promise to drive further advancements in personalized medicine and significantly improve patient outcomes.

Future Directions in AI and Radiomics for Neuroimaging

As the fields of radiomics and artificial intelligence in neuroimaging continue to evolve, several emerging technologies and methodologies promise to further revolutionize this area of medicine. These advancements aim to enhance the precision of diagnostics and treatments, fostering the development of personalized medicine while overcoming inherent challenges.

Integration of Multi-Omics Data with Radiomic Features

Combining radiomic characteristics with multi-omics data is one of the most intriguing advances in neuroimaging. This novel method improves our comprehension of the intricate biological foundations of neurological disorders by integrating genomic, proteomic, and radiomic data to produce a thorough, multi-layered analysis.

For instance, this integration can be especially enlightening in the case of glioblastoma, a prevalent and aggressive form of brain tumor. While proteomic analysis can shed light on the pathways that these mutations affect, such as altered cell cycle regulation or apoptosis, genomic data may identify particular mutations in genes that drive tumor growth, such as IDH1 or TP53. This is enhanced by radiomic analysis, which measures the physical features of the tumor that are evident on MRI, such as edge sharpness or textural heterogeneity, which can reveal tumor aggression and possible treatment response. When combined, these data layers can assist physicians in more precisely diagnosing the tumor and creating individualized treatment regimens based on the genetic profile and radiomic phenotype of the tumor.

AI models and tools are essential for enabling this intricate integration. Large volumes of heterogeneous data from proteomic, radiomic, and genomic research can be analyzed and synthesized by sophisticated machine learning methods like deep learning. These artificial intelligence (AI) algorithms are able to find patterns and correlations in these disparate data sets, offering useful insights that are not immediately visible using traditional analysis techniques. This skill makes it possible to create predictive models that can more precisely predict how a disease will advance and how well a therapy will work, which eventually results in more individualized and efficient patient care plans.

Federated Learning in Radiomic Neuroimaging

Federated learning represents a transformative approach in the field of radiomics, particularly within neuroimaging. This AI-driven methodology enables the collaborative development of models across multiple institutions without compromising the privacy of patient data. It's especially beneficial for radiomic analysis, where the need for large, diverse datasets is paramount to ensuring the robustness and accuracy of predictive models.

Federated learning in radiomic neuroimaging enables researchers and clinicians to share radiomic data from medical images, including CT and MRI scans, across various healthcare systems and geographical regions. By working together, the common problem of data silos is resolved, improving AI model training datasets without directly exchanging private patient data. Federated learning makes it easier to create more generalist AI models that can identify subtle radiomic signals of neurological disorders and tumor characteristics by combining radiomic data from a variety of patient groups.

In addition to increasing the precision of radiomic models in forecasting the course of a disease and the effectiveness of treatment, this wider data integration aids in the development of individualized treatment regimens based on radiomic biomarkers. In order to ensure that radiomic insights are fully utilized to improve patient outcomes, federated learning plays a crucial role in furthering the precision medicine approach in neuro-oncology and other neurodegenerative disease investigations.

Challenges and Opportunities

The potential for integrating AI and radiomics into neuroimaging is enormous, but in order to maximize tumor characterization and enhance prognostic models, a number of particular issues must be resolved. When handling the great variety and complexity of tumor imaging data, these difficulties become very apparent.

Standardization of Radiomic Features

Standardizing radiomic characteristics across many imaging platforms and methodologies is a major difficulty. The extraction and dependability of radiomic characteristics can be greatly impacted by the inconsistencies that frequently plague tumor imaging as a result of different imaging settings and procedures. For instance, variations in the resolutions and setups of MRI scanners might change the way tumor textures and forms look, which can cause disparities in radiomic analysis. Furthermore, while promising, the integration of multi-omics data with radiomics poses challenges in terms of data alignment and interpretation, necessitating advanced computational techniques to guarantee precise multi-dimensional data integration.

Validation and Reproducibility Issues

The validation and reliability of radiomic signals used for treatment response prediction and tumor prognosis represent another significant hurdle. For radiomic models to be used in a variety of clinical settings and patient populations, they must be sufficiently reliable. The lack of external validation and small sample sizes in many radiomic studies, however, cast doubt on the model's clinical applicability and generalizability. For radiomic techniques to be used in clinical practice, it is imperative that they yield consistent and trustworthy results in a variety of circumstances.

Collaborative Platforms and the Future of Tumor Characterization

Collaborative platforms that concentrate on the standardization and validation of radiomic procedures are crucial to overcoming these obstacles. To encourage top-notch radiomic research and guarantee that procedures are open and repeatable, initiatives like the Radiomics Quality Score (RQS) and the Quantitative Imaging Network (QIN) have been established. These systems assist in overcoming the challenges of limited sample sizes and improve the dependability of radiomic instruments in clinical settings by facilitating multi-center investigations that support the robust validation of radiomic signatures.

Moreover, collaborative federated learning programs, such as those led by international brain tumor consortia, are crucial. They make it possible for institutions to create shared AI models that can learn from a wide range of anonymized data without jeopardizing patient privacy. This method speeds up the development of precise and broadly applicable radiomic tools for tumor characterization and prognosis, in addition to increasing the robustness of AI models.

For the area to advance, it is essential to address the unique problems in radiomics and tumor characterization within neuroimaging through teamwork and sophisticated computational techniques. By focusing on these specific areas, the neuroimaging community can enhance the accuracy and reliability of tumor studies, paving the way for more precise and personalized patient treatment plans.

Conclusion

The field of medical diagnostics and customized treatment is undergoing a revolutionary change with the incorporation of AI and radiomics into neuroimaging. In addition to improving the accuracy and effectiveness of tumor characterization and prognosis, this convergence changes neuroimaging's capacity to profoundly impact clinical judgment and patient outcomes. Through the use of complex AI algorithms and modern radiomic techniques, physicians can now gain a deeper understanding of the biological activity of tumors, which helps them make more accurate predictions about how the disease will evolve and how well a treatment will work.

As we look to the future, continuous advancements in AI technologies and their application in radiomics will undoubtedly unlock even more potential, facilitating the development of more effective, tailored treatment regimens. However, for these advancements to realize their full potential, addressing challenges such as standardization, validation, and reproducibility of radiomic features is essential. The ongoing collaboration across clinical, technological, and research domains will be pivotal in overcoming these hurdles, promoting a more integrated and evidence-based approach to neuro-oncology.

Ultimately, as AI-driven tools become more refined and accessible, the promise of truly personalized medicine comes closer to reality, offering hope for improved survival rates and quality of life for patients with neurological conditions. The continued exploration and integration of multi-omics data, alongside sophisticated imaging analytics, heralds a new era of diagnostic precision and therapeutic effectiveness, marking a significant milestone in the evolution of neuroimaging and cancer care.

Suggested Reading

1. Ak M, Toll SA, Hein KZ, Colen RR, Khatua S. Evolving role and translation of radiomics and radiogenomics in adult and pediatric neuro-oncology. AJNR Am J Neuroradiol. 2022;43(6):792–801. https://doi.org/10.3174/ajnr.A7297.
2. O'Sullivan NJ, Kelly ME. Radiomics and radiogenomics in pelvic oncology: current applications and future directions. Curr Oncol. 2023;30(5):4936–45. Published 2023 May 11. https://doi.org/10.3390/curroncol30050372.
3. Abdel Razek AA, Alksas A, Shehata M, et al. Clinical applications of artificial intelligence and radiomics in neuro-oncology imaging. Insights Imaging. 2021;12(1):152. https://doi.org/10.1186/s13244-021-01102-6.
4. Beig N, Bera K, Tiwari P. Introduction to radiomics and radiogenomics in neuro-oncology: implications and challenges. Neurooncol Adv. 2021;2(Suppl 4):iv3–iv14. Published 2021 Jan 23. https://doi.org/10.1093/noajnl/vdaa148.
5. Yi Z, Long L, Zeng Y, Liu Z. Current advances and challenges in radiomics of brain tumors. Front Oncol. 2021;11:732196. Published 2021 Oct 14. https://doi.org/10.3389/fonc.2021.732196.
6. Stathopoulos I, Serio L, Karavasilis E, Kouri MA, Velonakis G, Kelekis N, Efstathopoulos E. Evaluating brain tumor detection with deep learning convolutional neural networks across multiple MRI modalities. J Imaging. 2024;10(12):296. https://doi.org/10.3390/jimaging10120296.
7. Alavanja A, Hooper GW, Hasse A, Carroll T, Ginat DT. A preliminary diagnostic accuracy study of quantitative MRI biomarkers for differentiating parotid tumor types. Gland Surg. 2023;12(2):134–9. https://doi.org/10.21037/gs-22-88.
8. Albalawi E, Thakur A, Dorai DR, et al. Enhancing brain tumor classification in MRI scans with a multi-layer customized convolutional neural network approach. Front Comput Neurosci. 2024;18:1418546. https://doi.org/10.3389/fncom.2024.1418546.
9. Bielak L, Wiedenmann N, Berlin A, et al. Convolutional neural networks for head and neck tumor segmentation on 7-channel multiparametric MRI: a leave-one-out analysis. Radiat Oncol. 2020;15:181. https://doi.org/10.1186/s13014-020-01618-z.
10. Hooper GW, Ansari S, Johnson JM, Ginat DT. Advances in the radiological evaluation of and theranostics for glioblastoma. Cancer. 2023;15(16):4162. https://doi.org/10.3390/cancers15164162.
11. Zhu G, Jiang B, Tong L, Xie Y, Zaharchuk G, Wintermark M. Applications of deep learning to neuro-imaging techniques. Front Neurol. 2019;10:869. Published 2019 Aug 14. https://doi.org/10.3389/fneur.2019.00869.

12. Avberšek LK, Repovš G. Deep learning in neuroimaging data analysis: applications, challenges, and solutions. Front Neuroimaging. 2022;1:981642. Published 2022 Oct 26. https://doi.org/10.3389/fnimg.2022.981642.
13. Choi KS, Sunwoo L. Artificial intelligence in neuroimaging: clinical applications. Investig Magn Reson Imaging. 2022;26(1):1. https://doi.org/10.13104/imri.2022.26.1.1.
14. Hoinkiss DC, Huber J, Plump C, Lüth C, Drechsler R, Günther M. AI-driven and automated MRI sequence optimization in scanner-independent MRI sequences formulated by a domain-specific language. Front Neuroimaging. 2023;2:1090054. Published 2023 May 12. https://doi.org/10.3389/fnimg.2023.1090054.
15. Wisnu Wardhana DP, Maliawan S, TGB M, Rosyidi RM, Wiranata S. Radiomic features as artificial intelligence prognostic models in glioblastoma: a systematic review and meta-analysis. Diagnostics (Basel). 2024;14(21):2354. Published 2024 Oct 22. https://doi.org/10.3390/diagnostics14212354.
16. Yoon JH, Lee H, Kwon D, et al. Integrative approach of omics and imaging data to discover new insights for understanding brain diseases. Brain Commun. 2024;6(4):fcae265. Published 2024 Aug 8. https://doi.org/10.1093/braincomms/fcae265cheng.

Chapter 5
Artificial Intelligence for the Assessment of Intracranial Hemorrhage and Cerebrovascular Disease

Grayson W. Hooper, Daniel Thomas Ginat, and Radhika Rajpurohit

Hemorrhage

Intracranial hemorrhage (ICH) has multiple etiologies that can be broken down by age and clinical scenario. For example, scant subarachnoid blood along the cerebral convexities in a young person could represent reversible cerebral vasoconstrictive syndrome or trauma, while a large volume of blood in the basal cisterns likely represents aneurysm rupture. Acute scenarios such as these are usually straightforward diagnoses. However, small volumes of acute blood along the tentorial leaflets, in the posterior fossa, or tangent to the dural venous sinuses may be difficult to detect. Further, subacute subdural hematomas, especially if bilateral, can be quite difficult to detect when the blood products are isoattenuating to gray matter.

ICH has significant prognostic and treatment implications, especially with respect to medication management (Fig. 5.1). AI efficacy in the setting of ICH has been found to be generally positive with respect to intracranial hemorrhage—though not universally—with studies indicating improvements in sensitivity, turnaround time, and scan view delay (Fig. 5.2a,b), while two more recent studies have indicated false positives and increased radiologist turnaround times.

G. W. Hooper
UH Cleveland Department of Radiology, Cleveland, OH, USA

D. T. Ginat (✉)
Co-founder, Rad-Lab.ai, Chicago, IL, USA

R. Rajpurohit
University of Delaware, Newark, DE, USA

D. T. Ginat (ed.), *Artificial Intelligence in Neuroradiology*,
https://doi.org/10.1007/978-3-032-24568-7_5

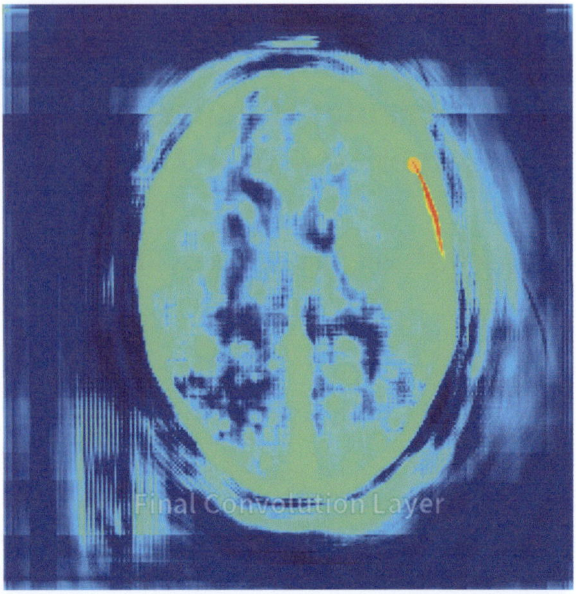

Fig. 5.1 AIDOC (Tel Aviv, Israel) CT heat map shows high probability of left cerebral convexity subdural hemorrhage

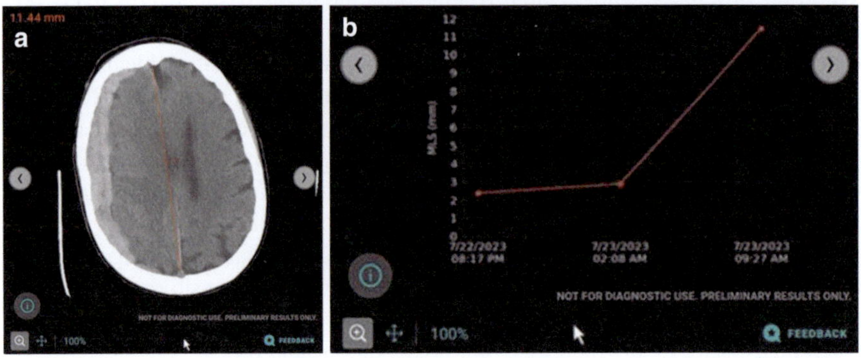

Fig. 5.2 (**a**) AIDOC automated midline shift assessment in the setting of a right holohemispheric subdural hematoma. (**b**) AIDOC midline shift tracker that can automatically notify staff at configurable threshold values

Vascular Occlusion

In essence, CVD is a group of conditions that affects blood flow to the brain. These diseases can be classified as ischemic or hemorrhagic, but also as chronic or acute. And given that the brain is an organ with extremely high metabolic demands, a catastrophic acute event tied to chronic CVD may ultimately progress to death or significant disability with little or no warning.

One of the most pressing scenarios in diagnostic radiology secondary to CVD is acute vascular occlusion. A thromboembolic event can lead to a large vessel

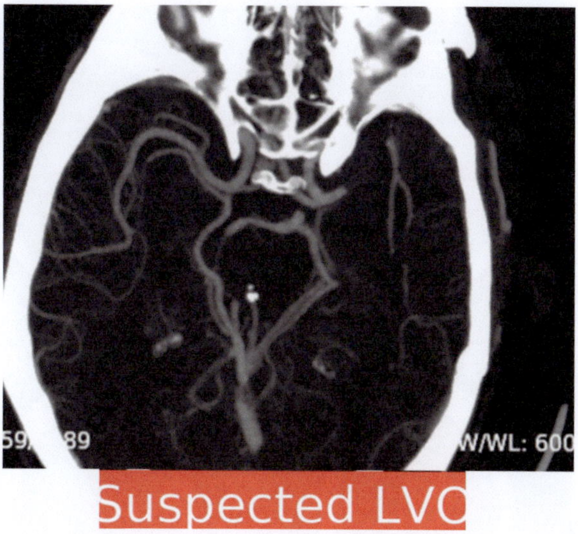

Fig. 5.3 VizAI (San Francisco, CA) CTA flags a left MCA occlusion

occlusion (LVO), defined commonly as the internal carotid artery, basilar artery, M1 segment of the MCA, and occasionally the proximal M2 segment of the MCA (Fig. 5.3). Prompt diagnosis is essential in triage and management, including mechanical thrombectomy. Unfortunately, radiology miss rates have held steady at approximately 3–5% while imaging volume, including advanced studies like CT angiography of the head and neck, continues to increase. It is in this scenario where AI holds significant promise.

Indeed, even as of 2021, AI has been credited with a 98% sensitivity and 98% specificity in finding LVOs with a number of platforms cleared by the FDA that can automatically triage studies as well as improve the turnaround time of LVO reporting by 22 min. Additionally, AIDOC has launched a proprietary platform—Full Brain Solution—as of July 2023 to not only seek LVOs, but also medium vessel occlusions (MVOs), which is unique among all platforms.

Ischemic Stroke

An ischemic infarct may occur without identifiable vascular occlusion. Therefore, stroke detection and patient triage can begin with (and may rely upon) the noncontrast head CT. The Alberta Stroke Program Early Computed Tomography Score (ASPECTS) is one such system.

In ASPECTS, the brain is topographically divided and scored 0–10 based on the amount of territory infarcted, with mechanical thrombectomy recommended for scores of 6 or higher. Unfortunately, interobserver variability is significant and manual calculation can be cumbersome. However, AI tools, including Avicenna's deep learning algorithm (La Ciotat, France), have been found to increase ASPECTS

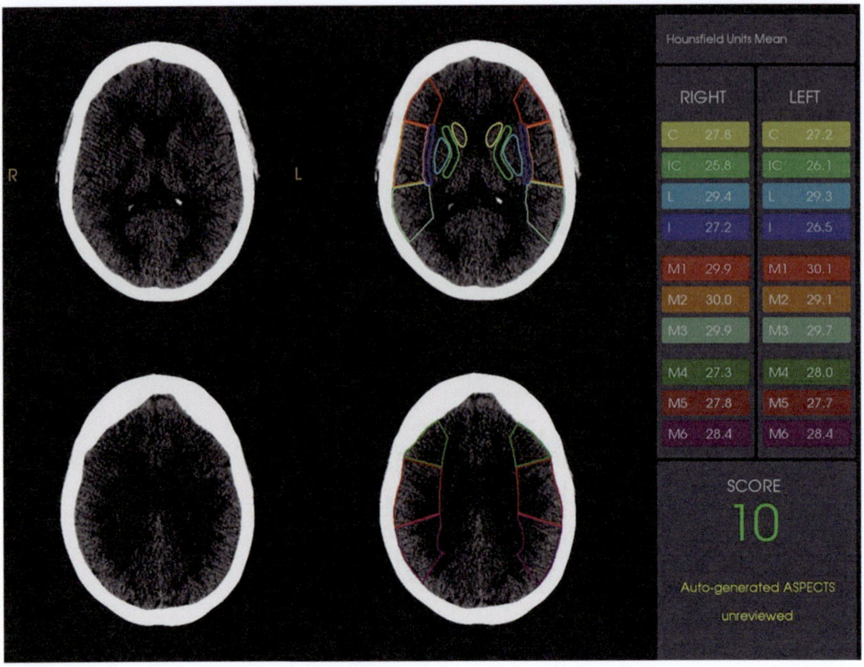

Fig. 5.4 RAPIDAI automatically assessed the brain topography based on Hounsfield Unit values and presented a score of 10, which is normal in this case

scoring accuracy, precision, and decrease case evaluation time. RAPIDAI's (San Mateo, CA) automated calculations were also found to be equal to or greater than those of experienced radiologists (Fig. 5.4).

CT perfusion imaging with contrast can also be obtained and quickly assessed on potential intervention candidates, as seen in Fig. 5.5 from RapidAI below.

As a chronic process, atherosclerosis results in a gradual reduction of arterial luminal diameter. This may result in ischemic phenomena itself; however, it is plaque rupture that delivers near-instantaneous, often catastrophic consequences. As a result, analysis of individual cerebral vascular plaques could provide valuable risk stratification. One study retrospectively reviewed MRI T1 and postcontrast T1 characteristics of basilar artery plaques and was able to extract useful features to create a model that could predict which plaques were symptomatic from the ones that were not, with an AUC of 0.936. But what of the propensity for an intracranial plaque to rupture? Though the data are sparse, sonographic and CT information has shown that certain imaging characteristics of atheromatous plaque do correlate with instability. For example, one 2016 study showed that plaques that are both homogeneous and anechoic in echotexture have a greater risk of rupture, even when accounting for the size/degree of stenosis they impart to a vessel. A more recent study used contrast-enhanced ultrasound to partition carotid artery plaques into vulnerable and

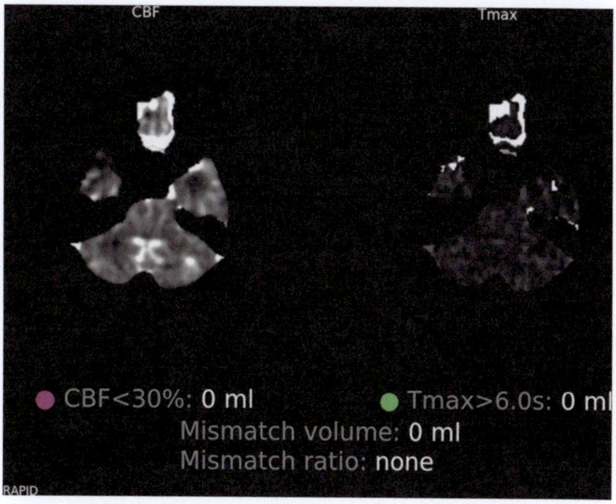

Fig. 5.5 RapidAI automated CT perfusion calculation

stable groups based on whether neovascularization was present. Subsequent retrospective analysis of CTA images on these same patients (and plaques) was performed. Features were extracted from both stable and unstable plaques, and the intraclass correlation coefficient (ICC) was applied to assess the reliability of these features. The selected features were then t-tested to identify those with statistically significant differences between the two groups. A total of 10 radiomics features were identified from the above analysis. These features were then used to construct models, one of which, model_RF, showed good performance (AUC: 0.933) in differentiating vulnerable from stable plaques in the training and validation sets.

Prediction of stroke outcomes is based upon clinical factors such as age, sex, history of prior stroke, baseline modified Rankin score, and diabetes. However, when combined with information obtained through radiomics analysis, the accuracy of these predictions increases, as one large retrospective study that combined clinical data and an MRI radiomics model built solely from DWI and ADC map features showed. Moreover, noncontrast CT has also shown promise in predicting prognoses of ischemic stroke patients (Fig. 5.6). And similar to the MRI study, the fusion model derived from both clinical information and CT radiomics parameters demonstrated greater value than either model independently (fusion model AUC: 0.857 vs. radiomics model AUC: 0.705 vs. clinical model AUC: 0.643).

Further, outcome prediction can also be linked, remarkably, to analysis of the brain as a whole. As Bretzner et al. demonstrated in a large retrospective study, radiomics features derived from T2-FLAIR sequences of the brain could be used to create a relative brain age (RBA) biomarker (Fig. 5.7). Independent from chronological age, RBA reflects patients' brain health relative to their peers, and advanced RBA was shown to be a significant, independent risk factor for worse outcomes in poststroke patients.

Aneurysm

Aneurysms are yet another manifestation of CVD that have severe consequences if they rupture. The prevalence of intracranial aneurysm is about 3% of the population, with 20% in that group having multiple. Unfortunately, predicting *when* an aneurysm will rupture is extremely difficult, as there are many variables such as location, size, concomitant patient medical risk factors, and even genetic variability for which to account.

Diagnosing aneurysms can also be a challenge in a high-volume practice, especially if the angiographic examinations are ordered for other purposes. AI has shown benefit in detecting and flagging suspected aneurysms on examinations, demonstrating a positive predictive value of 62%. Furthermore, manual measurement of aneurysms, which is important in risk stratification, can be a time consuming task for the radiologist with interobserver variability that can confound future management. It is here too that AI can be beneficial as some studies have shown improved sensitivity in automated aneurysm measurements.

AI has shown promise in predicting aneurysm rupture risk using digital subtraction angiography, CT angiography, and, more recently, MR angiography. However, given that the majority of studies on this topic are retrospective, there is no consensus on the clinical applicability of developed features and models. Indeed, there are even limitations on the type of features utilized to build models, as at least one study avoided including morphologic features in their predictive model because manual segmentation could have introduced interobserver variability, which would diminish reliability. However, another more recent study conducted at Tufts University (Boston, MA) performed a retrospective analysis of morphologic radiomics features exclusively and found that the elongation and flatness features possessed AUCs of 0.71 and 0.72, respectively, which underperformed against established size and shape parameters. More recent attempts to predict rupture risk utilize convolutional neural network analysis of wall shear stress and wall strain via computational fluid dynamics. Together, their AUC value was 0.883. Further, Li and colleagues were able to use CTA to devise a convolutional neural network that could analyze aneurysm structural patterns in order to predict the probability of rupture with 10-15% improvement over human neuroradiologists.

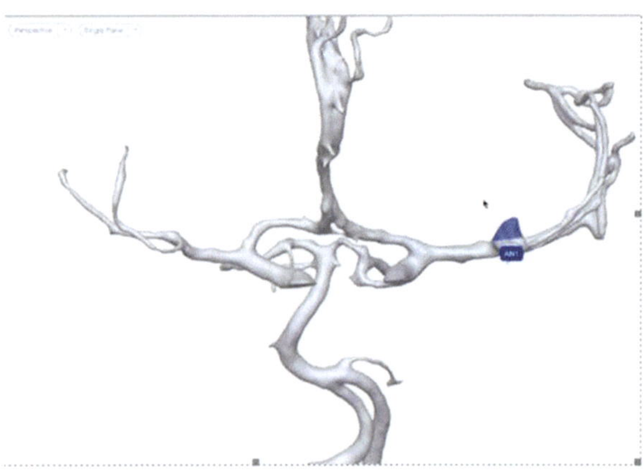

Fig. 5.6 A RAPID AI-flagged aneurysm at the M1-M2 junction

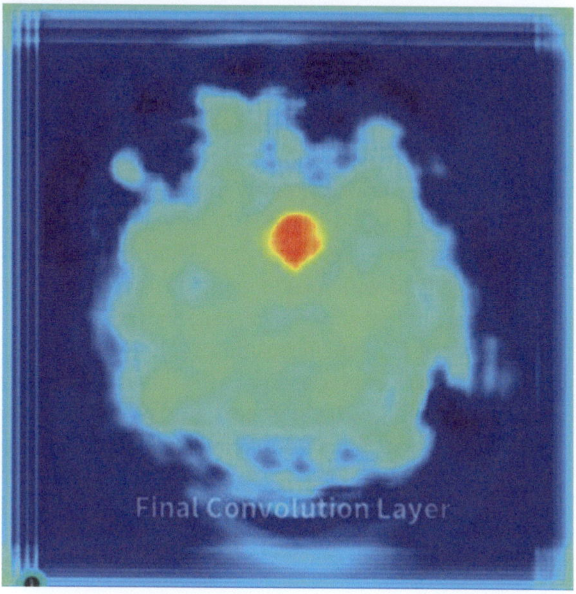

Fig. 5.7 AIDOC heat map showing a suspected aneurysm in the vicinity of the left paraclinoid ICA

AVM

Cerebral arteriovenous malformations (AVM) are abnormal tangled vessels in the brain parenchyma, which result in shunts between arteries and veins. This relatively rare disorder affects approximately 1% of the population and is a leading cause of spontaneous non-traumatic ICH in young adults. It is often discovered incidentally during CT or MRI imaging for other presentations such as acute hemorrhage. Radiomics may hold valuable potential in predicting clinical manifestations of this disease. In the unruptured state, AVMs may still cause seizures; being able to predict the probability of seizure would be useful. One such retrospective study by Zhao et al. combined three clinical features and 15 radiomics features based on time-of-flight MRA to predict epilepsy with an AUC of 0.82. Though the three clinical features that had undergone multivariate regression analysis and were found to be independent risk factors (patient age, lesion size, and frontal lobe involvement) are somewhat intuitive, the imaging features are not. Regardless, the combined model was shown to perform better than either clinical or radiomics alone—a testament to the potential utility of pixel-level analysis. With this model, a clinical nomogram was constructed to determine the probability of epilepsy based on total points. And while this nomogram was created with retrospective data, such a "theory-to-practice" leap acts as a tangible clinical starting point as opposed to an ethereal set of statistical-computational data, which could undergo later prospective validation.

Future Directions

Artificial intelligence will revolutionize the world. This will include medicine and radiology. As it stands now in late 2023, radiomics is in the "proof of concept" phase in which most studies are retrospective analyses. These analyses are conducted with high-powered software and statistics that simply did not exist 20 years ago. However, they are by their very nature limited as retrospective, in that data overfitting is a consistent concern. Even so, these studies are building the foundations that the field will need to begin the theory-to-practice transition. Coupled with a century of clinical experience, the models designed with the integrative information from modern medical imaging could change clinical practice as we know it. In a short time, multicenter prospective studies will undoubtedly address the lingering concerns, and within 10 years, advanced clinical-radiological radiomics models will guide most clinical decision-making and perhaps even obviate the need for biopsies.

Suggested Reading

1. Del Gaizo AJ, Osborne TF, Shahoumian T, Sherrier R. Deep learning to detect intracranial hemorrhage in a National Teleradiology Program and the impact on interpretation time. Radiology. 2024;6(5):e240067. https://doi.org/10.1148/ryai.240067.
2. Ginat D. Implementation of machine learning software on the radiology worklist decreases scan view delay for the detection of intracranial hemorrhage on CT. Brain Sci. 2021;11(7):832. https://doi.org/10.3390/brainsci11070832.
3. Savage CH, Tanwar M, Elkassem AA, Sturdivant A, Hamki O, Sotoudeh H, Sirineni G. Prospective evaluation of artificial intelligence triage of intracranial hemorrhage on non-contrast head CT examinations. AJR. 2024;27:1–13. https://doi.org/10.2214/AJR.24.31639.
4. Albers GW, Wald MJ, Mlynash M, Endres J, Bammer R, Straka M, Maier A, et al. Automated calculation of Alberta Stroke Program Early CT Score: validation in patients with large hemispheric infarct. Stroke. 2019;50(11):3277–9. https://doi.org/10.1161/STROKEAHA.119.026430.
5. Panch T, Szolovits P, Atun R. Artificial intelligence, machine learning and health systems. J Glob Health. 2018;8(2):020303. https://doi.org/10.7189/jogh.08.020303.
6. Zhang Y, Joshi J, Hadi M. AI in acute cerebrovascular disorders: what can the radiologist contribute? Semin Roentgenol. 2024;59(2):137–47. https://doi.org/10.1053/j.ro.2024.01.001.
7. Ayobi A, Davis A, Chang PD, Chow DS, Nael K, Tassy M, Quenet S, et al. Deep learning-based ASPECTS algorithm enhances reader performance and reduces interpretation time. AJNR. 2025;46(3):544–51. https://doi.org/10.3174/ajnr.A8491.
8. Kumar V, Gu Y, Basu S, Berglund A, Eschrich SA, Schabath MB, Forster K, et al. Radiomics: the process and the challenges. Magn Reson Imaging. 2012;30(9):1234–48. https://doi.org/10.1016/j.mri.2012.06.010.
9. Sakamoto Y, Okubo S, Nito C, Suda S, Matsumoto N, Abe A, Aoki J, et al. The prevalence of and factors related to vascular hyperintensity on T1-weighted imaging in acute ischemic stroke. Cerebrovasc Dis. 2017;44(3–4):203–9. https://doi.org/10.1159/000479593.
10. DeSai C, Hays Shapshak A. Cerebral Ischemia. In: StatPearls [Internet]. Treasure Island (FL): StatPearls Publishing; 2023.
11. Murakami T. Atherosclerosis and arteriosclerosis. Hypertens Res. 2023;46(7):1810–1. https://doi.org/10.1038/s41440-023-01284-0.

12. Doonan RJ, Gorgui J, Veinot JP, Lai C, Kyriacou E, Corriveau MM, Steinmetz OK, Daskalopoulou SS. Plaque echodensity and textural features are associated with histologic carotid plaque instability. J Vasc Surg. 2016;64(3):671–677.e8. https://doi.org/10.1016/j.jvs.2016.03.423.
13. Shan D, Wang S, Wang J, Lu J, Ren J, Chen J, Wang D, Qi P. Computed tomography angiography-based radiomics model for predicting carotid atherosclerotic plaque vulnerability. Front Neurol. 2023;14:1151326. https://doi.org/10.3389/fneur.2023.1151326.
14. Zhou Y, Wu D, Yan S, Xie Y, Zhang S, Lv W, Qin Y, et al. Feasibility of a clinical-Radiomics model to predict the outcomes of acute ischemic stroke. Korean J Radiol. 2022;23(8):811–20. https://doi.org/10.3348/kjr.2022.0160.
15. Zhang L, Wu J, Ruize Y, Ruoyu X, Jiawen Y, Qianrui F, Dawei W, Wei Z. Non-contrast CT radiomics and machine learning for outcomes prediction of patients with acute ischemic stroke receiving conventional treatment. EJR. 2023;165:110959. https://doi.org/10.1016/j.ejrad.2023.110959.
16. Bretzner M, Bonkhoff AK, Schirmer MD, Hong S, Dalca A, Donahue K, Giese AK, et al. Radiomics-derived brain age predicts functional outcome after acute ischemic stroke. Neurology. 2023;100(8):e822–33. https://doi.org/10.1212/WNL.0000000000201596.
17. Shi Z, Zhu C, Degnan AJ, Tian X, Li J, Chen L, Zhang X, et al. Identification of high-risk plaque features in intracranial atherosclerosis: initial experience using a radiomic approach. Eur Radiol. 2018;28(9):3912–21. https://doi.org/10.1007/s00330-018-5395-1.
18. Lyden P. Using the National Institutes of Health Stroke Scale: a cautionary tale. Stroke. 2017;48(2):513–9. https://doi.org/10.1161/STROKEAHA.116.015434.
19. Pagiola I, Mihalea C, Caroff J, Ikka L, Chalumeau V, Iacobucci M, Ozanne A, et al. The PHASES score: to treat or not to treat? Retrospective evaluation of the risk of rupture of intracranial aneurysms in patients with aneurysmal subarachnoid hemorrhage. J Neuroradiol. 2020;47(5):349–52. https://doi.org/10.1016/j.neurad.2019.06.003.
20. Ludwig CG, Lauric A, Malek JA, Mulligan R, Malek AM. Performance of Radiomics derived morphological features for prediction of aneurysm rupture status. J Neurointerv Surg. 2021;13(8):755–61. https://doi.org/10.1136/neurintsurg-2020-016808.
21. Yamanouchi M, Arimura H, Kodama T, Urakami A. Prediction of intracranial aneurysm rupture risk using non-invasive radiomics analysis based on follow-up magnetic resonance angiography images: a preliminary study. Appl Sci. 2022;12(17):8615. https://doi.org/10.3390/app12178615.
22. Zuurbier SM, Al-Shahi Salman R. Interventions for treating brain arteriovenous malformations in adults. Cochrane Database Syst Rev. 2019;9(9):CD003436. https://doi.org/10.1002/14651858.CD003436.pub4.
23. Zhao S, Zhao Q, Jiao Y, Li H, Weng J, Huo R, Wang J, et al. Radiomics analysis for predicting epilepsy in patients with unruptured brain arteriovenous malformations. Front Neurol. 2021;12:767165. https://doi.org/10.3389/fneur.2021.767165.

Chapter 6
Artificial Intelligence for Evaluating Neurodegenerative Diseases

Golnaz Lotfian and Daniel Thomas Ginat

Background

The development of AI techniques aimed at enhancing disease identification and progression tracking has been prompted by the growing complexity of neuroimaging data, as well as the requirement for early, precise diagnoses. This chapter will examine the specific AI developments in the diagnosis of neurodegenerative diseases, with an emphasis on the application of deep learning and machine learning to the analysis of neuroimaging data. We'll focus on the most exciting uses of AI in clinical contexts, such as its ability to identify Alzheimer's, Parkinson's, and other neurodegenerative diseases in their early stages. We will also look at the commercial AI technologies that are now on the market for neuroimaging, assessing their clinical application, efficacy, and limits. The application of AI in clinical practice is not without difficulties, despite its potential. Widespread adoption is still hampered by problems like data quality, model transparency, and ethical issues, particularly those pertaining to algorithmic bias and patient privacy. Furthermore, even though AI has shown a lot of promise, there are still obstacles to fully automating and standardizing diagnosis because of the complexity of human neurobiology and the heterogeneity of neuroimaging techniques. These issues will be covered in this chapter, along with potential future developments for AI in neuroradiology.

G. Lotfian (✉)
Department of Diagnostic Radiology and Nuclear Medicine, Rush University Medical Center, Chicago, IL, USA

D. T. Ginat (✉)
Co-founder, Rad-Lab.ai, Chicago, IL, USA

D. T. Ginat (ed.), *Artificial Intelligence in Neuroradiology*,
https://doi.org/10.1007/978-3-032-24568-7_6

Discussion

Convolutional Neural Networks (CNNs)

Convolutional neural networks represent one of the most significant advancements in deep learning, particularly in the field of neuroimaging. CNNs are designed to automatically extract and learn relevant features from grid-like input data, such as images, through a series of convolutional layers. This architecture allows CNNs to identify spatial hierarchies in the data, enabling them to detect subtle patterns and anomalies that may be challenging for traditional methods. Due to this capability, CNNs are particularly well-suited for neuroimaging tasks, where the analysis of complex, high-dimensional brain images is crucial for detecting early signs of neurodegenerative diseases. CNNs can detect a wide range of neurodegenerative disorders with excellent accuracy rates. For instance, a CNN was used in a study by Miah et al. [2] to distinguish between MRI images of healthy individuals and those of people suffering from Alzheimer's disease. The model successfully identified atrophic patterns in the entorhinal cortex and hippocampal regions, achieving an outstanding sensitivity of 90% and specificity of 92% in recognizing alterations associated with Alzheimer's disease. This level of accuracy helps in both diagnosis and tracking the course of the disease over time.

Transfer Learning

One of the most important tactics in the use of AI in neuroimaging is transfer learning. This method entails fine-tuning a pre-trained model that has been created on a big dataset for certain neuroimaging tasks. Transfer learning enables better performance on smaller, domain-specific datasets frequently seen in clinical settings by utilizing the knowledge acquired from broad imaging datasets. This approach is especially helpful for evaluating neurodegenerative disorders, as the complexity and diversity of these conditions can make it difficult to obtain sizable, annotated datasets. For example, in order to detect minor changes in the brain, such as atrophy or certain pattern modifications, illnesses like Parkinson's disease and Alzheimer's disease frequently need comprehensive imaging. It is now possible to integrate AI technologies into standard clinical practice by using transfer learning to improve model accuracy while lowering the time and resources required for training. Practically speaking, transfer learning can help with early diagnosis by making it possible for models to more accurately identify atrophic patterns in important brain regions even when patient data is scarce. A model developed on a smaller dataset of MRI scans from patients with early-stage Alzheimer's disease, for instance, would be able to recognize important characteristics of the condition and assist in prompt intervention techniques. In addition to increasing diagnostic precision, this feature helps track the course of the disease over time, enabling doctors to modify treatment regimens according to the unique needs of each patient.

Explainable AI (XAI)

The need for explainable AI has increased as AI technologies are incorporated more deeply into clinical operations. XAI seeks to increase transparency in the decision-making process of AI models. In neuroradiology, where diagnostic choices have a significant influence on patient care, this is particularly crucial. A practical example of XAI in action is its application in diagnosing Alzheimer's disease using MRI scans. For instance, a deep learning model trained to identify atrophic patterns in the hippocampus can generate predictions regarding the likelihood of Alzheimer's. XAI techniques, such as feature visualization, allow clinicians to see which specific aspects of the MRI influenced the model's decision. Radiologists can then assess whether the identified features, such as reduced hippocampal volume or changes in the entorhinal cortex, align with clinical knowledge and patient history. Recent developments in XAI approaches, like visual attention mapping, enable radiologists to evaluate the accuracy of AI model predictions. By highlighting areas of the brain that contribute most to the AI's conclusions, these techniques foster a collaborative dialogue between AI systems and healthcare professionals. XAI promotes trust between physicians and AI systems by offering insight into the decision-making process, making it easier for clinical practice to embrace AI more widely.

AI Application in Neurodegenerative Disease Evaluation

The application of artificial intelligence in the evaluation of neurodegenerative diseases is transforming clinical practice, providing tools that enhance diagnostic accuracy, facilitate early detection, and support personalized treatment strategies. This section explores key applications of AI in the assessment of conditions such as Alzheimer's disease, Parkinson's disease, Huntington's disease, and normal pressure hydrocephalus, highlighting how these technologies are integrated into clinical workflows.

Early Diagnosis and Risk Assessment

Early diagnosis is one of the most promising applications of AI in the assessment of neurodegenerative diseases. Imaging data from several modalities, such as MRI and PET scans, can be analyzed by AI algorithms to detect minute alterations that may be present long before clinical symptoms appear. For instance, deep learning models, particularly convolutional neural networks, have demonstrated efficacy in identifying early Alzheimer's disease biomarkers, such as amyloid plaque buildup and hippocampus atrophy, before cognitive deterioration is noticeable. In a recent study, a CNN model achieved a test accuracy of 91.7% and an impressive AUC value of 0.96, highlighting its high discriminative ability for positive-negative classification. This level of performance underscores the potential of deep learning models to assist in the non-invasive identification of amyloid deposition using 18F florapronol PET scans.

Recent advancements have also highlighted the substantial efficiency gains afforded by AI in neuroimaging. Studies have shown that AI-based image enhancement can significantly reduce MRI scan times—by as much as 45%—without sacrificing image quality. This reduction in scan duration not only improves patient throughput but also enhances the comfort of the patient, potentially leading to fewer motion artifacts and clearer imaging results.

By automating the image feature learning process, CNNs eliminate the need for manual feature engineering, enabling the simultaneous analysis of large datasets. This efficiency allows for rapid decision-making and facilitates earlier, more reliable diagnoses. These techniques could greatly influence therapy efficacy and patient outcomes by supporting earlier intervention and potentially improving treatment responses.

Image Segmentation and Quantification

AI has transformed the processes of image segmentation and quantification in neuroimaging, especially using deep learning approaches. Conventional techniques frequently depend on radiologists' manual delineation, which can be laborious and unpredictable depending on the examiner's training and experience. In addition to being time-consuming, this manual procedure is constrained by human variables, which could result in inconsistent measurements.

On the other hand, complicated imaging data from modalities like MRI, CT, and fMRI can be processed rapidly and accurately by AI-driven segmentation algorithms. These systems automatically recognize and define regions of interest, including the hippocampus, basal ganglia, and cortical areas affected by neurodegenerative conditions, using convolutional neural networks.

Deep learning models can effectively generalize across a variety of patient groups and imaging methods because they can extract complex patterns and features from vast datasets. This ability to capture subtle, often imperceptible changes—such as hippocampal atrophy, cortical thinning, or abnormal white matter changes—is particularly valuable in neurodegenerative diseases like Alzheimer's, where early alterations can precede clinical symptoms. These changes, which may be too subtle for conventional methods to detect, are critical for understanding the progression of the disease. As a result, AI-driven segmentation leads to extremely reproducible volumetric measurements with less inter-observer variability, making it an essential tool for longitudinal assessments.

AI also dramatically increases the speed of segmentation, processing large datasets in a fraction of the time it would take manually. For example, traditional manual segmentation of a single brain scan can take anywhere from 30 to 60 min, depending on the complexity and the number of regions being measured. In contrast, AI-based segmentation can process the same scan in as little as 2–5 min, representing a 5- to 10-fold reduction in time. AI can also rapidly measure changes in hippocampal volume over time in MRI-based Alzheimer's assessments, providing vital information about the disease's trajectory. This includes tracking the rate of atrophy—an important indicator of disease progression—that can be overlooked or inaccurately assessed with traditional techniques. AI algorithms can quantify the volume of different brain regions and detect even the smallest changes across successive scans in mere minutes, providing insights that would have taken hours with conventional methods.

Additionally, AI-assisted volumetric evaluations facilitate the precise tracking of atrophy rates and the accurate measurement of brain region changes over time.

Table 6.1 Example of AI utilization and accuracy in the detection and evaluation of neurodegenerative diseases

Neurodegenerative disease	AI technique	Shown accuracy in various studies
Alzheimer's disease	Deep learning on structural MRIs	90%+
Parkinson's disease	Deep neural nets on neuromelanin-sensitive MRI	80%+
Progressive supranuclear palsy	MRI planimetry measurements	80–90%
Huntington's disease	MRI volumetric analysis using AI software	95%

These automatic calculations from MRI and CT images make it easier to assess alterations over multiple scans, significantly improving the efficiency of longitudinal studies. For instance, where traditional methods may require several hours of expert radiologist input to manually trace and compare regions across multiple scans, AI can complete these tasks in minutes, allowing for much faster decision-making and treatment adjustments. This speed is particularly valuable for ongoing clinical trials and patient monitoring, where timely insights are crucial.

Anomaly Detection and Prediction

AI systems excel in anomaly detection, spotting minute and unusual changes in medical data that human observers would overlook. By utilizing advanced imaging techniques such as MRI and PET, artificial intelligence algorithms are especially skilled at spotting patterns linked to neurodegenerative diseases. To identify abnormalities like white matter hyperintensities and cortical thinning, which are signs of Alzheimer's disease, AI models can, for instance, examine MRI data. These abnormalities frequently show up before clinical symptoms do, allowing for early detection and treatment. Similarly, PET scans can identify metabolic alterations associated with dementia, including hypometabolism in particular brain regions, when combined with AI. (Table 6.1).

In a 2024 study, Sánchez-Rojas et al. used MRI volumetric analysis using AI software to identify early indicators of Huntington's disease in people who have not yet shown symptoms. This study serves as an exemplary illustration of the potential of AI in neuroimaging. Their study showed that AI could detect notable volumetric alterations in the brain that match up with genetic markers that are known to indicate the disease. In addition to demonstrating AI's potential to greatly aid in early diagnosis, this capacity also shows how AI may be able to limit the progression of disease by implementing therapeutic interventions earlier.

Integration with Clinical Data

In order to provide a comprehensive evaluation of neurodegenerative diseases, AI can combine neuroimaging data, such as fMRI, CT, and PET, with additional clinical data, including patient history and genetic factors. This multimodal approach enables AI to detect both structural and functional abnormalities, offering a more holistic view of the disease. For example, while CT and MRI scans reveal structural changes, fMRI and PET can detect functional alterations, such as disruptions in brain activity or metabolism, which may not be immediately apparent from imaging alone. By correlating these various data sources, AI enhances diagnostic precision, supports early detection, and allows for more individualized treatment plans tailored to each patient's unique condition.

AI's ability to combine imaging data with clinical markers becomes especially important when analyzing abnormal protein deposits, such as tau inclusions, which are hallmarks of Alzheimer's disease and other neurodegenerative conditions. Tau abnormalities are closely linked to clinical decline, yet validating these changes using traditional neuroimaging techniques can be challenging. This is where AI offers significant advantages. Recent work by Ushizima et al. [13] demonstrated how AI models can bridge the gap between neuroimaging (e.g., PET and MRI) and histological data to interpret abnormal tau inclusions.

Ushizima et al. developed a sophisticated computational pipeline that integrates large-scale voxel-to-voxel correlations between PET and high-resolution histological signals, leveraging advanced deep learning techniques. The pipeline enables the creation of 3D maps that quantify tau inclusions across the entire brain. By processing terabytes of data from hundreds of histology slides and co-registering this data to MRI scans, their AI model accurately segments tau deposits and generates high-resolution 3D density maps. For instance, their convolutional neural network demonstrated excellent performance in detecting tau inclusions, with receiver operating characteristic area under the curve scores of 0.87, 0.85, and 0.91 for three distinct tau antibodies (AT100, AT8, and MC1), indicating high accuracy in estimating the presence and density of tau protein.

This AI-driven pipeline facilitates the validation of PET tracers used to detect tau protein in vivo, offering an innovative way to accelerate the development of molecular neuroimaging techniques. By integrating neuroimaging with histological data through AI, the approach not only improves the detection of abnormal protein deposits but also provides a valuable tool for clinical validation, potentially speeding up the process of PET tracer development and approval. Combining neuroimaging with histological data in this way enhances our understanding of neurodegenerative diseases at a molecular level, improving diagnostic capabilities and offering new avenues for therapeutic strategies.

AI in Neurodegenerative and Demyelinating Diseases

Researchers have utilized artificial intelligence in the domain of multiple sclerosis (MS) to improve diagnosis accuracy and treatment administration. Employing sophisticated AI technologies like convolutional neural networks and support vector machines, researchers have attained notable precision in the analysis of MRI data for lesion identification and quantification, with accuracy rates nearing 90%. This accuracy is essential for both early detection and tracking disease advancement.

AI enhances the long-term management of MS by consolidating digitized patient data, encompassing electronic health records and outcomes from wearable sensors. These sensors, developed utilizing frameworks such as Sensor, Observation, Sample, and Actuator (SOSA) and the Web Annotation Data Model (WADM), provide continuous monitoring and data acquisition, hence improving decision-making in therapeutic environments. Furthermore, machine learning models have effectively processed speech recordings to identify small alterations suggestive of multiple sclerosis, demonstrating the promise of artificial intelligence in early diagnosis and monitoring disease progression.

AI has demonstrated potential in the realm of cognitive tests. The Integrated Cognitive Assessment (ICA), a language-neutral evaluation, has shown a high accuracy (95% AUC) in identifying cognitive impairments in multiple sclerosis patients, outperforming conventional assessments such as the Brief International Cognitive Assessment for MS (BICAMS). Furthermore, AI-driven analysis of the Brief Visuospatial Memory Test-Revised (BVMT-R) utilizing convolutional neural networks has demonstrated approximately 80% accuracy in detecting and monitoring cognitive and visuospatial impairments. These tools are essential for delivering a comprehensive strategy for managing MS, ensuring that both cognitive and physical health are considered. Researchers have utilized artificial intelligence in the domain of multiple sclerosis (MS) to improve diagnosis accuracy and treatment administration.

Commercially Available AI Software and Tools

A number of commercially available techniques have been developed to improve the assessment of neurodegenerative disorders as a result of the integration of AI and deep learning technology with neuroimaging. These solutions facilitate prompt and efficient patient treatment by streamlining workflows and increasing diagnostic accuracy. Here are some noteworthy AI-powered technologies that are currently in use.

NeuroQuant (NQ)

NeuroQuant (Cortech Solutions, San Diego, USA) is an advanced AI-powered program that leverages MRI scan analysis to produce detailed numerical evaluations of brain anatomy, particularly focusing on critical regions such as the cerebral cortex and hippocampal areas (Fig. 6.1). By automating the volumetric assessment process, NQ enhances the detection of atrophy patterns associated with neurodegenerative diseases like Alzheimer's. Recent studies have demonstrated that NQ can identify significant reductions in hippocampal volume, facilitating earlier diagnoses and timely interventions. Notably, NQ exhibits excellent inter-method reliability across a range of brain regions, making it a valuable tool for clinicians. Its rapid

MORPHOMETRY RESULTS

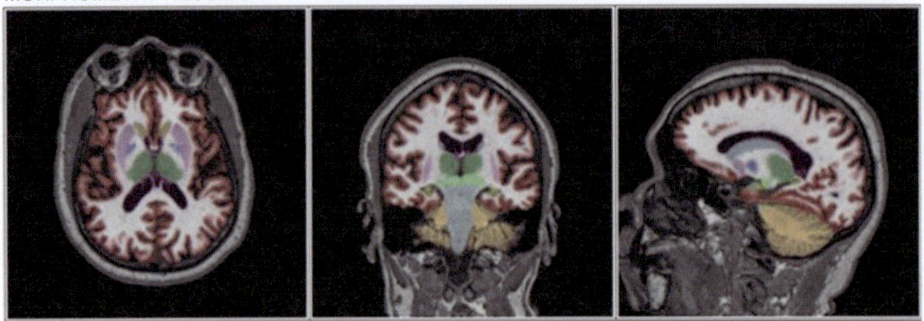

Intracranial Volume (ICV) (cm^2)		1666.86			
Brain Structure	LH Volume (cm^3)	LH Volume (% of ICV)	RH Volume (cm^3)	RH Volume (% of ICV)	Asymmetry Index (%)*
Forebrain Parenchyma	549.39	32.96	565.86	33.95	-2.95
Cortical Gray Matter	264.52	15.87	272.54	16.35	-2.99
Superior Lateral Ventricle	18.44	1.11	24.08	1.44	-26.52
Inferior Lateral Ventricle	1.16	0.07	1.06	0.06	9.38
Hippocampus	2.84	0.17	2.98	0.18	-4.78
Amygdala	1.04	0.06	1.23	0.07	-16.85
Caudate	3.09	0.19	3.64	0.22	-16.33
Putamen	5.51	0.33	5.73	0.34	-3.84
Pallidum	0.82	0.05	0.91	0.05	-11.11
Thalamus	7.79	0.47	8.38	0.50	-7.31
Cerebellum	71.48	4.29	69.39	4.16	2.97

Fig. 6.1 Example of NeuroQuant analysis of brain morphometry on MRI, including volume measurements of various structures

processing capabilities—approximately 5–10 min compared to the several hours required by traditional methods—allow for efficient integration into clinical workflows. Moreover, the consistent volume measurements obtained with NQ, regardless of slice thickness, reinforce its utility in monitoring disease progression and evaluating treatment efficacy.

FreeSurfer

FreeSurfer (Martinos Center for Biomedical Imaging, Boston, USA) is a robust open-source software suite renowned for its capabilities in the segmentation and visualization of neuroimaging data. Frequently utilized in assessing neurodegenerative conditions such as Huntington's disease, FreeSurfer excels in measuring cortical thickness and surface area (Fig. 6.2). Studies have shown that FreeSurfer effectively detects structural changes related to disease progression, thereby aiding clinicians in correlating imaging findings with cognitive decline. Although FreeSurfer is regarded as a gold standard for volumetric measurement, it requires more extensive processing time—typically around 4–6 h—and necessitates a level of technical expertise, such as familiarity with UNIX programming. This complexity can limit its accessibility in clinical settings.

While both NQ and FreeSurfer provide valuable insights into neurodegenerative diseases, their methodologies differ significantly. NQ employs a streamlined

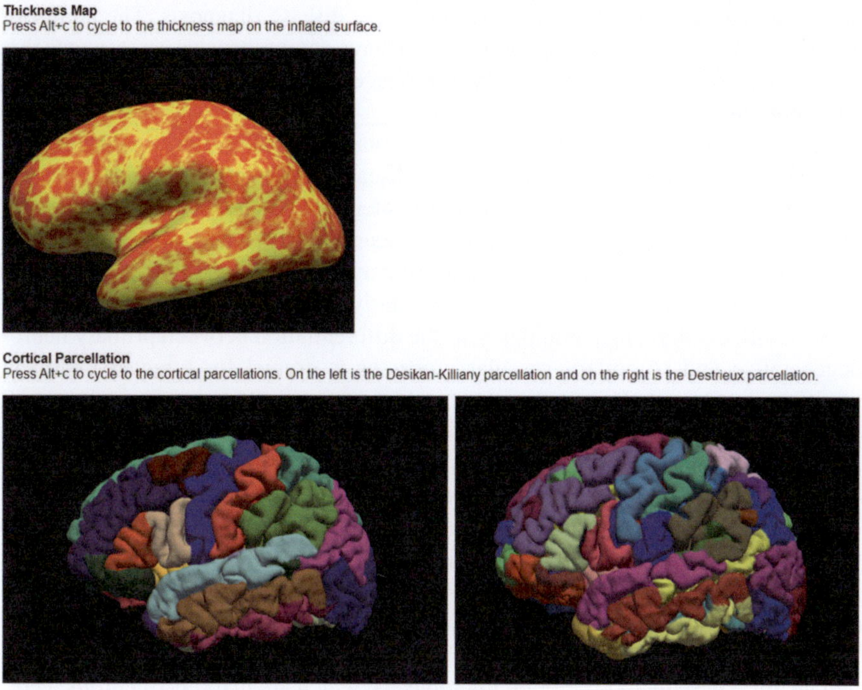

Fig. 6.2 Screenshot examples of cortical thickness and cortical parcellation from the FreeSurfer tutorial. (FsTutorial/OutputData_freeview, Free Surfer Wiki)

approach that prioritizes speed and efficiency, while FreeSurfer offers more granular control over segmentation at the cost of processing time. The choice of MRI protocol, including slice thickness, plays a crucial role in the reliability of volumetric measurements from both tools. Recent findings indicate that thinner slices (1 mm) yield slightly improved inter-method reliability compared to thicker slices (1.2 mm). However, both tools have shown excellent correlation in volume measurements, highlighting their complementary roles in clinical practice.

In light of these differences, careful consideration of the MRI parameters—such as slice thickness and scanning sequences—is essential when interpreting volumetric data. Consistency in these factors across clinical trials will enhance the reliability of findings and facilitate more accurate assessments of neurodegenerative disorders. Ultimately, the integration of both NQ and FreeSurfer into routine clinical workflows can provide comprehensive insights into brain health, aiding in the early diagnosis and management of neurodegenerative diseases.

Vascular Brain (VB)

Cerebrovascular health and its effects on cognitive decline are central topics addressed by the Vascular Brain (VB) AI tool developed by Vuno (Seoul, South Korea). VB utilizes advanced AI algorithms to analyze CT and MRI data, identifying cerebrovascular anomalies such as microbleeds, white matter lesions, and other critical alterations relevant to neurodegenerative disease diagnosis. The ability of VB to leverage various imaging modalities ensures comprehensive assessments that aid in the differentiation of primary neurodegenerative processes from vascular contributions.

Research indicates that vascular pathology plays a significant role in the development and progression of neurodegenerative diseases, including Parkinson's disease, vascular dementia, and mixed dementia. By integrating quantitative assessments of white matter hyperintensities, microbleeds, lacunar infarcts, and other microvascular changes, VB assists radiologists in accurately evaluating the vascular contributions to cognitive impairment. This is particularly beneficial in cases where patients present with overlapping pathologies, as the differentiation between primary neurodegenerative and secondary vascular processes is crucial for targeted treatment planning.

VB's utilization of MRI allows for the detection of microstructural changes, such as cerebral microbleeds and white matter damage, through high-resolution sequences (e.g., SWI, FLAIR). These findings are vital for characterizing chronic ischemic damage and assessing small vessel disease, both of which are associated with cognitive decline. Additionally, VB's analysis of CT imaging, while traditionally more focused on acute vascular events, complements MRI findings by identifying calcifications and larger infarcts that contribute to an overall vascular health profile.

The measurable alterations assessed by VB provide actionable insights into cerebral health. These include cerebral microbleeds, which are markers of chronic cerebral small vessel disease; white matter hyperintensities, indicative of chronic ischemia or demyelination; and lacunar infarcts, associated with subcortical vascular cognitive impairment. Furthermore, VB can quantify brain atrophy patterns, enhancing diagnostic accuracy in diseases such as Alzheimer's by mapping regional atrophy linked to neurodegeneration. The tool's ability to identify enlarged perivascular spaces (PVSs) further enriches its diagnostic utility, as these spaces are often seen in association with small vessel pathology and neurodegenerative conditions.

Compared to other AI-based neurodegenerative software, such as NeuroQuant and FreeSurfer, VB shares the goal of enhancing diagnostic precision through advanced imaging analysis. NeuroQuant and FreeSurfer are widely used for volumetric analysis and quantification of brain atrophy, providing critical metrics for diagnosing Alzheimer's disease and other forms of dementia. Like VB, these tools enable the measurement of brain volume and structural integrity. However, VB focuses specifically on cerebrovascular alterations, such as microbleeds and white matter lesions, which bridges the gap between vascular and neurodegenerative assessments. While NeuroQuant and FreeSurfer excel in detailed cortical thickness measurements and subcortical structure analysis, VB's integration of vascular insights provides a comprehensive approach that supports the evaluation of mixed pathology cases.

DeepBrain

DeepBrain (Vuno, Seoul, South Korea) is a cutting-edge artificial intelligence technology that analyzes MRI and PET images to evaluate neurodegenerative diseases. DeepBrain uses deep learning algorithms to detect minute morphological and metabolic alterations linked to diseases like Lewy body dementia. Given that prompt and precise diagnosis is essential for efficient management and action, this competence is especially important.

Following the best MRI and PET procedures is crucial to maximizing DeepBrain's effectiveness. High-resolution T1-weighted images with a slice thickness of 1 mm are advised for MRI in order to improve the identification of atrophic alterations in important brain areas such as the substantia nigra and hippocampal regions. Diffusion tensor imaging can also be used to help differentiate neurodegenerative diseases by offering useful information regarding white matter integrity.

The use of radiotracers such as fluorodeoxyglucose (FDG) and particular ligands for tau and amyloid disease is essential in PET imaging. FDG-PET is very useful for measuring metabolic activity and spotting patterns that are typical of Lewy body dementia, like decreased glucose metabolism in the temporoparietal and posterior cingulate cortex. By ensuring that the data supplied into DeepBrain is thorough and of excellent quality, this multimodal strategy enhances the algorithm's capacity to identify subtle neurodegenerative changes. High-quality imaging minimizes noise and artifacts, ensuring more accurate morphological and metabolic measurements. This, in turn, allows DeepBrain's deep learning models to detect small-scale atrophic changes and metabolic anomalies reliably, ultimately bolstering diagnostic precision.

Clinical studies have demonstrated that by identifying particular patterns of brain shrinkage and functional decline, such as reduced volume in the hippocampus, substantia nigra, and posterior cortical atrophy, DeepBrain dramatically increases the diagnostic accuracy for Lewy body dementia. Additionally, it can highlight metabolic reductions in the temporoparietal and posterior cingulate cortex, which are critical markers of neurodegenerative processes. According to studies, the instrument outperforms several traditional diagnostic techniques, achieving sensitivity rates as high as 92% and specificity close to 90%. This degree of precision is essential because it permits early diagnosis, which enables medical professionals to start personalized treatment strategies sooner and enhance patient outcomes and quality of life.

Automated Ventricular Measurement

An important development in the use of artificial intelligence in neurology is VizAI, a San Francisco, California-based company. VizAI's technology is excellent at automatically measuring ventricular volumes in brain imaging scans using complex AI algorithms. This is crucial for diagnosing illnesses like hydrocephalus and other neurodegenerative diseases. The software's ability to accurately measure volumetric changes over time gives doctors a useful tool for tracking the course of a disease and the effectiveness of treatment (Fig. 6.3).

It is advised to follow certain imaging protocols in order to take full advantage of VizAI's capabilities. The best images are MRI scans, especially high-resolution 3D T1-weighted pictures with a slice thickness of no more than 1 mm. These thorough scans guarantee that VizAI's algorithms can precisely evaluate the ventricles' shapes and compute volumes with little mistake, which is essential for trustworthy longitudinal research.

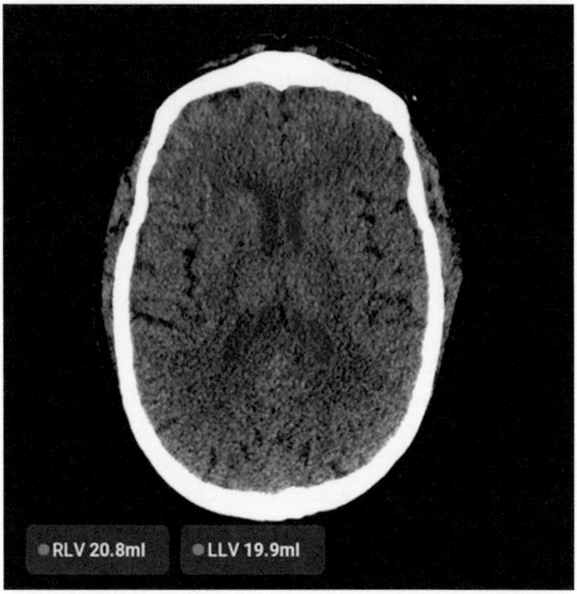

Fig. 6.3 VizAI automated ventricular volume measurements on head CT

VizAI's usefulness can be further increased by using additional MRI modalities, like T2-weighted FLAIR, which offer more information about the periventricular white matter alterations frequently linked to neurodegenerative diseases. VizAI can distinguish between normal age-related ventricular enlargement and disease-related changes in ventricular size thanks to this multimodal imaging technique, improving diagnostic precision and facilitating the exact customization of treatment regimens.

Challenges and Limitations

Even though AI technologies for assessing neurodegenerative disorders have advanced significantly, there are still a number of obstacles and restrictions that may affect their clinical usefulness and efficacy.

Data Quality and Availability
The availability and quality of data is one of the main obstacles to creating reliable AI models for neurodegenerative disease diagnosis. AI algorithm training and validation require high-quality, annotated neuroimaging datasets that capture a wide range of disease presentations. However, neuroimaging datasets specific to neurodegenerative diseases often suffer from limitations in sample size and diversity, particularly for less common conditions like frontotemporal dementia or atypical Parkinsonian disorders. This can result in AI models that do not generalize well when applied to patient populations outside the training set, affecting diagnostic reliability.

Furthermore, many neurodegenerative diseases, such as Alzheimer's and Lewy body dementia, exhibit subtle and gradual morphological changes that are difficult to detect without high-resolution, standardized imaging. The lack of datasets with consistent imaging protocols exacerbates this challenge, as models trained on heterogeneous data may struggle to accurately identify critical biomarkers like hippocampal atrophy or cortical thinning.

Longitudinal data is particularly vital for diagnosing and tracking the progression of neurodegenerative diseases, but such data is scarce due to the logistical difficulties of long-term patient follow-ups and the expense of repeated imaging. This limitation hinders the ability of AI to predict disease trajectory and assess treatment response over time.

Additionally, inconsistencies in imaging equipment and protocols, such as differences in MRI field strengths, coil types, and PET tracer selection, introduce variability that complicates data harmonization. These discrepancies can lead to AI models that fail to reliably detect and interpret the subtle metabolic and structural changes associated with early-stage disease, ultimately impacting the accuracy and utility of AI in real-world neurodegenerative diagnostics.

Interpretability and Transparency

Interpretability and Transparency: Deep learning-based AI models in particular frequently function as "black boxes," making it challenging for therapists to comprehend how they reach particular results. This issue is particularly relevant to the diagnosis of neurodegenerative conditions, where subtle morphological and metabolic changes detected by AI must align with established clinical and radiological knowledge for accurate interpretation. Because radiologists and neurologists must have faith in the AI's recommendations, this lack of interpretability may pose a serious obstacle to clinical adoption. For example, an AI tool's identification of early hippocampal atrophy or cortical thinning in MRI results without a clear explanation of the contributing features or rationale could make practitioners hesitant to trust its diagnostic outputs. Additionally, understanding how AI algorithms distinguish between overlapping pathologies, such as Alzheimer's and Lewy body dementia, is essential for guiding treatment decisions.

Ethical Considerations and Bias

Particularly in the context of diagnosing neurodegenerative diseases, the ethical concerns surrounding AI's use in neuroimaging are gaining increasing attention. Biases in AI systems resulting from the training datasets may cause differences in diagnosis and treatment. These biases may result in models for neurodegenerative diseases that perform poorly across a range of patient populations, possibly missing important diagnostic characteristics in underrepresented groups. For instance, datasets that mostly include elderly patients may underrepresent early-onset Alzheimer's disease, making it difficult for AI models to detect early-stage symptoms in younger populations. In a similar vein, research has demonstrated that neurodegenerative diseases such as Parkinson's disease can manifest differently in different ethnic groups, underscoring the significance of varied training data for precise AI performance. To guarantee fair and moral implementation in clinical practice, these biases must be addressed by employing broad and diversified training datasets and regularly assessing AI performance across a range of patient demographics.

Regulatory and Standardization Challenges
AI's use in identifying neurodegenerative diseases is particularly complicated by the constantly changing regulatory landscape in the healthcare industry. The absence of uniform and thorough laws specific to neuroimaging AI might cause ambiguity for both developers and medical professionals, even though many nations have set standards and guidelines for the approval and use of AI products. For instance, the FDA's approach to AI/ML-based medical devices and the European Union's Medical Device Regulation provide frameworks that may not yet fully address the nuances of AI used in neurodegenerative diagnosis, where early and precise detection is critical. Multi-center data variability is another difficulty because AI models frequently have to combine imaging data from various institutions with disparate protocols, such as different PET tracer types or MRI sequence parameters. Inconsistencies in biomarker measurement (e.g., hippocampus volume) might complicate validation, which can impact the models' effectiveness as well as their route to regulatory approval. In order to allow comparison and guarantee that these AI tools satisfy the strict requirements for clinical application in detecting illnesses like dementia and Parkinson's disease, it is imperative that performance indicators be standardized. AI adoption and integration into standard clinical practice may encounter major obstacles in the absence of explicit recommendations that address the particulars of neurodegenerative diagnosis.

Conclusion

A new age in the diagnostic assessment of neurodegenerative disorders has been ushered in by the developments in AI technology, especially in machine learning and deep learning. These technologies have greatly increased diagnostic accuracy by utilizing advanced algorithms that can analyze complex imaging data, allowing for early diagnosis and action. Convolutional neural networks and transfer learning are two examples of tools that have shown remarkable ability to detect small changes in the brain. This has made it possible to precisely track the evolution of diseases and customize treatment regimens. There are still issues, nevertheless, such as interpretability of the model, data quality, and ethical issues with bias and inequities in care. For AI in neuroimaging to be successfully implemented and accepted, several issues must be resolved. As we work through these challenges, it becomes evident that combining clinical knowledge with AI technologies has the potential to completely transform patient care by providing neurodegenerative disease patients with faster and more efficient treatments. Accepting this development will change the care of neurodegenerative diseases for years to come by improving patient outcomes and diagnostic accuracy.

Suggested Reading

1. Suzuki K, Yoshimura K, Kawataki T, Hanihara M, Takeda S, Kinouchi H. Prediction of pathological and radiological nature of glioma by mass spectrometry combined with machine learning. Neurosurgery Open. 2021;2(1). https://doi.org/10.1093/neuopn/okaa026.
2. Miah AS, Mamunur Rashid Md, Redwanur Rahman Md, et al. Alzheimer's disease detection using CNN based on effective dimensionality reduction approach. In: Advances in intelligent systems and computing. Published online 2021. pp. 801–811. https://doi.org/10.1007/978-3-030-68154-8_69.
3. Wang LX, Wang YZ, Han CG, Zhao L, He L, Li J. Revolutionizing early Alzheimer's disease and mild cognitive impairment diagnosis: a deep learning MRI meta-analysis. Arq Neuropsiquiatr. 2024;82(8):1–10. https://doi.org/10.1055/s-0044-1788657.
4. Li H, Yang Z, Qi W, Yu X, Wu J, Li H. Parkinson's image detection and classification based on deep learning. BMC Med Imaging. 2024;24(1):187. Published 2024 Jul 25. https://doi.org/10.1186/s12880-024-01364-8.
5. Sackl M, Tinauer C, Urschler M, Enzinger C, Stollberger R, Ropele S. Fully automated hippocampus segmentation using T2-informed deep convolutional neural networks. NeuroImage. 2024;298:120767. https://doi.org/10.1016/j.neuroimage.2024.120767.
6. Jung W, Jeong G, Kim S, et al. Reliability of brain volume measures of accelerated 3D T1-weighted images with deep learning-based reconstruction. Neuroradiology. Published online September 24, 2024. https://doi.org/10.1007/s00234-024-03461-5.
7. Amland R, Selbæk G, Brækhus A, et al. Clinically feasible automated MRI volumetry of the brain as a prognostic marker in subjective and mild cognitive impairment. Front Neurol. 2024;15:1425502. Published 2024 Jul 1. https://doi.org/10.3389/fneur.2024.1425502.
8. Koussis P, Toulas P, Glotsos D, Lamprou E, Kehagias D, Lavdas E. Reliability of automated brain volumetric analysis: a test by comparing NeuroQuant and volbrain software. Brain Behav. 2023;13(12). https://doi.org/10.1002/brb3.3320.
9. Yim Y, Lee JY, Oh SW, et al. Comparison of automated brain volume measures by NeuroQuant vs. Freesurfer in patients with mild cognitive impairment: effect of slice thickness. Yonsei Med J. 2021;62(3):255–61. https://doi.org/10.3349/ymj.2021.62.3.255.
10. Yang MH, Kim EH, Choi ES, Ko H. Comparison of normative percentiles of brain volume obtained from NeuroQuant® vs. DeepBrain® in the Korean population: correlation with cranial shape. J Korean Soc Radiol. 2023;84(5):1080–90. https://doi.org/10.3348/jksr.2023.0006.
11. An EJ, Kim JB, Son J, et al. Deep learning-based binary classification of beta-amyloid plaques using 18F florapronol PET. Nucl Med Commun. Published online September 27, 2024. https://doi.org/10.1097/MNM.0000000000001904.
12. Wang R, Wang H, Shi L, et al. A novel framework of MOPSO-GDM in recognition of Alzheimer's EEG-based functional network. Front Aging Neurosc. 2023;15:1160534. https://doi.org/10.3389/fnagi.2023.1160534.
13. Ushizima D, Chen Y, Alegro M, et al. Deep learning for Alzheimer's disease: mapping large-scale histological tau protein for neuroimaging biomarker validation. NeuroImage. 2022;248:118790. https://doi.org/10.1016/j.neuroimage.2021.118790.
14. Joo L, Shim WH, Suh CH, et al. Diagnostic performance of deep learning-based automatic white matter hyperintensity segmentation for classification of the Fazekas scale and differentiation of subcortical vascular dementia. PLoS One. 2022;17(9). https://doi.org/10.1371/journal.pone.0274562.
15. Rudie JD, Gleason T, Barkovich MJ, et al. Clinical assessment of deep learning-based super-resolution for 3D volumetric brain MRI. Radiol Artif Intell. 2022;4(2):e210059. Published 2022 Jan 12. https://doi.org/10.1148/ryai.210059.
16. Naji Y, Mahdaoui M, Klevor R, Kissani N. Artificial intelligence and multiple sclerosis: up-to-date review. Cureus. 2023;15(9):e45412. Published 2023 Sep 17. https://doi.org/10.7759/cureus.45412.

Chapter 7
Natural Language Processing for Neuroradiology

Golnaz Lotfian

Background

Natural language processing and its main objective of creating an intersection of computer science and human language in all its forms, verbal, written, and beyond, has undergone rapid advancement over the decades. Some of its early foundational work began in the mid-twentieth century with machines designed to translate Russian into English using rudimentary rule-based systems in the 1950s. By the 1980s, the introduction of statistical methods marked a significant shift from these rudimentary approaches to probabilistic models and larger data collections, laying the foundation for what would become deep learning. The 2010s witnessed advancements with the introduction of transformer architectures (e.g., GPT and BERT), which enabled a more precise language understanding and interpretation. Over the past 70 years, these advancements in natural language processing have created paths for the commercialization of NLP applications, including search engines, translation services, and virtual reality platforms, in a wide range of industries, including the expanding medical sector.

G. Lotfian (✉)
Department of Diagnostic Radiology and Nuclear Medicine, Rush University Medical Center, Chicago, IL, USA

D. T. Ginat (ed.), *Artificial Intelligence in Neuroradiology*,
https://doi.org/10.1007/978-3-032-24568-7_7

NLP Advancement in Neuroradiology

Automated and Structured Reporting

While advancements in voice-to-text technology are not unique to radiology, their impact on the medical industry is significant, particularly in terms of time efficiency and quality of reporting and note-taking. NLP's ability to translate voice into documented reports is increasingly utilized in hospitals and medical institutions worldwide. Today, many radiologists in the U.S. rely on PowerScribe 360, a cloud-based tool developed by Nuance Communications, which enables streamlined reporting with its advanced speech recognition capabilities (Fig. 7.1). PowerScribe utilizes algorithms that have the ability to recognize medical terminology, acronyms, and jargon. Additionally, this NLP tool comes fully integrated with electronic health records (EHR) and picture archiving and communication systems (PACS), allowing for streamlined access to patient data and imaging studies to assist radiologists in developing comprehensive reports efficiently.

Nuance is set to enhance its offerings beyond PowerScribe 360 with the launch of PowerScribe One. This advanced technology seeks to leverage AI to enhance speech recognition and deliver a "co-pilot" experience for radiologists. PowerScribe One incorporates predictive analytics and decision-support capabilities into the reporting process, potentially minimizing diagnostic errors and improving patient outcomes. This AI co-pilot will be proficient at proposing differential diagnoses and connecting them to pertinent case studies and guidelines, thereby serving as an interactive assistant in the diagnostic process. Furthermore, its improved interoperability with other health informatics systems ensures a smooth workflow, wherein AI-generated insights are directly integrated into clinical pathways, hence facilitating a more interconnected and intelligent healthcare environment.

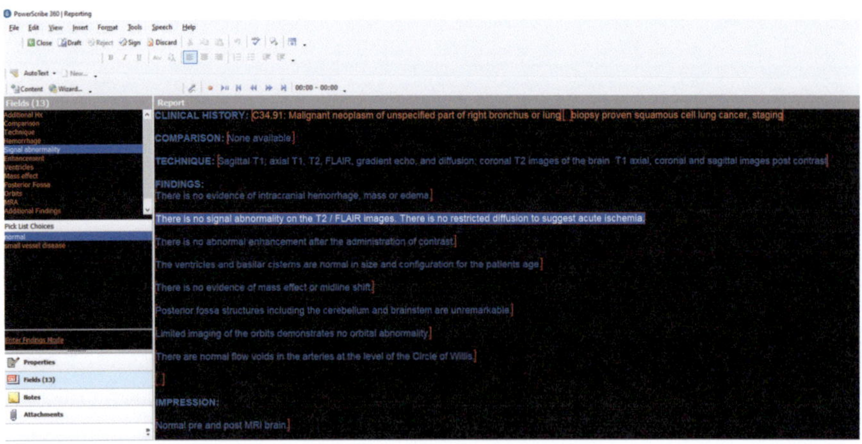

Fig. 7.1 Screenshot of PowerScribe 360 Auto Reporting

Enhancing Accuracy in Laterality Recognition

One of the critical aspects of ensuring the accuracy of automated radiology reports is the precise recognition of laterality, notably differentiating between the right and left sides of the body. Given the clinical significance of such details, it is crucial to minimize errors that could lead to misdiagnosis or incorrect treatment. PowerScribe incorporates advanced NLP algorithms designed to identify laterality—whether left, right, or bilateral—based on the proximity of descriptors to keywords and the overall context within the report.

While these algorithms perform well in most cases, challenges can arise in more complex sentence structures. For example, a statement such as "right-sided temporal lobe lesion with associated left-sided mass effect" might lead the software to misinterpret which descriptors correspond to which side. Similarly, redundancy or conflicting mentions in reports can also create confusion. In cases where a radiologist alternates between discussing the left and right hemispheres without clear transitions—for instance, "Right frontal lobe shows a cortical lesion, and left parietal lobe has a similar finding"—the software might incorrectly assign laterality to both findings if the term "left" is not explicitly tied to the second description.

To mitigate these risks, PowerScribe includes real-time alerts that detect potential right-left discrepancies and prompt radiologists to verify and correct any inconsistencies before final submission. This feature enhances report reliability and reduces the risk of laterality errors. However, the effectiveness of these safeguards depends significantly on clear and structured reporting. In neuroradiology, where subtle findings such as lateralized diffusion restriction or asymmetry in enhancement patterns can carry significant diagnostic weight, clarity is paramount. As automated systems continue to evolve, addressing the nuances of complex phrasing and encouraging standardized reporting protocols will be essential for optimizing the accuracy and clinical utility of radiology reports.

Furthermore, recent advances in natural language processing enable the possibility of rapid and accurate identification of critical information in narratives provided in radiology reports. In neuroradiology, there is ongoing research focusing on pre-training the T5 transformer, or Text-To-Text Transfer Transformer, to generate automatic MRI report conclusions. There are documented reports of these NLP-generated conclusions that closely match the quality of expert-written reports in as many as 75% of the cases. This capability not only helps reduce radiology workload and fatigue-related errors but also assists physicians in their diagnosis and decision-making process. Radiology reports are often stored as unstructured free text, but NLP's ability to extract key observations and measurements from both standardized templates and free text formats enables the opportunity to create accurate and coherent reports, improve communication between radiologists and clinicians, and expedite flagging of time-sensitive findings and observations.

Image Analysis

The integration of NLP and machine learning sets the foundation for cutting-edge advancement in interpreting and conceptualizing medical observations. The combination has a strong potential to enhance diagnostic accuracy, increase efficiency, and significantly improve patient care. Advancements in deep learning architectures, such as convolutional neural networks, have significantly enhanced the ability of computer-based models to classify images based on specific features, such as tumor type or cancer stage. These deep learning models can identify abnormalities, like fractures or tumors, with high precision. Additionally, the data segmentation capabilities of machine learning allow for both qualitative assessments and quantitative analysis, such as lesion size and volume. Another key application of machine learning in radiology is its ability to classify and analyze images, detect patterns, and monitor changes over time. When combined with NLP and its ability to organize and interpret both structured and free-text data, this integration opens numerous opportunities for advancement in patient care.

Firstly, the integration of NLP and ML can effectively identify discrepancies and inconsistencies in radiology and clinician reports. Secondly, it holds significant potential for enhancing diagnostic accuracy and increasing the reliability of radiology reports. Well-trained NLP models have demonstrated high accuracy in classifying head CT reports. Research involving large datasets of head CT neuroradiology reports has shown that finely tuned models can accurately differentiate between normal, pathological, and intracranial hemorrhage cases, achieving accuracy rates exceeding 90%. Additionally, computer-based analysis of radiology reports and automated reporting tools can streamline radiologists' workload, optimize report prioritization, and ultimately improve patient care. Another example of these advancements is GPT-4, a complex language model developed by OpenAI that offers several applications in radiology. GPT-4 can generate comprehensive radiology reports based on the input from imaging data, radiologist observations, and patient history. The model's ability to process natural language allows it to contextualize complex clinical data and narratives. Platforms like RadAI and Zebra Medical Vision leverage advanced NLP and ML techniques specifically tailored for radiology. These systems use pre-trained algorithms designed to interpret imaging reports and extract pertinent data effectively. Otherwise, CharGPT mini can be used as an assistant for formulating differential diagnosis, for example (Fig. 7.2). RadAI has demonstrated robust performance and high accuracy in detecting abnormalities within radiology reports. Both RadAI and Zebra Medical Vision have conducted comprehensive validation studies to confirm that their systems meet stringent clinical standards. Zebra Medical Vision has also published numerous clinical trials validating the accuracy and reliability of their models for detecting conditions such as pulmonary embolism, stroke, and diabetic retinopathy. The natural language processing capabilities of these complex platforms can be extremely useful in providing tools that improve accuracy and efficiency. Moreover, in educational settings, these readily available commercialized platforms can help generate case studies and

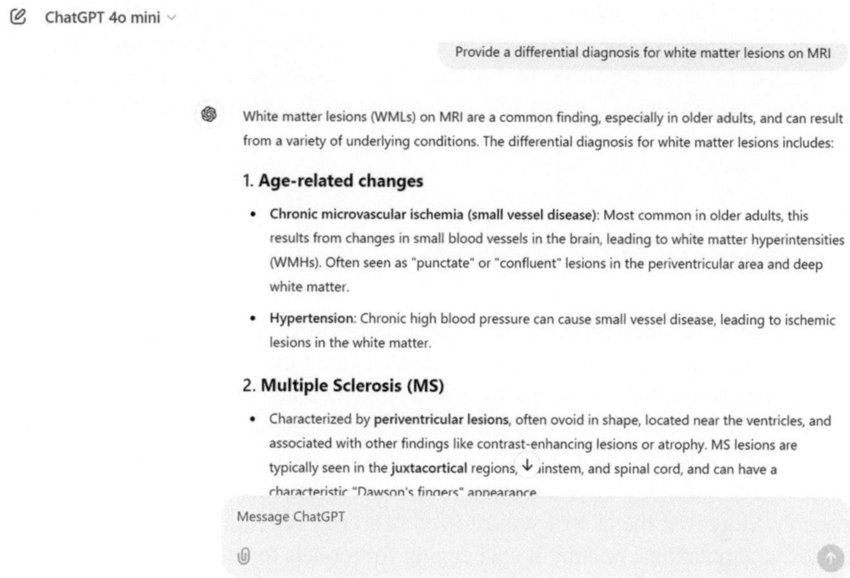

Fig. 7.2 Example of ChatGPT mini for differential diagnosis of white matter lesions

educational material for radiology trainees by simulating real-life scenarios and providing accurate feedback.

Research and Data Analysis

Radiology research often requires large cohorts and extensive datasets. NLP's ability to mine vast pools of data enhances research efficiency by identifying useful trends and correlations. In spine research, NLP has proven invaluable, particularly in the automated grading and labeling of spinal stenosis and vertebral segments. Recent studies have shown how deep learning can be integrated with NLP to automate the extraction of level-specific labels from free-text radiology reports, which are then used for precise vertebral segmentation and disc-level designation.

One approach uses a U-Net architecture combined with spine-curve fitting methods to accurately localize vertebrae and assign disc levels. Additionally, multi-input, multi-task, and multi-class convolutional neural networks have been employed to grade central canal and foraminal stenosis on axial and sagittal imaging series. This integration of technologies not only enhances the accuracy of pathology identification but also streamlines the workflow, significantly reducing both interpretation time and inter-reader variability among radiologists.

By leveraging large datasets of lumbar MRI images, these methodologies have demonstrated state-of-the-art performance in spinal stenosis classification, underscoring their potential to improve the efficiency and clinical value of radiological assessments. The predictive modeling capabilities of these tools also aid researchers by enabling more sophisticated analyses of imaging and textual data, thereby offering deeper insights into patient outcomes and demographic variations in spinal pathologies.

Limitations and Future Research

While there is vast potential for the adaptation of NLP in radiology, there are also several limitations that impact its effectiveness. One of the key limitations of NLP in radiology is the need for high-quality, well-annotated imaging data to effectively train robust NLP and ML models. Without sufficient and accurately labeled data, creating models that deliver reliable results is challenging. An accurate interpretation and annotation of radiology texts and images require manual, time-consuming, and costly research. Moreover, the lack of standardized radiology reporting can lead to inconsistencies in annotations, making it challenging for models to be universally applicable across different institutions. Additionally, due to the inherent self-learning nature of NLP, ongoing research and data validation are necessary to develop unbiased models that provide predictable outcomes. The complexity of machine learning algorithms can also obscure how decisions are made, making it difficult for radiologists to interpret and understand the reason behind the model's output. Most studies have primarily concentrated on proprietary models like ChatGPT, Google Gemini, and Anthropic Claude. The proprietary nature of these algorithms, combined with the use of programming interfaces that necessitate data transfer beyond the healthcare institution, raises significant privacy concerns. In an industry where data accuracy, privacy, and security are critical to delivering quality patient care, computer-based languages and models must undergo rigorous data quality checks and external validation. Recent developments in designing and evaluating open-source large language models (LLMs), such as Meta's Llama 3, offer greater control and transparency over the underlying algorithms used in natural language processing. This advancement holds promise for increasing the adoption of NLP in the medical industry. Ultimately, additional investment and support of ongoing research are required to ensure these technologies can effectively integrate into everyday healthcare practices and meet the high standards necessary for patient safety and care.

Suggested Reading

1. Casey A, Davidson E, Poon M, et al. A systematic review of natural language processing applied to radiology reports. BMC Med Inform Decis Mak. 2021;21(1):179. Published 2021 Jun 3.
2. Linna N, Kahn CE Jr. Applications of natural language processing in radiology: a systematic review. Int J Med Inform. 2022;163:104779.

3. López-Úbeda P, Martín-Noguerol T, Escartín J, Luna A. Automatic generation of conclusions from neuroradiology MRI reports through natural language processing. Neuroradiology. 2024;66(4):477–85.
4. Barash Y, Guralnik G, Tau N, et al. Comparison of deep learning models for natural language processing-based classification of non-English head CT reports. Neuroradiology. 2020;62(10):1247–56.
5. Travis Caton M Jr, Wiggins WF, Pomerantz SR, Andriole KP. Effects of age and sex on the distribution and symmetry of lumbar spinal and neural foraminal stenosis: a natural language processing analysis of 43,255 lumbar MRI reports. Neuroradiology. 2021;63(6):959–66.
6. Liu F, Zhou P, Baccei SJ, et al. Qualifying certainty in radiology reports through deep learning-based natural language processing. AJNR Am J Neuroradiol. 2021;42(10):1755–61.
7. Adams LC, Truhn D, Busch F, et al. Llama 3 challenges proprietary state-of-the-art large language models in Radiology Board–Style Examination questions. Radiology. 2024;312(2):e241191.

Chapter 8
AI for Quality Assurance, Imaging Quality Improvement, and Workflow Optimization

Asim Dhungana and Daniel Thomas Ginat

Image Enhancement Using AI

Noise Reduction

Noise can impair the identification of critical imaging signs, leading to reduced diagnostic accuracy. Deep learning methods have shown remarkable capabilities in the domain of noise reduction, improving signal enhancement and enabling clearer interpretation of images. In a retrospective study, Hales et al. developed a denoising autoencoder model using arterial spin labeling (ASL) sequences collected from 131 pediatric neuro-oncology patients and 11 healthy controls. The dataset included both pseudo-continuous ASL (pCASL) and multiple inflow-time (multi-TI) pulsed-ASL (PASL) scans collected on a 3T MRI scanner. Using the denoising model, researchers achieved an average signal-to-noise ratio (SNR) improvement of 62% when compared to the raw images.

Motion Artifact Correction

Subject head motion during MRI scanning can result in significant blurring and ghost artifacts, which may interfere with subsequent interpretation or downstream analysis. Concern for motion-induced artifacts can be particularly pronounced in

A. Dhungana (✉)
Pritzker School of Medicine, University of Chicago, Chicago, IL, USA
e-mail: asim.dhungana@uchicagomedicine.org

D. T. Ginat
Co-founder, Rad-Lab.ai, Chicago, IL, USA

D. T. Ginat (ed.), *Artificial Intelligence in Neuroradiology*,
https://doi.org/10.1007/978-3-032-24568-7_8

pediatric, cognitively impaired, and psychiatric populations, as well as in patients with neurological movement disorders (e.g., Parkinson's disease and Huntington's disease). Using motion-free MRI scans corrupted with simulated artifacts, researchers trained a 3D-CNN to reduce the severity of artifacts on data impacted by real motion in patients with Parkinson's disease, resulting in improved SNR and higher cortical surface reconstruction quality.

As another example, patient motion and resultant misregistration when performing digital subtraction angiography (DSA) may introduce artifacts due to misalignment, in some cases necessitating reimaging or possibly patient sedation. When starting from misregistered DSA images, a DL-based model developed by Ueda et al. was able to produce aligned angiograms, reducing or sometimes eliminating signs of artifact.

Device Artifact Correction

Artifacts may also arise from metallic devices in the patient, introducing significant distortions that may compromise imaging quality. Given their proximity, dental devices and implants may interfere with head and neck imaging as well as neuroimaging, including both MRI and CT. AI algorithms can assist in the detection and correction of such artifacts, facilitating better interpretation by radiologists.

Diffusion Imaging Distortion Correction

Diffusion-weighted imaging (DWI) can provide valuable information about tissue architecture and plays an important role in mapping white matter tracts. Despite its utility, DWI can suffer from susceptibility-induced spatial distortions, which may impair registration with structural images. Susceptibility corrections can be performed by various algorithms (e.g., TOPUP in FSL) but require repeated data acquisition with reverse phase encodings ("blip up, blip down"). In cases where protocol limitations do not allow use of these algorithms, Schilling et al. have developed Synb0-DisCo, a deep learning tool that results in distortion corrections practically identical to those produced by the aforementioned algorithms.

Spatial Enhancement and Super-Resolution

In addition to noise reduction and artifact correction, AI-driven techniques can also play an important role in enhancing the spatial resolution of images. In the field of so-called "super-resolution" methods, lower resolution raw images can be acquired and later enhanced, increasing patient comfort by decreasing the required scanning time, a significant limiting factor in the inclusion of various sequences in a scanning protocol In a prospective study of 32 patients undergoing standard-of-care brain MRI and 45% faster imaging with subsequent AI enhancement, Rudie et al. found no significant difference in the overall image quality of the two sets of sequences. These findings suggest that using the AI-based image enhancement software, subtleMR, may improve scanning efficiency without sacrificing quality. Another AI tool, SynthSR, has similarly been applied to convert clinical brain MRI scans to high-resolution T1 scans that can be readily used in research applications.

Synthetic Contrast Enhancement

Contrast-enhanced imaging is employed throughout radiology for the generation of images with improved clarity and sensitivity. Despite its widespread clinical utility, gadolinium-based contrast agents can be associated with notable safety risks, including kidney injury and rare but severe allergic responses. For this reason, alternative imaging approaches with substitute contrast material or reduced dosage are growing in popularity in order to expand patient eligibility for these imaging studies. Deep learning methods offer a promising opportunity to reduce or even eliminate contrast doses while still achieving a comparable enhancement in imaging quality. Using 10% of the standard contrast dose in T1-weighted MRIs, Pasumarthi et al. developed a deep learning model for image enhancement that predicted the full-dose contrast-enhanced images. These predicted images were found to have the same enhancing pattern as the full-dose images in 90% of cases when rated by 2 independent board-certified radiologists. Other studies of virtual contrast-enhanced low-dose MRIs have shown similar findings; however, smaller brain lesions (<10 mm) resulted in a significant reduction in one model's performance and another model tended to omit smaller vessels, suggesting that full-dose may still be necessary in certain contexts to avoid sacrificing testing sensitivity.

Multimodal Transformation and Generative AI

Synthetic MRI allows for the reconstruction of a variety of image contrasts using a single scan collected from a patient. Generative adversarial networks (GANs) may be applied to produce synthetic images using other sequences collected from a patient (Fig. 8.1). In the context of spinal imaging, Schlaeger et al. demonstrate the feasibility of GAN generation of high-quality synthetic T2-weighted, fat-saturated MRI from T1-weighted, non-fat-saturated MRI sequences collected from the same patient. They show improved assessment of spinal pathology, especially in settings where patients may not receive T2-weighted, fat-saturated imaging due to time constraints or motion artifacts. Other applications of generative networks include the generation of diffusion-weighted imaging and the enhancement of the quality of synthetic FLAIR images.

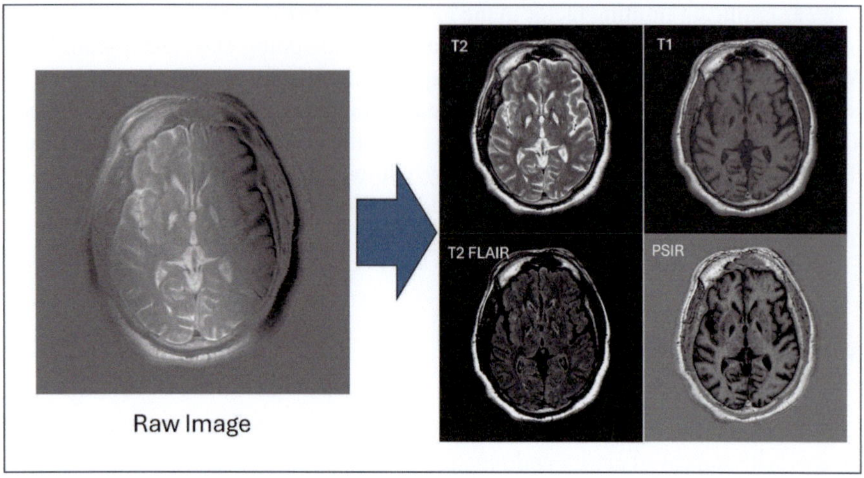

Fig. 8.1 Synthetic MRI. Multiple different sequences are derived from the initial raw images

MRI-guided radiotherapy planning requires the acquisition and co-registration of both MRI and CT scans. To save imaging time and reduce radiation exposure to the patient, there is great interest in generating synthetic CT images from MRI scans. Using a dataset of patients with paired MRI and CT scans, Ranjan et al. trained a GAN to generate a synthetic CT from a patient's T2-weighted MRI and compared these images with the patient's true CT, demonstrating high fidelity.

Scan Acceleration

Various approaches for AI-driven acceleration of imaging protocols have been developed utilizing many of the previously mentioned techniques for image enhancement, including noise reduction and synthetic image generation. Noise reduction methods allow image acquisition at a lower signal-to-noise ratio through raw MRI undersampling. These low-quality scans are then processed through denoising software to reconstruct high-quality images. This approach has been utilized by many tools, including SwiftMR, a deep-learning enterprise solution developed by AIRS Medical. SwiftMR has been shown to reduce scan times by up to 50% and has been validated in a variety of applications in neuroradiology, including lumbar spine MRI, epilepsy, brain metastasis detection, and MR angiography. Synthetic image generation methods acquire data in an abbreviated protocol and subsequently generate missing sequences using this limited data. A notable tool is SubtleSYNTH, which has shown success in producing spinal STIR images from sagittal T1- and T2-weighted images. In a multi-center, multi-reader trial by Tanenbaum et al., synthetic STIR was found to be diagnostically interchangeable with acquired STIR while offering superior image quality.

AI-driven acceleration of imaging improves the efficiency of healthcare delivery by increasing scan throughput, shortening appointment slots, and accommodating urgent add-on patients more effectively. Given the shortened scan time, sequences collected later in a scanning session are also less susceptible to motion degradation. Accelerated protocols also enhance patient experience, particularly in patients where claustrophobia, chronic pain, and anxiety may be barriers to image acquisition.

Automated Anomaly Detection and Worklist Prioritization

Introduction

The integration of AI methods into neuroimaging workflows offers the opportunity to automate the detection of various anomalies. Earlier detection of subtle imaging signs may inform worklist prioritization and facilitate rapid intervention. Rapid action is especially crucial in emergent scenarios such as intracerebral hemorrhage (ICH), where time-to-diagnosis and time-to-treatment are shown to be closely tied to patient outcomes. Similar urgency can be seen in other acute neurological conditions, including, but not limited to, acute infarction, large-vessel occlusion, aneurysm detection, and traumatic brain injury. In these cases, non-contrast head CTs often play an important role in the early triage of patients.

Automated Anomaly Detection

Titano et al. trained a 3D convolutional neural network (3D-CNN) to screen head CTs for the presence of acute neurological events, including intracerebral hemorrhage, hydrocephalus, and venous thrombosis, among other conditions. This model was validated in a randomized, double-blinded, prospective trial in a simulated clinical environment, demonstrating a significant reduction in the time to diagnosis from minutes to seconds.

Subarachnoid hemorrhage from aneurysmal rupture has a mortality rate of 44%, which underscores the importance of early detection and treatment of aneurysms. A systematic analysis of 43 prior studies examined the accuracy of AI methods in the detection of cerebral aneurysms, finding a high risk of bias with poor generalizability in the majority of studies, largely owing to their retrospective, single-center designs. To reduce the risk of bias in AI tools, it is critical to draw upon large, diverse datasets that represent the populations the tools will ultimately be applied to.

Worklist Prioritization in Emergent Neurovascular Cases

In recent years, various companies have emerged in the landscape of AI-guided worklist prioritization. Instead of reading imaging studies in the order they have been collected, this technology allows for the automated flagging of high-risk cases that may warrant expedited interpretation.

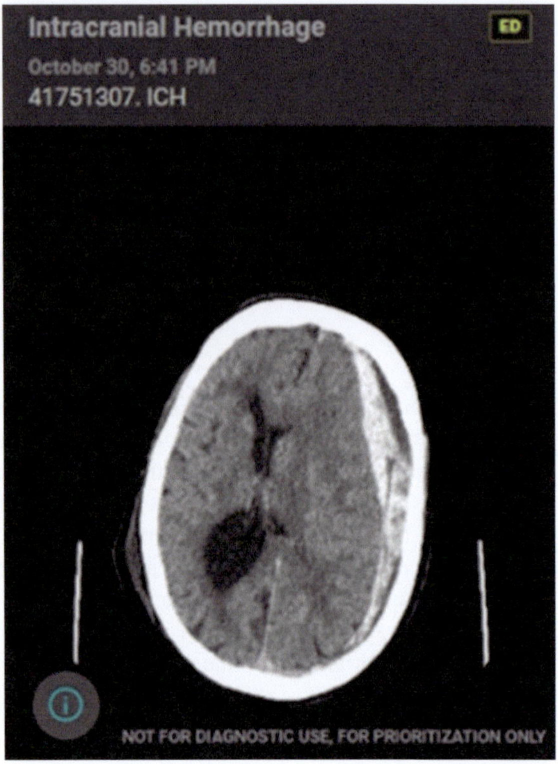

Fig. 8.2 Aidoc widget on the PACS worklist showing a case flagged for intracranial hemorrhage

Aidoc first received FDA approval for its commercial ICH detection software in 2018, which has since been shown to have strong accuracy in multiple settings. The software includes a widget on PACS that lists cases on the worklist flagged for acute intracranial hemorrhage (Fig. 8.2). In a retrospective, multi-center study by Kundisch et al., the Aidoc ICH detection software was applied on non-contrast head CTs to examine the discordance between model and radiologist detection. Researchers found that, although the software overcalled diagnoses 1.9% of the time, usage of the AI tool by an expert radiologist resulted in a 12.2% increase in ICH detection. Another study by Ginat demonstrated that the performance of the software also varied based on the clinical setting, with relatively higher accuracy in the trauma/emergency setting and relatively lower accuracy in the inpatient setting. Moreover, the software would also flag follow-up stability scans of inpatients with known prior ICH, which may not be as important to prioritize as undiagnosed ICH in a new patient. In addition, Aidoc notifies users if a suspected hemorrhage may have been overlooked and has not been included in the report via a no engagement alert (Fig. 8.3).

ICH detection software continues to be an area with active development. In February 2024, Viz.ai received FDA approval for ICH Plus. In a retrospective analysis of 4203 non-contrast head CTs from a single institution, Roshan et al.

Fig. 8.3 Aidoc no engagement alert email for intracranial hemorrhage

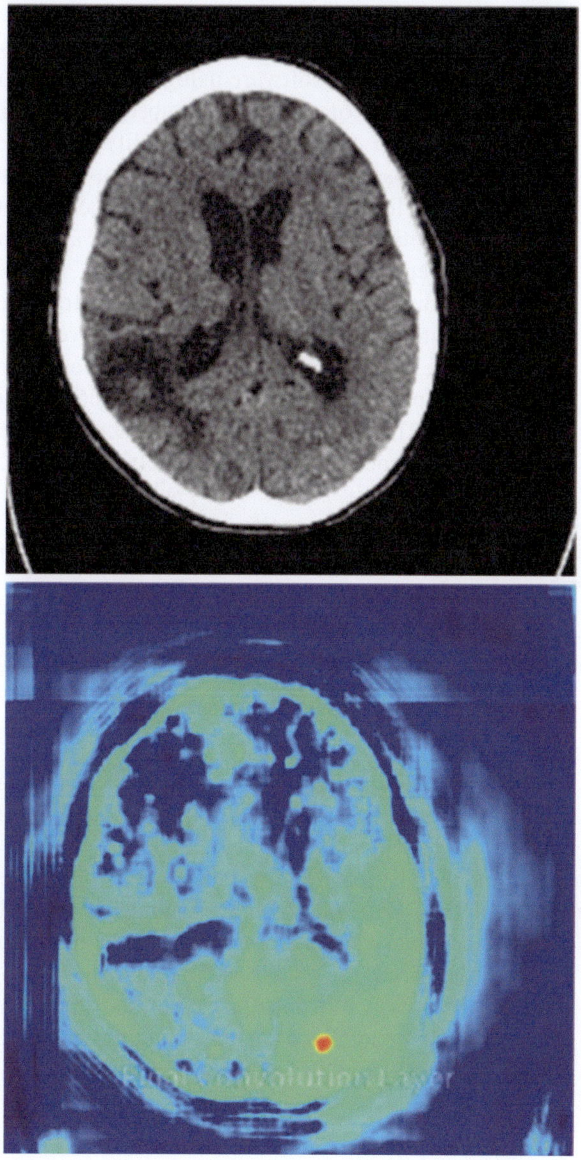

demonstrated strong model performance (sensitivity 85.3%, specificity 98.3%, PPV 81.3%, NPV 98.7%). In May 2024, Heuron received FDA approval for its ICH detection software, though extensive institutional validation studies remain to be performed.

Numerous other groups have also developed software to detect cervical spinal fractures, though many of these models still have yet to be thoroughly validated. In 2019, Aidoc received FDA clearance for a convolutional neural network called C-spine, which can help triage cervical spine fractures on non-contrast cervical spine CTs. Aidoc has reported a sensitivity of 91.7% and specificity of 88.6% for this software using data from its own retrospective, blinded, multinational study of 186 cases. Subsequent studies by outside researchers have demonstrated considerable variability in the performance of the C-spine model. In a retrospective study of 1904 non-contrast CT cervical spine studies at an academic-level I trauma center, Voter et al. found poor diagnostic accuracy, with sensitivity 54.9%, specificity 94.1%, positive predictive value (PPV) 38.7%, and negative predictive value (NPV) 96.8%. Model performance was noticeably worse in the detection of chronic fractures. The poor PPV was primarily attributed to the presence of degenerative irregularities, including degenerative ossicle, facet degeneration, and ossification of the ligamentum flavum. However, in another retrospective study of 665 non-contrast CT cervical spine studies with a 21% prevalence of spine fractures, Small et al. demonstrated reasonable performance of the Aidoc model (accuracy 92%, sensitivity 76%, specificity 97%, PPV 87%, NPV 94%) when compared to radiologistś (accuracy 95%, sensitivity 93%, specificity 96%, PPV 87%, NPV 98%). Additionally, there were seven cases in which the software detected a fracture that was missed by the radiologist on both CT and MRI.

Challenges and Considerations

Despite significant advances in automated detection of anomalies, a multitude of challenges remain before these tools can be freely applied in a clinical setting. The potential for false positives or negatives is a significant consideration in the implementation of AI tools for the detection of anomalies and the prioritization of worklists. The risk of false positives should be carefully weighed against the risks of delayed diagnosis, but excessive false positives may ultimately prove counterproductive if they divert the radiologist's attention away from more pertinent studies. In addition, the presence of false negatives and the variable performance of models across different cohorts and contexts highlight the importance of vigilance by radiologists when utilizing these tools in a clinical setting.

Quantitative Image Analysis

Introduction

The inherently quantitative nature of imaging data lends itself to the development of AI tools for the precise measurement of imaging findings, including both structural and functional values. By leveraging AI, annotation and quantification of imaging data can be performed more rapidly and with greater fidelity.

Automated Segmentation and Volumetric Analysis

A fundamental component of quantitative image analysis is automated segmentation and volumetric analysis. Automated brain segmentation and volumetric analysis can be performed with high fidelity using various research software products, including FSL, FreeSurfer, and SPM. Precise volumetric measurements can help quantify the extent of atrophy in neurodegenerative diseases, such as hippocampal atrophy in Alzheimer's disease. This automated approach may expedite the interpretation of images while also minimizing the potential for inconsistencies in manual segmentation of regions of interest by individual radiologists. In patients with longitudinal imaging, quantitative image analysis may be able to more accurately track the progression of pathology over time.

Moreover, similar measurements may aid in the quantification of tumor size and progression as well as treatment. Stereotactic radiotherapy of brain metastases delivers a high dose of radiation per tissue volume, requiring precise segmentation of cancerous lesions. Automated detection and segmentation of brain metastases using the DeepMedic deep convolutional neural network achieved 98% sensitivity, with only 7 false-positive metastases detected per patient when employing multimodal integration of two different MRI sequences.

Challenges in Data Standardization and Harmonization

The utility and reproducibility of imaging studies can be hindered by variations in acquisition protocols across different scanners and imaging sites, which may interfere with the interpretation of longitudinal imaging collected for a patient in either a clinical or research context. Harmonization techniques can facilitate the comparison of these studies despite discrepancies in acquisition. In a longitudinal MRI dataset from multiple sclerosis patients, contrast harmonization performed by the CNN DeepHarmony algorithm was shown to improve the consistency of volume atrophy quantification between scanning protocols. Another group applied harmonization using an attention-guided deep domain adaptation framework to classify the T1-weighted MRI scans of patients with dementia or mild cognitive impairment from the Alzheimer's Disease Neuroimaging Initiative (ADNI) database.

Clinical Decision Support

AI-driven clinical decision support systems can incorporate imaging and clinical data to guide further management. For example, machine learning software has been used to classify and provide thyroid cancer risk assessment for thyroid nodules on ultrasound (Fig. 8.4). This approach has been found to decrease interpration time by 24%, increase specificity by 37%, and increase cancer detection, while reducing biopsy of benign nodules.

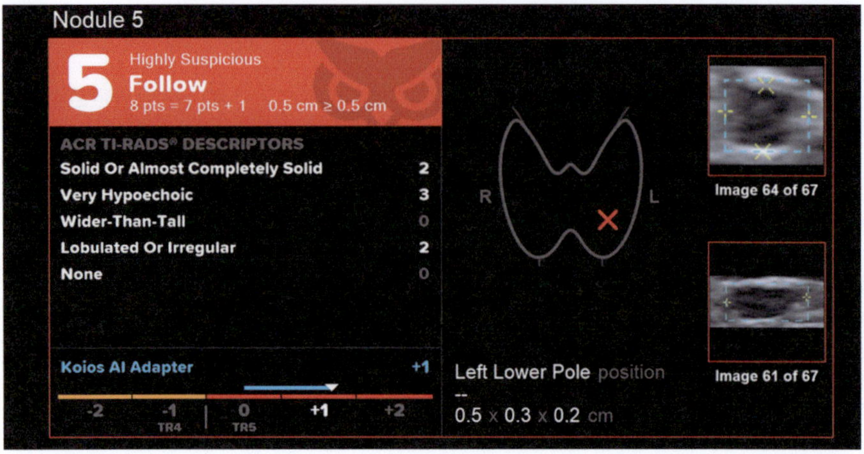

Fig. 8.4 Example of Koios Smart Ultrasound software for automated thyroid nodule characterization with suggestion for follow up

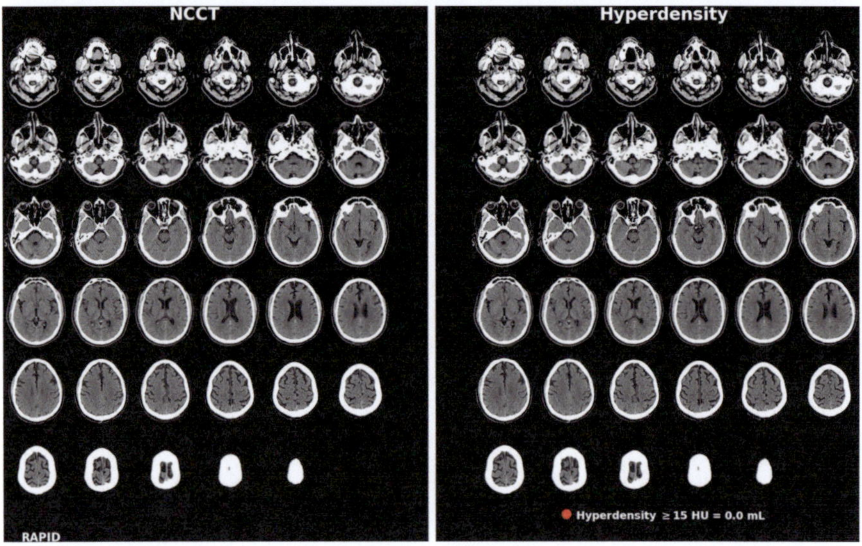

Fig. 8.5 Example of RAPID hyperdensity software output that is eligible for reimbursement

Reimbursements

Several imaging AI products are eligible for reimbursement from insurance providers. Payment mechanisms include the Common Procedural Terminology (CPT) code and the creation of the first New Technology Add-On Payment (NTAP). Reimbursement may be contingent upon including a statement such as the following in the radiology report with reference to RAPID CT hyperdensity analysis (Fig. 8.5): "Quantitative computed tomography (CT) tissue characterization using

RAPID AI (Hyperdensity, Hypodensity and/or ASPECTS), including interpretation and report, obtained with concurrent Non-contrast head CT examination. This was performed and medically necessary in order to facilitate accurate detection and expedite triage of intracranial hemorrhage and cerebral edema. Rapid AI analysis was performed, personally reviewed, and saved for inclusion in the patient's medical record."

Conclusions

As of June 2024, there are over 900 FDA-cleared AI algorithms in medicine, with over 700 classified in the field of radiology alone. Many AI tools have emerged in the field of neuroradiology in recent years, hoping to enhance image quality, improve diagnostic accuracy, optimize workflows, and reduce the burden of time-consuming, rote tasks. Given this growing landscape, practicing neuroradiologists will inevitably encounter these algorithms being applied in the clinical setting. Familiarity with the strengths and limitations of this software will encourage better integration into clinical workflows, with the goal of ultimately improving patient outcomes.

Suggested Reading

1. Gondara, L. Medical image denoising using convolutional denoising autoencoders. In: 2016 IEEE 16th international conference on data mining workshops (ICDMW). 2016. pp. 241–246. https://doi.org/10.1109/ICDMW.2016.0041.
2. Jifara W, Jiang F, Rho S, Cheng M, Liu S. Medical image denoising using convolutional neural network: a residual learning approach. J Supercomput. 2019;75:704–18.
3. Hales PW, Pfeuffer J, Clark A, C. Combined denoising and suppression of transient artifacts in arterial spin labeling MRI using deep learning. J Magn Reson Imaging JMRI. 2020;52:1413–26.
4. Duffy BA, et al. Retrospective motion artifact correction of structural MRI images using deep learning improves the quality of cortical surface reconstructions. NeuroImage. 2021;230:117756.
5. Ueda D, et al. Deep learning-based angiogram generation model for cerebral angiography without misregistration artifacts. Radiology. 2021;299:675–81.
6. Klinke T, et al. Artifacts in magnetic resonance imaging and computed tomography caused by dental materials. PLoS One. 2012;7:e31766.
7. De Crop A, et al. Analysis of metal artifact reduction tools for dental hardware in CT scans of the oral cavity: kVp, iterative reconstruction, dual-energy CT, metal artifact reduction software: does it make a difference? Neuroradiology. 2015;57:841–9.
8. Schilling KG, et al. Synthesized b0 for diffusion distortion correction (Synb0-DisCo). Magn Reson Imaging. 2019;64:62–70.
9. A fast medical image super resolution method based on deep learning network-web of science core collection. https://www.webofscience.com/wos/woscc/full-record/WOS:000458177800012?SID=USW2EC0ABCYCwLwIX3tiCI5DXBx61
10. Pham C-H, et al. Multiscale brain MRI super-resolution using deep 3D convolutional networks. Comput Med Imaging Graph. 2019;77:101647.
11. Rudie JD, et al. Clinical assessment of deep learning-based super-resolution for 3D volumetric brain MRI. Radiol Artif Intell. 2022;4:e210059.

12. Iglesias JE, et al. SynthSR: a public AI tool to turn heterogeneous clinical brain scans into high-resolution T1-weighted images for 3D morphometry. Sci Adv. 2023;9:eadd3607.
13. McDonald JS, et al. Acute adverse events following gadolinium-based contrast agent administration: a single-center retrospective study of 281 945 injections. Radiology. 2019;292:620–7.
14. Pasumarthi S, et al. A generic deep learning model for reduced gadolinium dose in contrast-enhanced brain MRI. Magn Reson Med. 2021;86:1687–700.
15. Ammari S, et al. Can deep learning replace gadolinium in neuro-oncology?: a reader study. Investig Radiol. 2022;57:99–107.
16. Kleesiek J, et al. Can virtual contrast enhancement in brain MRI replace gadolinium?: a feasibility study. Investig Radiol. 2019;54:653–60.
17. Tanenbaum LN, et al. Synthetic MRI for clinical neuroimaging: results of the magnetic resonance image compilation (MAGiC) prospective, multicenter, Multireader Trial. AJNR Am J Neuroradiol. 2017;38:1103–10.
18. Schlaeger S, et al. Implementation of GAN-based, synthetic T2-weighted fat saturated images in the routine radiological workflow improves spinal pathology detection. Diagn Basel Switz. 2023;13:974.
19. Schlaeger S, et al. Synthetic T2-weighted fat sat based on a generative adversarial network shows potential for scan time reduction in spine imaging in a multicenter test dataset. Eur Radiol. 2023;33:5882–93.
20. Hirte AU, et al. Realistic generation of diffusion-weighted magnetic resonance brain images with deep generative models. Magn Reson Imaging. 2021;81:60–6.
21. Hagiwara A, et al. Improving the quality of synthetic FLAIR images with deep learning using a conditional generative adversarial network for pixel-by-pixel image translation. Am J Neuroradiol. 2019;40:224–30.
22. Ranjan A, Lalwani D, Misra R. GAN for synthesizing CT from T2-weighted MRI data towards MR-guided radiation treatment. Magn Reson Mater Phys Biol Med. 2022;35:449–57.
23. Lui YW, et al. Artificial intelligence in neuroradiology: current status and future directions. AJNR Am J Neuroradiol. 2020;41:E52–9.
24. Yafasova A, et al. Time to thrombolysis and long-term outcomes in patients with acute ischemic stroke: a nationwide study. Stroke. 2021;52:1724–32.
25. Titano JJ, et al. Automated deep-neural-network surveillance of cranial images for acute neurologic events. Nat Med. 2018;24:1337–41.
26. Nieuwkamp DJ, et al. Changes in case fatality of aneurysmal subarachnoid haemorrhage over time, according to age, sex, and region: a meta-analysis. Lancet Neurol. 2009;8:635–42.
27. Din M, et al. Detection of cerebral aneurysms using artificial intelligence: a systematic review and meta-analysis. J Neurointerventional Surg. 2023;15:262–71.
28. Kundisch A, et al. Deep learning algorithm in detecting intracranial hemorrhages on emergency computed tomographies. PLoS One. 2021;16:e0260560.
29. Ginat DT. Analysis of head CT scans flagged by deep learning software for acute intracranial hemorrhage. Neuroradiology. 2020;62:335–40.
30. Burns JE, Yao J, Muñoz H, Summers RM. Automated detection, localization, and classification of traumatic vertebral body fractures in the thoracic and lumbar spine at CT. Radiology. 2016;278:64–73.
31. Burns JE, Yao J, Summers RM. Vertebral body compression fractures and bone density: automated detection and classification on CT images. Radiology. 2017;284:788–97.
32. Tomita N, Cheung YY, Hassanpour S. Deep neural networks for automatic detection of osteoporotic vertebral fractures on CT scans. Comput Biol Med. 2018;98:8–15.
33. Voter AF, Larson ME, Garrett JW, Yu J-PJ. Diagnostic accuracy and failure mode analysis of a deep learning algorithm for the detection of cervical spine fractures. AJNR Am J Neuroradiol. 2021;42:1550–6.
34. Small JE, Osler P, Paul AB, Kunst M. CT cervical spine fracture detection using a convolutional neural network. Am J Neuroradiol. 2021;42:1341–7.
35. Woolrich MW, et al. Bayesian analysis of neuroimaging data in FSL. NeuroImage. 2009;45:S173–86.

36. Dale AM, Fischl B, Sereno MI. Cortical surface-based analysis. I Segmentation and surface reconstruction. NeuroImage. 1999;9:179–94.
37. Ashburner J. SPM: a history. NeuroImage. 2012;62–248:791–800.
38. Li F, Liu M. A hybrid convolutional and recurrent neural network for hippocampus analysis in Alzheimer's disease. J Neurosci Methods. 2019;323:108–18.
39. Zhou M, et al. Radiomics in brain tumor: image assessment, quantitative feature descriptors, and machine-learning approaches. Am J Neuroradiol. 2018;39:208–16.
40. Charron O, et al. Automatic detection and segmentation of brain metastases on multimodal MR images with a deep convolutional neural network. Comput Biol Med. 2018;95:43–54.
41. Dewey BE, et al. DeepHarmony: a deep learning approach to contrast harmonization across scanner changes. Magn Reson Imaging. 2019;64:160–70.
42. Guan H, et al. Multi-site MRI harmonization via attention-guided deep domain adaptation for brain disorder identification. Med Image Anal. 2021;71:102076.
43. Artificial Intelligence and Machine Learning (AI/ML)-enabled medical devices. FDA. 2024. https://www.fda.gov/medical-devices/software-medical-device-samd/artificial-intelligence-and-machine-learning-aiml-enabled-medical-devices
44. Parikh RB, Helmchen LA. Paying for artificial intelligence in medicine. NPJ Digit Med. 2022;5(1):63. https://doi.org/10.1038/s41746-022-00609-6. PMID: 35595986; PMCID: PMC9123184.
45. Tanenbaum LN, et al. Deep learning–generated synthetic MR imaging STIR spine images are superior in image quality and diagnostically equivalent to conventional STIR: a multicenter, multireader trial. AJNR Am J Neuroradiol. 2023;44:987–93.
46. Yoo H, et al. Deep learning–based reconstruction for acceleration of lumbar spine MRI: a prospective comparison with standard MRI. Eur Radiol. 2023;33:8656–68.
47. Suh PS, et al. Improving diagnostic performance of MRI for temporal lobe epilepsy with deep learning-based image reconstruction in patients with suspected focal epilepsy. Korean J Radiol. 2024;25:374–83.
48. Oh G, et al. Deep learning-based image enhancement for improved black blood imaging in brain metastasis. Eur Radiol. 2025;36:928–38. https://doi.org/10.1007/s00330-025-11920-7.
49. Kim BK, You S-H, Kim B, Shin JH. Deep learning-based high-resolution magnetic resonance angiography (MRA) generation model for 4D time-resolved angiography with interleaved stochastic trajectories (TWIST) MRA in fast stroke imaging. Diagnostics. 2024;14:1199.
50. Barnes A, White R, Venables H, Lam V, Vaidhyanath R. Investigation of artificial intelligence-based clinical decision support system's performance in reducing the fine needle aspiration rate of thyroid nodules: A pilot study. Ultrasound. 2024;33(4):282–90. https://doi.org/10.1177/1742271X241299220. PMID: 39654847; PMCID: PMC11625399

Chapter 9
Legal, Regulatory, and Quality Considerations

Vrushab Gowda and Harlan Benjamin Harvey

Introduction

For the past two decades, artificial intelligence (AI) products, founders, and companies have captured headlines and found their way into common parlance. By 2030, the sector will be on track to contribute nearly $15 trillion to the global economy. It is no exaggeration to state that we are in the midst of an AI revolution. Among medical specialties, nowhere is this more acutely felt than in radiology, which features over 100 United States Food and Drug Administration (FDA) authorized products. This is logical, given that it is an intensely data-driven field marked by rich imagery, synthesis of visual and text-based input, standardized report generation, and heavy emphasis on pattern recognition, accuracy, and speed. These features are particularly accentuated within neuroradiology. Imaging is the first, and frequently the only, diagnostic modality for detecting intracranial pathology. AI applications in neuroradiology span the field, and include those in interpretive (e.g., stroke detection), non-interpretive (e.g., MRI Brain auto-protocoling), quasi-interpretative (e.g., radiologic-pathologic correlation tools), quality improvement (e.g., AI-enhanced peer review), and administrative (e.g., billing and image transfer) functions. Their unique role in the clinical space in turn prompts novel approaches to regulation and legal risk management, which together form the subject of this chapter.

V. Gowda (✉)
Department of Radiology, Massachusetts General Hospital, Boston, MA, USA

Harvard Medical School, Boston, MA, USA
e-mail: vgowda@mgh.harvard.edu

H. B. Harvey
Radiology Physicians, Inc., Dayton, OH, USA

D. T. Ginat (ed.), *Artificial Intelligence in Neuroradiology*,
https://doi.org/10.1007/978-3-032-24568-7_9

Regulatory Issues

The Role of the FDA

No dedicated pathway for regulating clinical AI yet exists in the United States. Further complicating matters, AI tools do not neatly fit into a single product category given the range of their applications. Naturally, those acting upon image data will be held to more stringent regulatory standards than those applied in back-office settings. Generally, interpretive tools deployed in the neuroradiology practice space represent some variant of a medical device.

The following discussion pertains to AI products deemed devices by the FDA and regulated as such. According to the federal Food, Drug & Cosmetic Act, this refers to "an instrument . . . intended for use in the diagnosis. . .or in the cure, mitigation, treatment, or prevention of disease . . . which does not achieve its primary intended purposes through chemical action."[1] The operative term here is "diagnosis;" neuroradiology AI tools which do not offer this functionality are not captured by this definition. It is separately worth noting that software products have long been held to constitute medical devices, even if they are wholly detached from physical hardware components. These "Software as a Medical Device" (SaMD) tools capture "software intended to be used for one or more medical purposes that perform these purposes without being part of a hardware medical device." Such products must obtain specific marketing clearance from the federal Food and Drug Administration (FDA) prior to clinical use, although limited exceptions exist for tools applied in research contexts. This is relevant, as FDA authorization effectively functions as a prerequisite not only for deployment at scale, but also for reimbursement, clinical integration, and even overseas expansion (as a number of foreign jurisdictions accept FDA review decisions in lieu of authorization from domestic healthcare regulators).

Conventional Regulatory Approaches

Standard FDA premarket review of medical devices looks to their intended use before stratifying them according to the level of risk they pose to patients. Candidate devices are categorized into Classes I-III in order of increasing risk; they are then subject to one of three discrete review pathways, where they are evaluated with an eye to safety and efficacy. The FDA has provided specific guidance on point for radiology products, establishing a distinction between computer-assisted detection tools (CADe) which "identify, mark, highlight, or in any other manner direct attention" to imaging findings, which it considers a Class II product, as opposed to

[1] 21 U.S.C. §321(h).

computer-assisted diagnosis (CADx) tools which can designate specific disease states, deeming them Class III devices.[2]

The De Novo pathway is reserved for low-risk Class I and II products without a precursor on the market. For novel AI tools with routine clinical stakes, such as those used to estimate brain parenchymal volume on CT, the De Novo classification route may be most appropriate. The 510(k) pathway is designed for low- to medium-risk products analogous to a "predicate" device previously cleared by the FDA. This offers an abridged route to premarket authorization if "substantial equivalence" to this preexisting predicate can be demonstrated. The lighter burden of performance data required in a 510(k) submission (vis-à-vis the other pathways) renders this an attractive avenue toward marketing clearance. The third pathway, Premarket Approval (PMA), is the most rigorous avenue for high-risk products and entails the most extensive regulatory submission.

Given the growing number of AI tools receiving FDA authorization, many developers are increasingly resorting to the 510(k) pathway for their products, effectively "tagging on" their product to previously successful submissions. Even still, the federal government has recognized the inherent limitations of the traditional risk class-based approach, which was designed for hardware medical devices. The 21st Century Cures Act established a series of exemptions for SaMD in 2016, carving out several functions from the statutory definition of "medical device." According to its section 3060(a), this excepts products (1) intended for administrative support, or used in (2) the maintenance of a healthy lifestyle, (3) electronic patient records, (4) storage or display of clinical data, and (5) "unless the function is intended to acquire, process, or analyze a medical image . . . for the purpose of (i) displaying, analyzing, or printing medical information . . . (ii) supporting or providing recommendations to a health care professional about prevention, diagnosis, or treatment and . . . (iii) enabling such health care professional to *independently review* (emphasis added) the basis for such recommendations to make a clinical diagnosis or treatment decision regarding an individual patient," collectively referred to as clinical decision support (CDS) products.[3]

In other words, neuroradiology AI tools serving back-office functions may no longer be subject to FDA premarket review, provided they do not directly act on imaging data to fulfill interpretive functions. At first glance, this language appears to codify what was already widely known: a tool that is not used in a clinical diagnostic or curative capacity should not trigger an extensive regulatory process. There is, however, a subtle wrinkle buried in the Cures Act's phrasing—an explicit reference to the clinician's ability to "independently review the basis" of a software tool's output. The FDA has shed light on its interpretation of this language in a pair of guidance documents.

In the first, "Clinical Decision Support Software" (CDS Guidance), the agency underscores that healthcare professionals must "be able to reach the same

[2] Radiology devices; reclassification of medical image analyzers. 83 Fed. Reg. 25598.

[3] 21 U.S.C. §360j(o).

recommendation . . . without relying primarily on the software function," while also requiring developers to demonstrate the "purpose or intended use of the software function, the intended user (e.g., ultrasound technicians, vascular surgeons), the inputs used to generate the recommendation (e.g., patient age and gender), and the rationale or support for the recommendation." The CDS Guidance does so without defining "rationale or support;" this leaves open the question of whether the FDA will evaluate an algorithm's input or internal logic to test the sufficiency of said "rationale," thereby creating a vague regulatory standard. This language also serves as an implicit check against black-box algorithms, which by their very structure may lack the ability to "explain" their findings. These deep learning programs are characterized by their opaque internal mechanisms, in many cases constantly changing and escaping precise description. Moreover, even in cases of transparent "white box" algorithms, a developer may face competitive disincentives to sharing this information with the FDA. It can contain proprietary information related to the product in question; mandating disclosure may exert a chilling effect on the industry.

The second guidance document, entitled "Changes to Existing Medical Software Policies" (Changes Guidance), underscores the FDA's position with respect to the remainder of 3060(a) exempt products. Namely, it continues to view the majority of CDS as falling outside the purview of premarket review pathways, with the exceptions of those tools which "alert a caregiver to take immediate clinical action." Generative AI tools may occupy a key niche as CDS products, particularly if they rely upon text inputs. For example, an application can synthesize data from the electronic health record, integrating prior studies and pathology reports to facilitate neuroradiologic-pathologic correlation at a glance. Despite its technical sophistication, this use case would meet the definition of CDS and likely not require formal FDA evaluation. The same likely holds true for other noninterpretive functions, such as AI tools used in peer review, quality improvement, and other workflow optimization settings.

Others may blur the line between traditional SaMD and CDS. Auto-protocoling software may operate on text inputs (e.g., clinical indication, labeled previous studies, allergy lists) from the patient's chart to fulfill an arguably administrative function, but one that can directly lead to patient harm. Take the case of an AI-powered program that erroneously administers MRI contrast to a patient with renal impairment or a gadolinium allergy. Even if a human operator were to review its output before making a clinical decision based on this information, classification of this tool as a premarket review-exempt CDS or a traditional SaMD is not straightforward. Developers would be well-advised to contact the FDA in advance of a formal application to clarify regulatory ambiguity. The agency offers a pre-submission meeting, otherwise known as a "q-sub," to medical device applicants, where they are permitted to ask questions, share preliminary data, and receive feedback on their products prior to formal review.

Future Direction

Product risk categorization is far from the only unique regulatory issue facing AI products. By definition, machine learning enables a manmade device to modulate its output by "training" on new datasets. As a function of time, the same algorithm, when presented with the same input, can produce drastically different outputs; a continuously learning stroke detection tool can grow increasingly sensitive with adequate training. This dynamic property of AI tools exposes the limits of traditional regulatory paradigms. When would a product's characteristics diverge so significantly from the point of initial FDA review that it could be held to constitute a new device? For a product that has already received a 510(k) clearance, when would it cease to be "substantially equivalent" to its predicate? For others, at which point could its inherent risk warrant a reclassification from a Class I to a Class II device? Should these changes prompt renewed FDA submissions? How would the agency monitor them in the real world?

Clearly, a dedicated governance scheme for AI products is needed. However, in the absence of statutory authorization from Congress, the FDA is unable to create a purpose-built regulatory framework for its premarket review. Congressional gridlock may render this the case for the foreseeable future; as with other federal agencies, the FDA can only issue regulations if granted the power to do so via legislation. It has instead resorted to a series of pilot programs and action plans which, although limited in scope, sketch a possible image of the future.

The Pre-Cert program figures prominently among them. In 2017, the FDA invited nine industry volunteers (including Apple, Verily, Samsung, and Johnson & Johnson) to participate in a longitudinal pilot, predominantly focused on novel digital therapeutics. Rather than look solely to technical features of the product itself, Pre-Cert advanced a total product lifecycle approach (TPLC) to regulation. Emphasis was instead applied to the quality and stewardship of data involved across the span of development. Such a process-based approach is not without precedent; it is closely patterned after the current good manufacturing practices (cGMP) prevalent in the pharmaceutical and hardware medical device sectors. More specifically, the FDA considered data generalizability and storage as they relate to algorithmic training, fine-tuning, and testing. This did not end with product development; once a device was in use, manufacturers would then routinely provide the FDA with performance data to facilitate postmarket surveillance in real time. In this way, TPLC paradigms offer a lighter regulatory touch than traditional product-based review pathways and are furthermore able to capture the structural dynamism inherent to AI products.

In addition, the FDA has floated some product-centric guardrails centered on intended use and change controls. With regard to the former, the FDA has hinted that it may undertake risk assessments with a view to (1) how the product will be integrated into clinical workflow, incorporating the importance of output to the healthcare decision-making process, (2) the severity of the disease state in question, and (3) the status of the product as either a locked or adaptive algorithm. In addition, it required developers to anticipate potential changes to their algorithm in advance and create standardized procedures for governing them. These changes can then be classified into one of three categories which would trigger their own premarket review pathway: (1) performance modifications without changes to input or intended use (e.g., a tumor volumetric tool training on glioblastoma-specific data), input modifications with no change to intended use (e.g., a stroke detection algorithm drawing upon both CT and MRI data), and (3) modifications to intended use (e.g., extending a cerebral vessel mapping algorithm's functions to include aneurysm detection). This tailored approach reflects the FDA's acknowledgement that existing regulatory frameworks may be inadequate for AI tools. Here, it aims to preserve its overarching goal of promoting safety and efficacy, while retaining a level of built-in plasticity to enable the industry to grow.

Nongovernmental Approaches

For their part, nongovernmental entities have stepped in to provide a measure of oversight. Quality management systems (QMS) form an essential component of postmarket governance. Indeed, the FDA requires manufacturers to maintain design controls, processes for corrective actions, and extensive recordkeeping procedures.[4] These are typically established according to International Organization for Standardization (ISO) criteria, traditionally ISO 13485 for medical devices. ISO has recently developed a new system specifically for AI products—ISO 42001. This global standard creates a continuous process improvement cycle for developers to follow, incorporating routine risk assessments, audits, and procedures to support responsible use. Developers may increasingly adhere to ISO 42001, among other nongovernmental standards, on their own accord. The benefits are manifold; obtaining an international stamp of approval would confer a degree of legitimacy, enhance interoperability, and promote public trust, all of which can boost sales and access to training data.

There has been a broader push toward self-regulation by nonprofit and industry groups. The Coalition for Health AI (CHAI) represents perhaps the largest, bringing together integrated academic institutions (MassGeneral Brigham, University of California Health), big tech (Google, Microsoft), professional societies (the National Academy of Medicine), and subject matter experts to develop a set of AI best practices. CHAI has published a growing number of reports that resemble guidance documents, including the Blueprint for Trustworthy AI and a proposal for a national network of AI assurance laboratories. In this regard it has been followed by a number of similar large partnerships aiming to fulfill much the same purpose, such as TRAIN and VALID AI. Whether these nonbinding initiatives will gain broader traction in the industry remains to be determined.

[4] 21 C.F.R. 820.

Liability Issues

Medical Professional Liability

Neuroradiology AI tools face an unclear liability landscape. In part, this is owing to the paucity of relevant caselaw on point; at the time of writing, there has been no case involving physician liability incurred from the use of an AI tool. However, it is highly likely that traditional medical professional liability frameworks will apply, operating according to conventional negligence theories, although even these will be hard-pressed to account for algorithmically-driven harm. Take the case of a neuroradiologist who, in relying exclusively on an automated stroke detection tool, misses calling a subtle ischemic penumbra on an early CT Head. The patient does not receive adequate care and develops a major stroke with lasting neurologic impairment. When confronting the radiologist in a malpractice case, the plaintiff bears the burden of proving (1) that the radiologist owed them a duty of care, (2) breached it, and (3) sustained damages as a result (4) through a causal relationship of said breach of duty.

A court would generally look to standards established by radiology professional societies, community practices (the "locality rule"), as well as the radiology department's operative procedures in determining both the scope of duty of care and whether it was breached.[5] Today, as neuroradiology AI products have not yet entered into the standard of care, it is plausible that the radiologist in question would be found liable for malpractice. Now, imagine two slightly different scenarios.

Assume that in this particular hospital's workflow, the AI tool was commonly used to screen for early ischemia and *was* held to represent the standard of care. Furthermore, radiologist expert witnesses called to trial would likewise demonstrate difficulty identifying the region of early ischemia. Would the defendant physician's actions, relying on the program, still constitute malpractice? This is a closer question. In a field as heavily dependent on digital tools as radiology, technical limitations can overshadow nuances in clinical judgment. A court may treat an AI device's (assuming it received FDA authorization and was being used appropriately) failure to identify a subtle or ambiguous finding in a similar vein to how it evaluates a CT or MRI artifact-degraded study. The net effect may be a relative diminution of liability risk falling on the individual neuroradiologist.

In a second scenario, imagine that the AI tool is incorporated within both professional and institutional protocols, successfully detects the hypoperfused area, and flags the region of interest to the neuroradiologist, who then chooses to disregard the finding in their report. This presents a unique scenario wherein the human radiologist, in exercising their individual clinical judgment, finds themselves at odds with a tool purporting to represent ground truth. Would it constitute a deviation from the standard of care? Courts and legal scholars have yet to offer an answer, but the physician's independent judgment can offer a compelling defense.

[5] Hall v. Hilbun, 466 So. 2d 856 (Miss. 1985).

Edge cases such as this will likely be decided on the basis of the suit's factual context. How subtle was the finding (relative to other human radiologists)? In this situation, what is the AI tool's sensitivity and specificity? How often do other radiologists elect to dispense with the AI program's output to substitute their personal clinical decision-making? This also leaves the issue of causation. Would a court interrogate the inner workings of an AI algorithm to evaluate whether reliance on the tool "caused" patient harm? Likely not; it is more plausible that a court would instead turn to an analysis of practice workflow. If the AI product was blindly relied upon to detect an impression-worthy finding, but the interpreting radiologist failed to independently confirm its validity, there may indeed be an argument for causation.

Although these vignettes suggest three different outcomes, two common threads unite them: (1) the importance of clearly articulated guidelines for the use of AI tools and (2) adequate training on their appropriate use. In both routine clinical practice and legal proceedings, departmental standard operating procedures and professional best practices are critical. There is a vital role to be played by radiological professional societies. The Radiological Society of North America and American College of Radiology, together with several of their counterparts overseas, have articulated a joint statement on AI development and process improvement. In the coming years, the American Society of Neuroradiology should follow with a complementary set of guidelines on clinical integration. In recent years, these same institutions, neuroradiology training programs, individual departments, and state medical societies have invested heavily in AI education, both as it applies to development and clinical use. The American College of Radiology has created the online ACR AI-LAB, which offers an open-access resource for providers to familiarize themselves with the practical points of AI deployment in an easy-to-use interface. These and other initiatives are increasingly becoming fixtures of formal radiology education, better informing future generations as they emerge into a digitally driven future.

Product Liability

Neuroradiologists are not merely the end-users of AI tools in their profession; in growing numbers, they are also participating in their development. This may expose them to elements of liability as they attach to developers. Picture a neuroradiologist who creates a novel diagnostic tool for the rapid quantification of amyloid PET studies. Over time, it underdiagnoses Alzheimer's disease and occasionally underestimates its progression. The caretaker of a patient who received a "normal" reading on the algorithm-enhanced study seeks a second opinion with a human radiologist, who identifies extensive disease. Separate from the issue of interpretation, could the developer-neuroradiologist face a viable lawsuit?

This chain of liability is likewise unclear. Although AI tools are products in a commercial sense, courts have historically not considered software "products" under product liability frameworks.[6] This may relate to the traditional notion that software cannot cause harm (in the same manner as a physical device). It is highly likely that this view will change over time, particularly as a distinct AI jurisprudence develops, and AI firmware merges into hardware products posing a risk of corporeal harm, such as autonomous vehicles and cerebrovascular disease localizers.

Under product liability structures, a court may apply one of two theories: negligence, similar to that described in the case study above, and strict liability. If a negligence argument is advanced, the threshold question relates to duty of care. Who does the developer owe this to, if anyone at all? Should the neuroradiologist-developer consider their obligation as attached to the interpreting neuroradiologist as end user, or should it extend all the way to the patients whose studies will be analyzed? Moreover, which professional standards should even be applied? There is no unified set of ethical principles that computer scientists and AI designers adhere to. And how would the institution that purchased and deployed the AI tool deflect liability for not detecting these errors prior to clinical use? These remain open questions at the time of writing.

Strict liability principles look not to the developer and their industry, but to the product itself. The key question is whether the AI tool contained a "manufacturing defect," which directly led to the patient's misdiagnosis and ensuing harm. This may prove a thornier avenue for plaintiffs to seek recovery, in part owing to the technical complexity of AI tools, many of which lack the ability to clearly explain their findings. A greater obstacle stems from the product's prior FDA authorization; courts have previously held that premarket review can act as a shield against questions of defective design.[7,8]

Data Privacy

Given the sheer volume of patient data contained within training datasets (not to mention real-world clinical information for continuously learning models), the algorithmic learning process implicates significant data privacy concerns. This is the province of the Health Insurance Portability and Accountability Act (HIPAA), which governs protected health information (PHI) as defined by 18 discrete identifiers (e.g., name, date of birth, medical record number, headshot, etc.).[9] To this end, HIPAA establishes a series of broad guidelines, among them the aptly named Security and Breach Notification Rules. Most relevant to the discussion at hand is the Privacy Rule, which covers disclosure. This requires healthcare entities to

[6] Restatement (Third) of Torts §19(a).

[7] Riegel v. Medtronic, Inc., 552 U.S. 312 (2008).

[8] Medtronic, Inc. v. Lohr, 518 U.S. 470 (1996).

[9] Health Insurance Portability and Accountability Act of 1996. Public Law 104–191.

notify individuals of any use or transfer of their PHI. Should a hospital choose to share unprocessed patient data with a third-party research institute or AI developer, it is legally obligated to (1) contact the affected individuals, (2) inform them of the disclosure in lay terms, and (3) to the extent possible, only share the minimum necessary PHI with the receiving entity. It is briefly worth noting that although patients may receive full access to their healthcare data, it is generally established that healthcare institutions hold a property interest in the medical imaging they produce.

Healthcare institutions can bypass these restrictions via deidentification. By stripping data of the 18 aforementioned PHI identifiers, they can altogether avoid the need to alert individual patients prior to data sharing, which can include a broader swath of information (e.g., not merely a single study, but an entire imaging record). However, this is not a foolproof avenue for neuroradiology image sharing. Many radiological studies contain "burned-in PHI" included on each image slice, often featuring the patient's name, date of birth, medical record number, and study location. Redacting this information may require an image editor to obscure it. Face reconstruction presents perhaps a greater issue; advanced multi-planar reformatting tools permit visualization of a patient's face from head and neck CT and MR data. A number of "defacing" tools are available, but they may adversely affect image fidelity.

Synthetic training data offers one route forward and is a key niche that the latest generative AI tools may fill. Rather than pore through technically fraught and highly sensitive patient data, AI tools can instead train on algorithmically generated "CT" models simulating neuropathology. Federated learning presents another. Here, an AI algorithm can be distributed across several institutions, each of which trains it on local data and shares targeted updates of the algorithm itself with its counterparts. This obviates the need for data to cross institutional boundaries while facilitating algorithmic learning simultaneously.

Conclusion

Neuroradiology is characterized by its diagnostic precision, the subtlety of its findings, and high clinical stakes involved. These factors readily lend themselves to AI deployment in the field.

As we have discussed, the regulatory landscape reflects the diversity of AI tools and capabilities; there is no one-size-fits-all approach to governance. Those assisting neuroradiologists with their image interpretive functions, including segmentation, lesion detection, and volumetric analysis, are held to high standards of premarket review. Absent major legislative changes, they will continue to require formal FDA authorization through the 510(k) or PMA pathways. Others that assist in the neuroradiologist's chart review, process improvement, research, and administrative functions may feature a lighter touch or fall outside of the scope of FDA jurisdiction altogether. Still others fall into a grey area between the two, which may face an intermediate level of regulatory scrutiny; these include workflow optimization tools that have a direct patient impact, such as auto-protocoling algorithms.

Similarly, the liability environment is fluid and heavily dependent on how AI tools are integrated within the neuroradiology workflow. If they are eventually incorporated into the standard of care, malpractice suits may take on an entirely different bent. What is clear is that best practice guidelines, adequate quality management frameworks, and training are essential to minimizing legal risk. No one is better placed to design these programs than neuroradiologists themselves, with the support of their divisions, practices, and professional societies.

Suggested Reading

1. McKinsey & Company. Applied AI: six growth considerations for private markets. 2023. https://www.mckinsey.com/industries/private-equity-and-principal-investors/our-insights/applied-ai-six-growth-considerations-for-private-markets.
2. van Leeuwen KG, Schalekamp S, Rutten MJCM, van Ginneken B, de Rooij M. Artificial intelligence in radiology: 100 commercially available products and their scientific evidence. Eur Radiol. 2021;31(6):3797–804.
3. Duong MT, Rauschecker AM, Mohan S. Diverse applications of artificial intelligence in neuroradiology. Neuroimaging Clin N Am. 2020;30(4):505–16.
4. Harvey HB, Gowda V. Regulatory issues and challenges to artificial intelligence adoption. Radiol Clin North Am. 2021;59(6):1075–83.
5. U.S. Food and Drug Administration. Software as a Medical Device (SAMD): clinical evaluation. 2017. https://www.fda.gov/media/100714/download
6. U.S. Food and Drug Administration. Investigational Device Exemption (IDE). 2022. https://www.fda.gov/medical-devices/premarket-submissions-selecting-and-preparing-correct-submission/investigational-device-exemption-ide
7. Van Raamsdonk A. Swiss regulators set to recognize US FDA-cleared or approved medical devices. 2022. https://www.emergobyul.com/news/swiss-regulators-set-recognize-us-fda-cleared-or-approved-medical-devices
8. Harvey HB, Gowda V. How the FDA regulates AI. Acad Radiol. 2020;27(1):58–61.
9. U.S. Food and Drug Administration. Clinical performance assessment: considerations for computer-assisted detection devices applied to radiology images and radiology device data in premarket notification (510(k)) submissions. 2020. https://www.fda.gov/media/77642/download
10. U.S. Food and Drug Administration. Clinical and patient decision support software: draft guidance for industry and food and drug administration staff. 2020. https://www.fda.gov/media/109618/download
11. Selbst AD, Powles J. Meaningful information and the right to explanation. Int Data Privacy Law. 2017;7(4):233–42.
12. Price WN. Big data and black-box medical algorithms. Sci Transl Med. 2018;10(471)
13. Price WN. Black-box medicine. Harv J Law Technol. 2015;28:419–67.
14. U.S. Food and Drug Administration. Changes to existing medical software policies resulting from section 3060 of the 21st Century Cures Act. 2019. https://www.fda.gov/media/109622/download
15. U.S. Food and Drug Administration. Requests for feedback and meetings for medical device submissions: the Q-Submission Program. 2023. https://www.fda.gov/regulatory-information/search-fda-guidance-documents/requests-feedback-and-meetings-medical-device-submissions-q-submission-program

16. U.S. Food and Drug Administration. Artificial intelligence/machine learning (AI/ML)-based Software as a Medical Device (SaMD) action plan. 2021. https://www.fda.gov/media/145022/download
17. U.S. Food and Drug Administration. Digital Health Software Precertification (Pre-Cert) program. 2022. https://www.fda.gov/medical-devices/digital-health/digital-health-software-precertification-pre-cert-program
18. U.S. Food and Drug Administration. Good machine learning practice for medical device development: guiding principles. 2021. https://www.fda.gov/medical-devices/software-medical-device-samd/good-machine-learning-practice-medical-device-development-guiding-principles
19. U.S. Food and Drug Administration. Current Good Manufacturing Practices cCGMPs) for food and dietary supplements. 2020. https://www.fda.gov/food/guidance-regulation-food-and-dietary-supplements/current-good-manufacturing-practices-cgmps-food-and-dietary-supplements
20. U.S. Food and Drug Administration. Proposed regulatory framework for modifications to artificial intelligence/machine learning (AI/ML)-based software as a medical device (SaMD)—discussion paper and request for feedback. 2019. https://www.fda.gov/media/122535/download
21. U.S. Food and Drug Administration. Marketing submission recommendations for a predetermined change control plan for artificial intelligence/machine learning (AI/ML)-enabled device software functions. 2023. https://www.fda.gov/regulatory-information/search-fda-guidance-documents/marketing-submission-recommendations-predetermined-change-control-plan-artificial
22. International Organization for Standardization. ISO/IEC 42001:2023(en). Information technology—artificial intelligence—management system. https://www.iso.org/obp/ui/#iso:std:iso-iec:42001:ed-1:v1:en
23. Coalition for Health AI. https://www.coalitionforhealthai.org/
24. PR Newswire. Coalition for Health AI (CHAI) announces founding partners. 2024. https://www.prnewswire.com/news-releases/coalition-for-health-ai-chai-announces-founding-partners-302089460.html
25. Coalition for Health AI. Blueprint for trustworthy AI: implementation guidance and assurance for healthcare. 2023. https://www.coalitionforhealthai.org/papers/blueprint-for-trustworthy-ai_V1.0.pdf
26. Shah NH, Halamka JD, Saria S, Pencina M, Tazbaz T, Tripathi M, Callahan A, Hildahl H, Anderson B. A nationwide network of health AI assurance laboratories. JAMA. 2024;331(3):245–9.
27. Harvey HB, Tomov E, Babayan A, Dwyer K, Boland S, Pandharipande PV, Halpern EF, Alkasab TK, Hirsch JA, Schaefer PW, Boland GW, Choy G. Radiology malpractice claims in the United States from 2008 to 2012: characteristics and implications. J Am Coll Radiol. 2016;13(2):124–30.
28. Sullivan HR, Schweikart SJ. Are current tort liability doctrines adequate for addressing injury caused by AI? AMA J Ethics. 2019;21(2):E160–6.
29. Harvey HB, Gowda V. Clinical applications of AI in MSK imaging: a liability perspective. Skeletal Radiol. 2022;51(2):235–8.
30. Gerke S, Minssen T, Cohen G. Ethical and legal challenges of artificial intelligence-driven healthcare. Artif Intell Healthcare. 2020:295–336.
31. Price WN, Gerke S, Cohen IG. Potential liability for physicians using artificial intelligence. JAMA. 2019;322(18):1765–6.
32. Mello M. Of swords and shields: the role of clinical practice guidelines in medical malpractice litigation. Univ Pa Law Rev. 2001;149(3)
33. Brady AP, Allen B, Chong J, Kotter E, Kottler N, Mongan J, Oakden-Rayner L, Pinto Dos Santos D, Tang A, Wald C, Slavotinek J. Developing, purchasing, implementing and monitoring AI tools in radiology: practical considerations. A multi-society statement from the ACR, CAR, ESR, RANZCR & RSNA. J Med Imaging Radiat Oncol. 2024;68(1):7–26.

34. Duong MT, Rauschecker AM, Rudie JD, Chen PH, Cook TS, Bryan RN, Mohan S. Artificial intelligence for precision education in radiology. Br J Radiol. 2019;92(1103):20190389.
35. Tejani AS, Elhalawani H, Moy L, Kohli M, Kahn CE Jr. Artificial intelligence and radiology education. Radiol Artif Intell. 2022;5(1):e220084.
36. American College of Radiology Data Science Institute. ACR AI-LAB. https://www.acrdsi.org/Get-Involved/AI-LAB
37. Gowda V, Jordan SG, Awan OA. Artificial intelligence in radiology education: a longitudinal approach. Acad Radiol. 2022;29(5):788–90.
38. Villasenor J. Products liability law as a way to address AI harms. Brookings. 2019. https://www.brookings.edu/research/products-liability-law-as-a-way-to-address-ai-harms
39. Harned Z, Lungren MP, Rajpurkar P. Machine vision, medical AI, and malpractice. Harv J L Tech Dig. 2019. https://jolt.law.harvard.edu/digest/machine-vision-medical-ai-and-malpractice
40. Kim S. Crashed software: assessing product liability for software defects in automated vehicles, 16 Duke Law Technol Rev. 2018;300–317.
41. Mezrich JL, Siegel E. Who owns the image? Archiving and retention issues in the digital age. J Am Coll Radiol. 2014;11(4):384–6.
42. White T, Blok E, Calhoun VD. Data sharing and privacy issues in neuroimaging research: opportunities, obstacles, challenges, and monsters under the bed. Hum Brain Mapp. 2022;43(1):278–91.
43. Hedderich DM, Weisstanner C, Van Cauter S, Federau C, Edjlali M, Radbruch A, Gerke S, Haller S. Artificial intelligence tools in clinical neuroradiology: essential medico-legal aspects. Neuroradiology. 2023;65(7):1091–9.
44. Schwarz CG, Kremers WK, Therneau TM, Sharp RR, Gunter JL, Vemuri P, Arani A, Spychalla AJ, Kantarci K, Knopman DS, Petersen RC, Jack CR Jr. Identification of anonymous MRI research participants with face-recognition software. N Engl J Med. 2019;381(17):1684–6.
45. Bhalerao GV, Parekh P, Saini J, Venkatasubramanian G, John JP, ADBS Consortium. Systematic evaluation of the impact of defacing on quality and volumetric assessments on T1-weighted MR-images. J Neuroradiol. 2022;49(3):250–7.
46. Tracey J, Moss L, Ashmore J. Application of synthetic data in the training of artificial intelligence for automated quality assurance in magnetic resonance imaging. Med Phys. 2023;50(9):5621–9.
47. Rehman MHU, Hugo Lopez Pinaya W, Nachev P, Teo JT, Ourselin S, Cardoso MJ. Federated learning for medical imaging radiology. Br J Radiol. 2023;96(1150):20220890

Index

D. T. Ginat (ed.), *Artificial Intelligence in Neuroradiology*,
https://doi.org/10.1007/978-3-032-24568-7

MIX
Papier aus verantwortungsvollen Quellen
Paper from responsible sources
FSC® C105338

If you have any concerns about our products,
you can contact us on
ProductSafety@springernature.com

In case Publisher is established outside the EU,
the EU authorized representative is:
Springer Nature Customer Service Center GmbH
Europaplatz 3, 69115 Heidelberg, Germany

Printed by Libri Plureos GmbH
in Hamburg, Germany